MODERN APPLICATIONS OF PLANT BIOTECHNOLOGY IN PHARMACEUTICAL SCIENCES

MODERN APPLICATIONS OF PLANT BIOTECHNOLOGY IN PHARMACEUTICAL SCIENCES

Lead Author

SAURABH BHATIA

PDM College of Pharmacy,
Bahadurgarh, Haryana, India

Co-Authors

KIRAN SHARMA

Department of Pharmaceutical Sciences, Jamia Hamdard,
New Delhi, India

RANDHIR DAHIYA

Department of Pharmacology, Maharishi Markandeshwar College of Pharmacy,
Mullana, Ambala, Haryana, India

TANMOY BERA

Department of Pharmaceutical Technology, Jadavpur University,
Kolkata, West Bengal, India

AMSTERDAM • BOSTON • HEIDELBERG • LONDON
NEW YORK • OXFORD • PARIS • SAN DIEGO
SAN FRANCISCO • SINGAPORE • SYDNEY • TOKYO

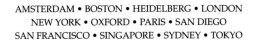
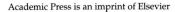

Academic Press is an imprint of Elsevier

Academic Press is an imprint of Elsevier
125, London Wall, EC2Y 5AS, UK
525 B Street, Suite 1800, San Diego, CA 92101-4495, USA
225 Wyman Street, Waltham, MA 02451, USA
The Boulevard, Langford Lane, Kidlington, Oxford OX5 1GB, UK

Notices
Knowledge and best practice in this field are constantly changing. As new research and experience broaden
our understanding, changes in research methods, professional practices, or medical treatment may become
necessary.

Practitioners and researchers must always rely on their own experience and knowledge in evaluating and
using any information, methods, compounds, or experiments described herein. In using such information
or methods they should be mindful of their own safety and the safety of others, including parties for whom
they have a professional responsibility.

To the fullest extent of the law, neither the Publisher nor the authors, contributors, or editors, assume any
liability for any injury and/or damage to persons or property as a matter of products liability, negligence
or otherwise, or from any use or operation of any methods, products, instructions, or ideas contained in
the material herein.

British Library Cataloguing-in-Publication Data
A catalogue record for this book is available from the British Library

Library of Congress Cataloging-in-Publication Data
A catalog record for this book is available from the Library of Congress

ISBN: 978-0-12-802221-4

For information on all Academic Press publications
visit our website at http://store.elsevier.com/

Typeset by Thomson Digital

Publisher: Mica Haley
Senior Acquisition Editor: Kristine Jones
Editorial Project Manager: Molly McLaughlin
Production Project Manager: Lucía Pérez
Designer: Mark Rogers

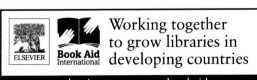

Working together
to grow libraries in
developing countries

www.elsevier.com • www.bookaid.org

Contents

About the Lead Author

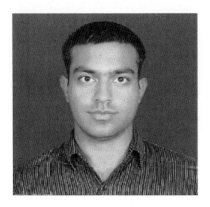

Dr. Saurabh Bhatia has six years of teaching experience at U.G. levels. He has worked as an assistant professor in four different organizations. Currently, he is working as an assistant professor in PDM College of Pharmacy, Haryana, India. Dr. Saurabh Bhatia did his post graduation from Bharati Vidya Peeth, Pune, India, followed by a PhD from Jadavpur University, Kolkata, India. He has around 30 research publications to his credit published in national and international journals. Besides publishing in reputed journals, Dr. Saurabh Bhatia is an author of four other books that are currently in press. His research interest extends from pharmacognosy to plant tissue culture, and he has done extensive work on various *in vitro* cultures of plants. In addition, he was the first person from India who has explored the medicinal values of various natural polymers isolated from marine red algae.

Preface

Plant tissue culture, a branch of plant science, stems from the totipotency of plant cells, a unique feature that now has been exploited extensively for the cause of human welfare. Nowadays plant tissue culture in one form or another has become one of the most promising branches of plant science. The techniques of tissue culture exist academically as well as for commercial production. Modern plant biotechnology is equipped with advance tools for the manipulation of plant-based biological systems. For deriving more applications a wide range of plant cells are manipulated by novel techniques. Plant tissue culture is now the major component of technologies that are applied in plant biotechnology.

The recent introduction of plant tissue culture in pharmaceutical science helps to understand the production and mechanism of plant-derived products more clearly. Products like edible vaccines and plant-made pharmaceuticals are still widely discussed for their merits and demerits. Regulation and dispensing of these products require the recruitment of defined professionals such as pharmacists or biotechnologists. The role of such professionals or future pharmacists can also be discussed for providing maximum safety to patients undergoing plant-made pharmaceutical therapy. These and many other modern studies require profound knowledge of key techniques such as genetic engineering and its associated applications. Cell and plant tissue culture constitutes an important aspect of plant biotechnology. For understanding the developmental stage during *in vitro* plant tissue culture, successful culturing and maintenance of protoplast, cell, tissue, and organ culture is required. This establishment helps in the regeneration of plants from their cultivated plant material. Such knowledge of tissue culture has contributed greatly to our understanding of the factors responsible for growth, metabolism, and differentiation of plants.

There is a dire need to have a book on plant tissue culture that especially focuses on the pharmaceutical applications and aspects of practical procedures and protocols of tissue culture. Students are acutely aware of the unavailability of a book on such topics, hence the attempt is to fill the void.

In addition to its focus toward modern techniques and pharmaceutical applications, this book deals with fundamental aspects of theory and practice of the *in vitro* culture of plants. It also presents historical accounts, basic principles, and modern-day applications of plant cell, tissue, and organ culture, which are essential for learning the art and science of plant cell culture. I am sure this book will serve as an important primer for students, researchers, and teachers who wish to learn plant tissue culture in a simple way. It is my hope that this book will prove useful for all undergraduate, graduate, and post-graduate students, as well as researchers and industrialists.

Modern Applications of Plant Biotechnology in Pharmaceutical Sciences was written primarily to share the up-to-date available knowledge with students, professors, researchers, and industrialists. The book has 14 chapters. All chapters are written in a lucid way with necessary illustrations and up-to-date information, so that readers can build a clear concept of the basic and applied aspects of plant tissue culture. Errors and inaccuracies, if any, will be corrected through feedback and suggestion from readers. We earnestly believe that the book will be valuable for undergraduate and post-graduate students. Editors at Elsevier Science, Kristine Jones (Senior Acquisitions Editor), Molly M. McLaughlin (Editorial Project Manager), Lucia Perez (Production Project Manager), and others, must be praised for their active work and support in our efforts. We are sure readers of this book, the students, the researchers, and industrialists, will find it interesting.

The publication of this book would not have been possible without the valuable work of earlier researchers. This book would not have seen the light of the day without the moral support and patience of my parents. I am highly thankful to my brother Sanjay Bhatia for his valuable suggestions and timely inputs. I am thankful also to PDM College of Pharmacy for providing me with a platform to work day and night.

Dr. Saurabh Bhatia
MPharm, PhD
Assistant Professor,
PDM College of Pharmacy,
Bahadurgarh, Haryana, India

1

History and Scope of Plant Biotechnology

Saurabh Bhatia

1.1 INTRODUCTION

Biotechnology has flourished since prehistoric times. When *Homo sapiens* realized that they could plant their crops and breed their own animals they learned to use biotechnology. From nearly 10,000 years ago, our ancestors were producing wine, beer, and bread, using fermentation. In this process microorganisms such as bacteria, yeast, and molds fed on provided food and released two main by-products: carbon dioxide and alcohol. Several discoveries such as fermentation of fruits into wine, malt into beers, and milk into yoghurt or curd or cheese

Modern Applications of Plant Biotechnology in Pharmaceutical Sciences. http://dx.doi.org/10.1016/B978-0-12-802221-4.00001-7

1

began the era of biotechnology. In prehistoric times bakers found that they could make soft and spongy bread rather than firm bread, and animal breeders realized that physical traits of various animal breeds could be magnified or lost by mating appropriate animals of different traits. From such discoveries some think of biotechnology as a tool to develop new types of plants and animals and others treat it as a source of human therapeutic drugs [1]. These thoughts give birth to one of the oldest and purest definitions of biotechnology:

Bio: *The use of biological process*

Technology: *To solve problems or make useful products*

Collectively, biotechnology refers to use of living organisms or their products to modify human health and the human environment.

After the end of the classical and ancient biotechnology era, modern biotechnology appears accompanied by the latest genetic techniques. This modern genetic era brings various techniques such as recombinant DNA technology and gene splicing. These lead to a modification of the earlier definition and give a few new definitions of biotechnology:

Biotechnology is a collection of new technologies that capitalize on the attributes of cells, such as the manufacturing capabilities, and put biological molecules, such as proteins and DNA, to work for us.

OR

Modern biotechnology refers to the use of cellular and bimolecular processes to solve problems or make useful products.

Subsequently, biotechnology started contributing in other fields such as agriculture, horticulture, etc. Since biotechnology has become the major tool for the production of therapeutic drugs, a recent emerging branch, "pharmaceutical biotechnology," covers its major applications. This provides a new definition of biotechnology:

A field that uses micro- and macroorganisms and hybridomas to create biopharmaceuticals that are safer and more cost-effective than conventionally produced pharmaceuticals, known as pharmaceutical biotechnology.

Thus, biopharmaceuticals are defined as pharmaceuticals manufactured by biotechnology methods, with the products obviously having biological sources, usually involving live organisms or their active components.

General applications of modern biotechnology involve production of hormones, genes, antibiotics, vaccines, interferons, alcohols, vitamins, organic acids, transgenic animals, immunological proteins, probes, monoclonal antibodies, and an antenatal diagnosis cure in preventing genetic disease. Biotechnology is the name given to the methods and techniques that involve the use of living organisms like bacteria, yeast, plant cells, etc., or their parts or products as tools (e.g., genes and enzymes). Biological techniques, which deal with plant cells to produce useful plants and their products, usually come under the domain of plant biotechnology or plant science [1,2].

Plant science is a relatively current discipline though its fundamental techniques have been applied throughout human history. For 12,000 years humans have been controlling crops and breeding plants to improve their desirable characteristics. Primitive farmers identified the crops for cultivation and explored their importance for human survival. These farmers found that they could increase the yield and improve the traits of crops by selecting seeds from particularly desirable plants. Initially they were unaware of the basic principles involved in improving the characteristics of plants. Over many years, they realized the importance of selection of seeds in maintaining the desirable traits of plants. Thus, in ancient plant biotechnology humans have domesticated crops and bred plants to further improve their desirable characteristics, whereas classical plant biotechnology (George Mendel, 1860s) originated the science of genetics and cross-breeding techniques to strengthen the characteristics of plants [1–5].

After George Mendel's discovery in the mid-1860s, the benefits of cross-breeding or hybridization became apparent, which explores the opportunities to cultivate the desirable plant traits up to several generations. This great discovery ends the classical breeding era and begins new era of modern plant breeding, which includes mutation breeding, green revolution, and plant tissue culture breeding [4,5].

Among the various branches, plant biotechnology is one of the most emerging disciplines of biotechnology. Plant biotechnology achievement depends on the basic techniques of plant tissue culture. Profound knowledge of plant biology is a primary requirement for its proper utilization in biotechnology. Plant tissue culture offers a basic understanding of physico-chemical requirements of cell, tissue, and organ culture, and their growth and development. According to the Council for Biotechnology Information:

> Plant biotechnology describes a precise process in which scientific techniques are used to develop useful and beneficial plants.

Plant cell, tissue, and organ culture establishment and plantlet regeneration under *in vitro* conditions has opened up new opportunities in plant biotechnology.

> Plant tissue culture is defined as culturing plant seeds, organs, explants, tissues, cells, or protoplasts on a chemically defined synthetic nutrient media under sterile and controlled conditions of light, temperature, and humidity.

Plant cell potential was initially proposed by Schleiden and Schwann in 1838–39 [5]. The first attempt at plant tissue culture was made by Harberlandt in 1902 [6]. Some of the earliest plant tissue culture media, for example, the root culture medium of White [7] and callus culture medium of Gautheret [8], were developed from nutrient solution used for whole plant culture. White evolved the medium from Upsenski and Upsenskaja's medium for algae [9], whereas Gautheret's medium is based on the Knop's salt solution [10]. All subsequent media are based on White and Gautheret's medium. Some explants may grow easily on simple media containing inorganic salts and utilizable sugar; for most others it is essential to add vitamins, amino acids, and growth substances in different qualitative and quantitative combinations. Sometimes nutritive mixtures have been added to plant tissue culture media.

> A medium containing only chemically defined compounds is referred to as synthetic media.

Ball raised whole plants of *Lupinus* by shoot tip culture [11]. Muir was first to break callus tissues into single cells [12]. Plant growth and development largely depends on nature, concentration, and ratios of plant growth hormones and vitamins supplemented into the culture media. Therefore in 1955 Skoog and Miller discovered kinetin as a cell division hormone [13,14], and after 2 years gave the concept of hormonal control (auxin:cytokinin) of organ formation [15]. Cocking was first to isolate protoplast by enzymatic degradation of the cell wall [16]. In 1962 Murashige and Skoog developed MS medium with higher salt concentration [17]. Thus, the ancient era was replaced by the classical era, which was further replaced by the modern era of plant biotechnology. This modern era developed a number of genetic tools and techniques to study the plant cell in a more elaborative manner. These achievements present a wide application of plant tissue culture in generating various therapeutic compounds. Out of these therapeutic compounds, pharmaceuticals made from plants are highly acknowledged [18].

Therefore plant tissue culture is a procedure to yield high-value secondary metabolites, which forms the basis of many practical applications in agriculture, horticulture, industrial chemistry, and pharmaceutical sciences, and is an essential requirement for plant genetic engineering. Moreover, it also prevents the extinction of certain elite species of plants from nature by preserving their germplasm or callus under *in vitro* conditions for many years [19].

1.2 HISTORY OF PLANT BIOTECHNOLOGY

The history of plant biotechnology explores the organized record of various researchers and events involved in culturing plant tissue and monitoring its growth and development in a controlled environment. Ancient biotechnology begins with early civilization where the primary focus has been on the development of agriculture and food production. By utilizing ancient science classical biotechnology makes widespread use of methods adapted to industrial production. Many methods developed through classical biotechnology are widely used even today. Various initiatives like the better understanding of microscopy, biochemical methods, and manipulation of genetic material within organisms by using their related sciences and technologies have been developed. This gives birth to new era called the modern era [18,19], more often known as the genetic era. This modern era plays a major contribution toward plant biotechnology. The major historical events (Table 1.1) and their prominent contributors (Figure 1.1) that play important roles in plant biotechnology are as follows.

1.2.1 Cell Theory

The cell was discovered by Robert Hooke in 1665. The first person to make a compound microscope was Zacharias Jansen, while the first to witness a live cell under a microscope was Anton van Leeuwenhoek. The observations of Hooke, Leeuwenhoek, Schleiden, Schwann, Virchow, and others led to the development of cell theory, which forms the foundations of modern plant biotechnology. In 1939, Schleiden and Schwann suggested that cells were the basic unit of life. They observed the independent nature of cells and thus explored their possibilities to regenerate into whole plant in a given environment [116]. Thus, cell theory is a widely accepted explanation of the relationship between cells and living things. Cell theory states:

- All living things or organisms are made of cells and their products.
- New cells are created by old cells dividing into two.
- Cells are the basic building units of life.

1.2.2 Concept of *In Vitro* Cell Culture

Plant tissue culture is an important tool in both basic and applied studies as well as in commercial application. In the nineteenth century the idea of experimenting with tissue and organs of plants under controlled laboratory conditions was born. For the first time in 1902, a German physiologist, Gottlieb Haberlandt, developed the concept of *in vitro* cell culture [6].

TABLE 1.1   Historical Achievements of Plant Biotechnology

Year	Discoverer	Discovery	References
1839	Schleiden M.J.	Cell theory and totipotency of cells	[20]
1865	Knop	Knop's solution, inorganic salt nutrition	[10]
1882	Sachs J.	Plants synthesize organ-forming substances that are polarly distributed	[20]
1902	Haberlandt (Austria)	Concept of "Totipotency" (first but unsuccessful attempt at tissue culture using monocots)	[6]
1904	Hannig B.	First attempt at development of embryo culture of selected crucifers	[20]
1907	Smith and Townsend	Reported the tumors on several plants that were later called crown gall disease	[21]
1909	Kuster E.	Demonstrated protoplast fusion though the products failed to survive	[20]
1921	Molliard M.	Cultivation of fragments of plant embryos	[20]
1922	Kotte (student of Haberlandt)	Improved medium: sugar, organic N-compounds	[22,23]
1922	Robbins W.J. (USA)	Root tip culture – *Pisum*, *Zea*, and *Gossypium*	[24,25]
1922	Knudson L.	Asymbiotic germination of orchid seeds	[20]
1923	Robbins and Maneval	Maintained maize roots for 20 weeks with the aid of subcultures	[26]
1924	Blumenthal F. and Meyer P.Z.	Lactic acid-induced callus formation on carrot root	[20]
1925	Laibach F.	Interspecific crosses in *Linum* spp. for the development of embryo culture	[20]
1925	Knudson L.	Developed orchid seeds by symbiotic germination	[20]
1926	Went	Discovery of auxin	[27]
1929	Laibach F.	Developed embryo culture to circumvent cross-incompatibility in *Linum* spp.	[20]
1933	Kogl, Haagen-Smit and Erxleben	Isolation of IAA (indo-3-acetic acid)	[28]
1932–1939	Gautheret	Root tip and root fragment culture, cambium culture, IAA promotes root growth, carrot explants, and repeated subculture	[8,29–32]
1932–1942	White (in the Rockefeller Institute)	Root tip culture – triticum, indefinite culture of isolated roots, importance of vitamin B complex in root culture (use yeast extract), procambial tissue culture (small leaf and shoot), tumor culture (callus without plant hormone), successful long-term culture of tomato roots	[33–39]
1936	LaRue C.R.	Developed embryo culture from different gymnosperms	[20]
1945	Loo S.W.	*In vitro* cultivation of excised stem tips of *Asparagus*	[40]

(Continued)

TABLE 1.1   Historical Achievements of Plant Biotechnology *(cont.)*

Year	Discoverer	Discovery	References
1946	Ball E.	First whole plants from shoot tips of *Lupinus* and *Tropaeolum*	[20]
1948	Skoog F. and Tsui C.	Reported the formation of adventitious shoots and roots in tobacco	[20]
1949	Nitsch J.P.	Reported the *in vitro* culture of fruits	[20]
1950	Ball E.	Regenerated the organs from callus of *Sequoia*	[20]
1950	Morel G.C.R.	Reported the first successful cultures of monocots using coconut milk	[20]
1951	Nitsch J.P.	Developed the *in vitro* culture of excised ovaries	[20]
1951	Skoog F.	Demonstrated the chemical control of growth and organ formation in culture	[20]
1951	Steward F.C. and Caplin S.M.	Developed tissue culture from potato tuber: the synergistic action of 2,4-D and coconut milk	[41]
1952	Morel and Martin	First virus-free plant through shoot tips culture (*Dahlia*) (propagation of many plants from one plant)	[42]
1952	Morel G. and Martin C.	First successful micrografts	[20]
1953	Tulecke W.R.	Haploid callus from pollen grain of *Ginkgo biloba*	[20]
1954	Muir, Hildebrandt and Riker (in Wisconsin)	Suspension culture by reciprocal shaker (*Nicotiana*), single cell clone by nurse cell culture method, first calli produced from a single cell by use of nurse cultures	[43]
1955	Steward and Shantz (in Cornell)	Discovered carrot root phloem in liquid medium and single suspension culture	[44]
1955	Miller, Skoog et al.	Discovery, structure, and synthesis of kinetin	[13,14]
1956	Reinert J. and White P.R.	*In vitro* cultivation of normal and tumor tissues of *Picea glauca*	[20]
1956	Routien J.B. and Nickell L.G.	Production of substances from plant tissue culture of *Phaseolus vulgaris*	[20]
1956	Nickell (Chas, Pfizer & Co. NY)	Single cell suspension culture of *Phaseolus vulgaris* (idea of producing plant alkaloids from tissue culture)	[45]
1957	Vasil I.K.	Culture of excised anthers of *Allium cepa*	[20]
1957	Skoog and Miller	Auxin/cytokinin balance (high kinetin → shoot; high auxin → root)	[15]
1958	Steward	Quantitative analysis of carrot culture and discovered embryogenesis *in vitro* (proved the concept of totipotency)	[46]
1958	Maheshwari N.	*In vitro* culture of excised ovules of *Papaver somniferum*	[20]
1958	Maheshwari P. and Rangaswamy N.S.	Regeneration of somatic embryos from nucellus of *Citrus ovules*	[20]
1958	Reinert J. and Steward F.C.	Pro-embryo formation in callus clumps and cell suspension of carrot	[20]

TABLE 1.1   Historical Achievements of Plant Biotechnology (*cont.*)

Year	Discoverer	Discovery	References
1958	Steward F.C. et al.	Growth and development in suspension cultures	[20]
1959	Tulecke W. and Nickell L.G.	Production of large amounts (134 L) of plant tissue by submerged culture	[20]
1960	Morel G.	Vegetative propagation of orchids by meristem culture	[20]
1960	Bergmann	Filtration of cell suspension and isolation of single cells by plating culture (*Nicotiana tabacum* and *Phaseolus vulgaris*)	[47]
1960	Jones et al.	Use of microculture method for growing single cells in hanging drops in a conditioned medium	[48]
1960	Cocking (UK)	Enzymatic isolation and culture of protoplast	[16]
1960	Kanta and Maheshwari	Developed test tube fertilization technique	[49]
1964	Guha and Maheshwari	Produced first haploid plants from pollen grains of *Datura*	[50]
1964	Mathes M.C.	Regeneration of roots and shoots on callus of *Populus tremuloides*	[20]
1965	Vasil V. and Hildebrandt A.C.	Developed protocol for the differentiation of tobacco plants from a single isolated cell in microculture	[20]
1965	Morel G.	Flower induction in *Lunaria annua* by vernalization *in vitro*	[20]
1967	Pierik R.L.M.	Successfully achieved protoplast fusion	[20]
1970	Power et al.	Plant regeneration from tobacco protoplast	[20,51]
1971	Nagata and Takebe	Development of two-stage culture medium for suspension cell cultures	[20]
1972	Carlson	Somatic hybridization of tomato and potato	[52]
1977	Chilton M.D. et al.	Development of alginate beads used for plant cell immobilization	[20]
1977	Noguchi M. et al.	Co-cultivation procedure developed for the *Agrobacterium*-mediated transformation of protoplasts	[20]
1975–1977	Zenk M.H. et al.	The use of immobilized cells for biotransformation of digitoxin into digoxin	[53,54]
1978	Melchers G. et al.	Ti plasmid DNA was present in the crown gall cell nucleus and not in plastids or mitochondria	[55]
1979	Brodelius P. et al.	Introduced the term somaclonal variation	[20]
1979	Marton L. et al.	Isolation of auxotrophs by cell colony screening in haploid protoplasts of *Nicotiana plumbaginifolia*	[56]
1980	Alfermann A.W. et al.	Use of a hollow fiber reactor for secondary metabolite production	[57]
1980	Chilton et al. and Willmitzer et al.	Naked DNA transformation of protoplasts	[58,59]

(Continued)

TABLE 1.1   Historical Achievements of Plant Biotechnology *(cont.)*

Year	Discoverer	Discovery	References
1981	Larkin P.J. and Scowcroft W.R.	Electrofusion of protoplasts	[60]
1981	Sidorov V. et al.	Intergeneric cybrid in radish and rape	[20]
1981	Shuler M.L.	First industrial production of secondary metabolites by suspension cultures of *Lithospermum* spp.	[61]
1982	Krens F.A. et al.	Co-integrate type of vectors designed for *Agrobacterium* transformation	[62]
1982	Zimmermann U.	Transformation of *Nicotiana* protoplasts with plasmid DNA and regeneration of transformed plants	[63,64]
1983	Pelletier G. et al.	Cryopreservation of alkaloid-producing cell culture of *Catharanthus*	[20]
1983	Mitsui Petrochemicals	Expression of foreign genes in regenerated plants and in their progeny	[20]
1983	Zambryski P. et al.	An Agrobacterium-transformed cell culture from the monocot *Asparagus officinalis*	[65]
1984	Paszkowski J. et al.	Industrial-scale fermentation of plant cells for production of shikonin (selection of cell lines with higher yield of secondary products)	[66]
1984	Chen et al.	Infection and transformation of leaf discs with *A. tumefaciens* and regeneration of transformed plants	[67]
1984	Block et al.	Development of disarmed Ti plasmid vector system for plant transformation	[68]
1984	Hernalsteens et al.	Development of binary vector system for plant transformation	[69]
1985	Tabata M. et al.	Gene transfer in protoplasts of dicot and monocot plants by electroporation	[70]
1985	Horsch R.B. et al.	Hairy root production for the first time in *Hyoscyamus muticus*. These roots produced more hyoscyamine than in planta	[71]
1985	Fraley R.T. et al.	The discovery of polymerase chain reaction	[72]
1985	An G. et al.	Transformation of tobacco protoplasts by direct DNA microinjection	[73]
1985	Fromm M.E. et al.	Biolistic gene transfer method for plant transformation	[74]
1985	Flores H.E. and Filner P.	Bt gene was isolated from *Bacillus thuringiensis*	[75]
1986	Mullis K. et al.	First monocot (asparagus) transformation by *Agrobacterium tumefaciens*	[76]
1986	Crossway A. et al.	Microinjection for direct DNA delivery into plant cells	[77]
1987	Sanford	Transformation of cotton (*Gossypium hirsutum* L.) by *A. tumefaciens* and regeneration of transgenic plants	[78]
1987	Barton	Use of microprojectile gun for particle bombardment for genetic transformation	[79]

TABLE 1.1 Historical Achievements of Plant Biotechnology *(cont.)*

Year	Discoverer	Discovery	References
1987	Bytebier B. et al.	Development of an embryogenic suspension culture of soybean (*Glycine max* Merrill.)	[80]
1987	Miki B.L.A. et al.	Automated mass propagation with organogenesis and embryogenesis	[81]
1987	Firoozabady et al.	Stable genetic transformation of intact *Nicotiana* cells by the particle bombardment process	[82]
1988	Klein T.M. et al.	Microinjection of cells and protoplasts for integration of foreign DNA	[83]
1988	Finer and Nagasawa	A procedure for the microinjection of plant cells and protoplasts	[84]
1988	Levin R. et al.	Recovery of stable transformants through particle bombardment	[85]
1988	Klein et al.	Development of random amplified polymorphic DNA	[86]
1989	Crossway A.	Transformation of soyabean through particle bombardment of embryogenic suspension culture	[87]
1989	Miki B. et al.	Plant transformation by microinjection of intact plant cells	[88]
1989	Klein T.M. et al.	Electroporation of intact plant tissues for direct DNA delivery	[89]
1990	Williams et al.	Silicon carbide fiber-mediated DNA delivery in plant cells	[90]
1990	Neuhaus G. and Spangenberg G.	Successful metabolic engineering of *Atropa belladonna* for increased alkaloid production	[91]
1990	Dekeyser R.A. et al.	Development of herbicide-resistant rice plants through PEG-mediated transformation	[92]
1990	Kaeppler H.F. et al.	The effect of several parameters on the suspension cultures of *Catharanthus roseus* cells	[93]
1991	Finner J.J. and McMullen M.D.	Production of first transgenic plants of a conifer (*Larix decidua*)	[94]
1991	Huang Y. et al.	Jasmonic acid is a signal transducer in elicitor-induced plant cell cultures	[95]
1992	Yun D.J. et al.	Zygotic embryogenesis for the recovery of fertile maize plants	[96]
1992	Datta S.K. et al.	Green hairy roots showing photoautotrophy due to development of photosynthetic ability	[97]
1992	Toivonen et al.	Improved plant transformation through electrophoresis	[98]
1992	Gundlach et al.	Genetic transformation of peach tissues by particle bombardment	[99]
1993	Kranz E. and Lorz H.	Established normal and transformed root cultures of *Artemisia annua* L. for artemisinin production	[100]
1993	Flores H.E. et al.	Amplified fragment length polymorphism was developed	[101]
1994	Griesbach R.J.	Development of "agrolistic" method of plant transformation	[102]

(Continued)

TABLE 1.1   Historical Achievements of Plant Biotechnology *(cont.)*

Year	Discoverer	Discovery	References
1994	Xiaojian and Brown	*E. coli* genome sequencing	[103]
1995	Jaziri et al.	Development of microarray	[104]
1995	Vos et al.	Genetic transformation of wheat mediated by *Agrobacterium tumefaciens*	[105]
1996	Hansen G. and Chilton M.D.	Developed the protocol of flavonoid metabolic engineering to modify flower color	[106]
1997	Blattener et al.	Sequenced human genome successfully	[107]
1997	Fodor	The first transgenic food crop to be commercialized was Flavr Savr	[108]
1997	Cheng et al.	Draft sequence of *Oryza sativa* L. (rice)	[109]
1998	Tanaka et al.	For transgenic plant development, eight of the most frequently tested species (maize, canola, potato, tomato, tobacco, soybean, cotton, and melon) were explored	[110]
2001	Venter et al.	Genetically engineered crop safety (1848 records up to 2006)	[111]
2001	Martineau	*A. tumefaciens* mediated transformation with virus-derived hairpin RNA constructs	[112]
2005	Yu et al.	Reported the improved whole-genome shotgun sequences for the genomes of *Indica* and *Japonica* rice, both with multimegabase contiguity, or almost 1,000-fold improvement over the drafts of 2002	[113]
2007	James	It was estimated that ~140 species of angiosperms had been genetically transformed	[114]
2007	Vain	Demonstrated advancements in plant genetic engineering regarding transferring genes into crop plants	[115]
2007	Thorpe	Demonstrated historical achievements in plant tissue culture	[116]
2008	Clarke J.L. et al.	Reported the *Agrobacterium*-mediated transformation for poinsettia for the first time	[117]

Haberlandt predicted that the cultured plant cells could grow, divide, and develop into embryos and then into whole plants. He isolated differentiated plant cells and was the first to culture them in Knop's salt solution [10], enriched with glucose (Figure 1.2). In his cultures, cells increased in size but failed to divide. Therefore, Haberlandt succeeded in maintaining isolated leaf cells alive for long periods but the cells failed to divide because the simple nutrient media lacked the necessary plant hormones. For his great efforts, to achieve continued cell division for the production of somatic embryos from vegetative cells, he is considered the father of plant tissue culture [6].

1.2.2.1 Totipotency of Plant Cells

From Haberlandt's postulates, Steward in 1968 coined a word to acknowledge the regeneration power: totipotency.

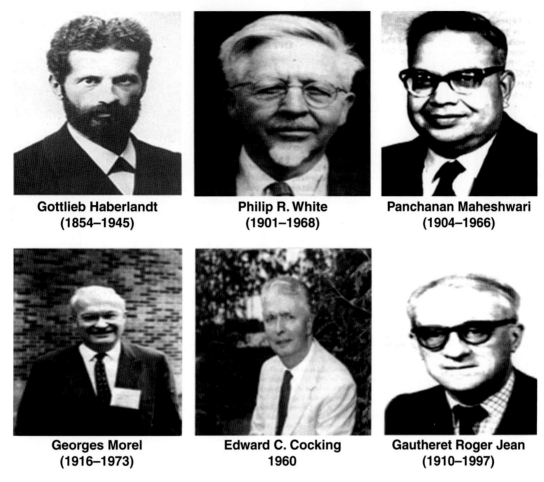

FIGURE 1.1 Popular contributors of plant tissue culture.

1.2.2.2 Improvement in Quality of Media

After the failure to grow perpetual tissue culture, the 1930s saw the development of plant tissue culture accelerated rapidly due to the discovery of vitamin B and natural auxins. Thus, from the 1930s the focus on improving the quality of media was begun. The pioneering root culture came to fruition when White established actively growing clones of tomato roots [35]. The first plant tissue culture synthetic media having defined chemical composition is the root culture medium of White [36].

1.2.2.3 Development of Plant Growth Regulators

During this period several plant growth hormones and their substitutes were discovered. Fritz Went discovered indoleacetic acid (IAA) [27]; Dutch plant physiologist Johannes Van Overbeek discovered the addition of coconut milk causes a drastic increase in the growth of plant embryos and tissue cultures [116]; Skoog and Tsui demonstrated induction of cell

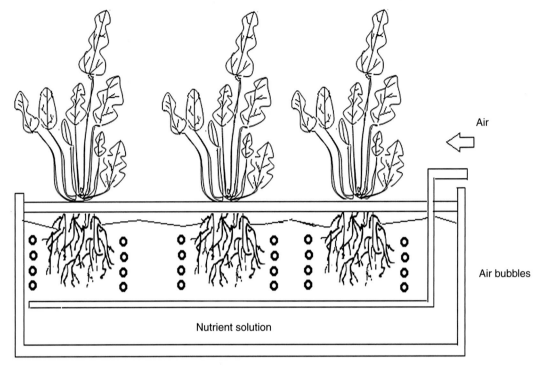

FIGURE 1.2   Knop's solution, inorganic salt nutrition.

division and bud formation due to adenine administration [118]; and Miller et al. isolated "kinetin"-adenine derivative (6-furyl aminopurine) [13,14]. They proposed the concept of hormonal control for organ formation. Some hormones were grouped together in one classification such as kinetin and many similar functioning compounds, which show bud-promoting activities are collectively classified as cytokinins [13,14]. In 1957, Skoog and Miller proved that the ratio of cytokinin to auxin in nutrient media greatly influences the morphogenesis of roots and shoots in plant tissue culture (Figure 1.3) [15]. This led to the discovery of several plant growth regulators (PGRs), which are widely used today.

1.2.2.4 Emergence of Certain Standard Synthetic Media

After the great discoveries of White's medium and several PGRs, various other standard media were discovered such as Murashige and Skoog (MS) medium [17], later revised by Linsmaier and Skoog [119], Gamborg et al. or B_5 medium [120], and Schenk and Hildbrandt medium [121].

1.2.2.5 Cell Suspension Culture and Plating Technique

After great success and expertise in callus culture, attention was now directed toward single cell cultures. Muir's observations regarding the homogeneous dispersion of callus in liquid medium to form single cell suspension were greatly appreciated [122,123]. This finding was further developed by Bergmann for cloning isolated single protoplasts, which is nowadays widely used as a plating technique [47].

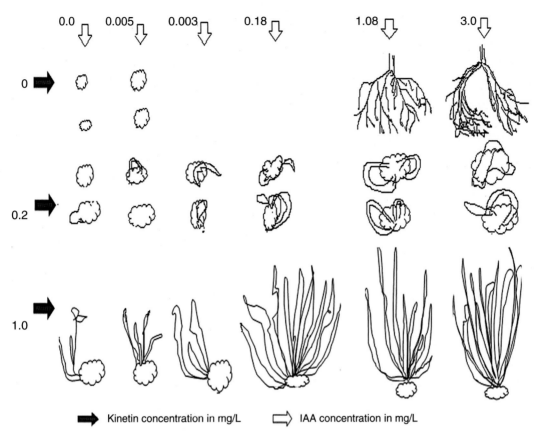

FIGURE 1.3 **Auxin/cytokinin balance [organogenesis in tobacco (Wisconsin no. 38) callus].** Effect of increasing IAA concentration at different kinetin levels and in the presence of casein hydrolysate (3 mg/L) on the growth and organ formation in tobacco callus cultured on semisolid White's medium. Age of cultures, 62 days. Note root formation in the absence of kinetin and in the presence of 0.18–3.0 mg/L kinetin with IAA concentrations in the range 0.005–0.18 mg/L. *From Skoog and Miller [15].*

1.2.2.6 Somatic Hybrid and Somatic Embryos

The first report of somatic embryo formation of carrot tissue appeared in 1958–1959 by Steward et al. and Reinert [46,124]. Later on, protoplast fusion by using various cell degrade enzymes to form a somatic hybrid was first demonstrated by Prof. Edward C. Cocking in the 1960s [16].

1.2.2.7 Test Tube Fertilization

To explore the role of tissue culture in plant genetic engineering, test tube fertilization involving excised ovules and pollen grains in the same medium was first conducted by Kanta and Maheshwari [49].

1.2.2.8 Period Between the 1940s and the 1960s

These early studies led to the development of root cultures, embryo cultures, and the first true callus/tissue cultures. The period between the 1940s and the 1960s was marked by the development of new techniques and the improvement of those already in use. It was the availability of these techniques that led to the application of tissue culture to five broad areas, namely:

1. Cell behavior (including cytology, nutrition, metabolism, morphogenesis, embryogenesis, and pathology)
2. Plant modification and improvement, pathogen-free plants
3. Germplasm storage
4. Clonal propagation
5. Product (mainly secondary metabolite) formation, in the mid-1960s

1.2.2.9 From the 1970s to the 1980s

In the early 1970s after arrival of several restriction enzymes, the genetic interferences with plant cells were started. The next breakthrough in the application of tissue culture came in 1974 when Zaenen et al. discovered that Ti plasmid is the tumor-inducing principle of *Agrobacterium tumefaciens* [125]. This crown gall disease-inducing bacterium, which was earlier recognized by Smith and Townsend in 1907, was later studied by Zambryski et al. in 1980 [126]. Larkin, in 1981, demonstrated somaclonal variation. After the discovery of the first automated DNA sequences, in 1985, the first transgenic plant was discovered [59]. This led to the discovery of the first genetically engineered crop, a tobacco, approved for release by the EPA (Environmental Protection Agency). With the advent of further advances in the 1990s, the transformation of gene in corn with a gene gun was announced. In 1994, Calgene, after having patented (1987) for the process to extend the shelf-life of tomato (by producing antisense RNA that silences the polygalacturonase gene), won approval from the US Food and Drug Administration (FDA) for the Flavr Savr® tomato [111].

1.2.2.10 Historical Research on Tobacco

Tobacco (*Nicotiana tabaccum* L.), has become a model system for tissue culture and genetic engineering over the past several decades and continues to remain the "Cinderella of plant biotechnology." *In vitro* tissue culture medium based on the studies associated with plant tissue culture has now been widely used as culture medium formulations for hundreds of plant species. Studies of growth and development, induction of haploids, microspore-derived embryos, and selection of mutant cell lines have been achieved successfully. Tobacco has been also employed for protoplast fusion, providing invaluable information on the way to explore the potential of somatic hybridization in other crops (Figure 1.4). Optimization of genetic transformation using *A. tumefaciens* and *Agrobacterium rhizogenes* has opened the opportunities in the area of transgenic plants for the production of recombinant proteins, vaccines, and antibodies. Horsh et al., in 1984, produced the first transgenic plants of tobacco by co-culture of leaf discs with *A. tumefaciens* [127]. In 1986, Abel et al. produced the first transgenic tobacco plant with useful agronomic traits [128].

1.2.2.11 After the 1990s

The 1990s saw continued expansion in the application of *in vitro* technologies to an increasing number of plant species. Major achievements are mentioned in Figure 1.5.

In 1944, Skoog demonstrated growth and organ formation in tobacco tissue culture

In 1962, Murashige and Skoog developed rapid growth and bioassays with tobacco tissue culture

In 1965, Murashige and Nakano demonstrated the morphogenetic behavior of tobacco and implications of plant senescence was studied

In 1972, Nagata and Takabe demonstrated plant regeneration from tobacco protoplast

In 1972, Carlson developed somatic hybrid (2n = 42) plant from protoplast fusion *Nicotiana glauca* (2n = 24) and *Nicotiana langsdorffii* (2n = 18)

In 1986, transgenic tobacco plant was developed

In 1989, Streber and Willmitzer transgenic tobacco plants expressing a bacterial detoxifying enzyme resistant to 2,4-D were developed

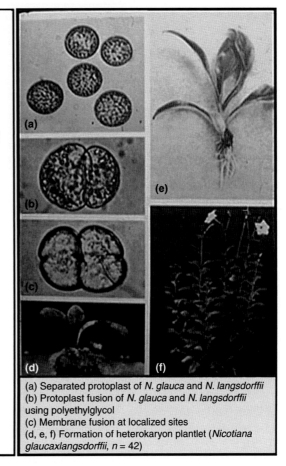

(a) Separated protoplast of *N. glauca* and *N. langsdorffii*
(b) Protoplast fusion of *N. glauca* and *N. langsdorffii* using polyethylglycol
(c) Membrane fusion at localized sites
(d, e, f) Formation of heterokaryon plantlet (*Nicotiana glaucaxlangsdorffii, n = 42*)

FIGURE 1.4 **Historical representation and development stages during somatic hybridization of *Nicotiana* sp.** [17,51,129–132].

1. Cell cultures have remained an important tool in the study of basic areas of plant biology and biochemistry and have assumed major significance in studies in molecular biology and agricultural biotechnology. Thus, progress is being made in the following areas in cell biology, e.g.:
   a. In cytoskeleton study
   b. Chromosomal changes in cultured cells
   c. Cell-cycle studies
   d. Neoplastic growth in cell cultures
   e. Primary metabolism studies in plants, for example, the regulation of carbohydrate metabolism in transgenics
   f. Identification of more than 80 enzymes of alkaloid biosynthesis
   g. Studies related to metabolic engineering for the production of secondary metabolites
   h. In the study of morphogenesis particularly of *Arabidopsis*
   i. In cytodifferentiation, mainly tracheary element formation

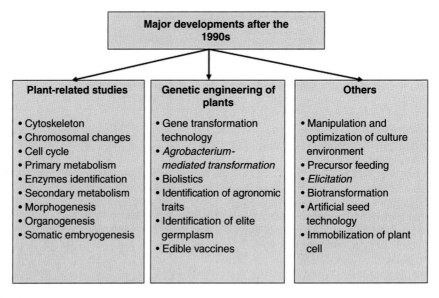

FIGURE 1.5   Illustration of major developments after the 1990s [133,134].

2. Organogenesis and somatic embryogenesis: Continued expansion in the application of *in vitro* technologies to an increasing number of plant species was observed such as including cereals and grasses, legumes, vegetable crops, potato and other root and tuber crops, oilseeds, temperate and tropical fruits, plantation crops, forest trees, and, of course, ornamentals.

3. Substantial progress has been made in extending cryopreservation technology for germplasm storage and in artificial seed technology.

4. Some novel approaches for culturing cells such as on rafts, membranes, and glass rods, as well as manipulation of the culture environment by use of nonionic surfactants, have been successfully developed.

5. Major breakthroughs after advancement in molecular biology are as follows:
   a. Genetic engineering of plants
   b. Development in gene transformation technologies
   c. Development of transport vectors for harnessing the natural gene transfer capability of *Agrobacterium*
   d. Methods to utilize these vectors for the direct transformation of regenerable explants
   e. Development of selectable markers
   f. Plant species not amenable to *Agrobacterium*-mediated transformation, physical, chemical, and mechanical means are used to get the DNA into the cells
   g. Biolistics to transform virtually any plant species and genotype
   h. Identification of agronomic traits of direct relevance to these industries, namely the control of insects, weeds, and plant diseases
   i. Technical improvements for increasing transformation efficiency
   j. Extending transformation to elite commercial germplasm
   k. Lowering transgenic plant production costs

6. At present, over 100 species of plants have been genetically engineered, including nearly all the major dicotyledonous crops and an increasing number of monocotyledonous ones, as well as some woody plants.

The current emphasis of plant biotechnology is toward the areas of plant tissue culture and molecular biology and their impact on plant improvement and biotechnology. In fact, progress in applied plant biotechnology is fully dependent on achieving sustainable and environmentally stable agriculture.

1.3 SCOPE AND IMPORTANCE OF BIOTECHNOLOGY

Plant biotechnology provides various scopes in different areas. Genetic alteration (resistance to biotic stress such as viral, fungal, bacterial, nematode, insect, and herbicide resistance) and abiotic stress with plants (transgenic plants) for either crop improvement or to improve the secondary metabolite production cover major possibilities in plant biotechnology, whereas germplasm preservation and artificial seed production contribute well in environmental conservation. Edible vaccines and production of high-value secondary metabolites explore its major role in pharmaceutical sciences. Some of the major opportunities are highlighted in Figure 1.6.

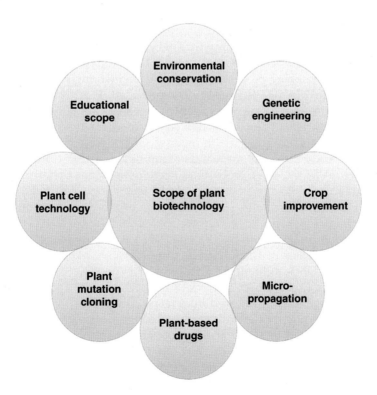

FIGURE 1.6   Different scopes of plant biotechnology.

Plant biotechnology has vast scope in the area of agriculture especially in crop improvement. In agriculture, production of transgenic plants with better resistance to pesticides (Bt toxin) and herbicides generates wide scope for plant biotechnology in agro-based industries. It is useful for understanding plant-associated nitrogen fixing bacteria, and to learn how these bacteria are key players in biogeochemical, ecological, and agricultural process and have adapted to carry out their activity under unfavorable conditions. It is also used for the utilization/effective production of cheap foods with a long shelf-life. Therefore, plant biotechnology has emerged as a science with immense potential for human welfare ranging from food processing and human health to environment protection [133–136]. There are many applications of plant biotechnology in the fields of industry, agriculture, pharmaceuticals, health care, food, energy, the environment, etc. The importance of this field of science in different streams will be evident from the following examples.

1.3.1 Biotechnology in Pharmaceutical Sciences

Biotechnology in pharmaceutical sciences has brought about the production of monoclonal antibody, DNA, RNA probes for the diagnosis of various diseases; valuable drugs; edible vaccines like human hepatitis B; therapeutic drugs such as alkaloids, glycosides, steroids, flavonoids, tannins, proteins, enzymes, antibiotics, metabolites, etc. Interference with the plant genotype leads to the expression of various recombinant proteins, which forms antibodies, vaccines, and several other proteins having various pharmaceutical applications. Development of hairy root culture by means of *Agrobacterium* infection makes plants less dependent on growth hormones for their future growth. This genetic transformation of tumor in plants also gives a better yield of secondary metabolites. Even today, a variety of pharmaceutical drugs and chemicals are being produced by genetic engineering with better quality and increased quantity. Thus, plant biotechnology has provided us with a very efficient and economic technique for the production of a variety of biochemicals [133–136].

In industrial applications, plant biotechnology is used for the production of transgenic drugs. The major benefits are expected in medical, pharmaceutical, and health sciences. In medical sciences, it is used for the production of antibiotics, insulin, growth hormone, interferon, clotting factor VIII, vaccines, probes for infectious and gene therapy, etc. A major breakthrough in plant biotechnology was through rDNA technology, which led to the production of therapeutic recombinant proteins. The basis of the production of recombinant proteins is molecular pharming of therapeutic plants by rDNA technology, which is depicted in Fig 1.7. Genetic manipulation of DNA to form the final DNA construct is the initial step of rDNA technology. Further transfer of DNA construct in respective plants to conduct trangenesis is the second step of rDNA technology. This transfer is possible by using a suitable vector (medium) such as *Agrobacterium* sp. Successful transfer may lead to production of various transgenes. This transgenesis is followed by screening of plants. In this step, plants having the suitable gene expression for the desired recombinant protein are selected. Finally, recombinant proteins are purified to form various biopharmaceuticals and vaccines. Some of the popular plant-derived biopharmaceuticals are human growth hormone, enkephalin, IgG, human lactoferrin (antimicrobial), human serum albumin, human α- and β-interferon, human α1-antitrypsin, erythropoietin, hirudin, human α and β hemoglobin, etc. Some important vaccines such as envelope surface protein (hepatitis b virus (humans), glycoprotein (rabies

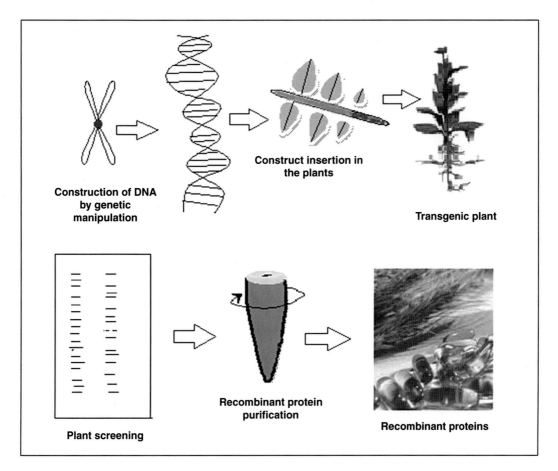

FIGURE 1.7 Production of recombinant proteins by rDNA technology.

virus), malarial B-cell epitope (malaria), and *Escherichia coli* Lt-B toxin (enterotoxigenic *E. coli*)) are also produced by rDNA technology [133–136].

1.3.2 Industrial Biotechnology

The biopharmaceutical era began with the production of the first transgenic drug, insulin in 1982 [137]. There are presently 84 biopharmaceuticals in the market helping 60 million patients worldwide with a cumulative market value of $20 billion (Figure 1.8) [137].

According to a recent survey it was found that the therapeutic protein market constituted 137 marketed products, with another 350 in Phase III clinical development. It was also predicted that in 2005 these figures would turn into 20,000 and their estimated sales by 2008 would be $20 billion (R-Pharma Report 2001 and DMD Monoclonal Antibody Report 2001) [133–137].

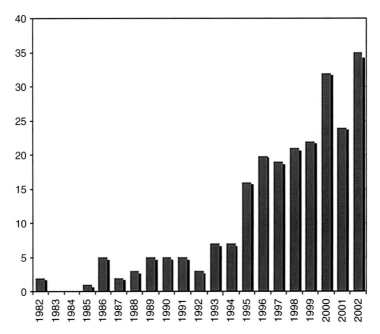

FIGURE 1.8   **Number of novel biotechnology drugs and vaccines approved during 1982–2002.** *Source: Information Systems for Biotechnology (2005).*

In comparison to bacteria, yeast, insect cells, and mammalian cells, plant systems, especially transgenic plant systems, act as a simple host to study the protein engineering, which is an important area where existing proteins and enzymes are remodeled for a specific function or for increasing the efficiency of their function [133–137].

Production of genetically modified food from transgenic plants generates various opportunities in commercial markets, though horticulture practices still need further understanding of the genetic traits of plants. Production of compounds like anticancer, antimicrobial, and flavanoids using this technique increases the demands of these elite cultivars in their commercial market.

Currently plant-made pharmaceuticals and their specified regulatory bodies are defined as follows:

- *USDA APHIS* (United States Department of Agriculture, Animal and Plant Health Inspection Service): Regulates plant growth, and defines the appropriate safeguards for regulated products and the transport of product constituents.
- *FDA CBER* (Center for Biologics Evaluation and Research) and *CDER* (Center for Drug Evaluation and Research): Regulates biologic products, their manufacture and distribution.
- *FDA CFSAN* (Center for Food Safety and Applied Nutrition) and *CMV* (Center for Veterinary Medicine): Regulates food and feed safety.
- Monsanto Protein Technologies: Provides safety assessments, drug master files, chemistry manufacturing controls, and biologics license agreement for client's drug registration and field production.

These regulatory bodies, especially APHIS, regulate field testing of the pharmaceutical (and industrial) crops [133–137]. These trials were approved for the production of safe

TABLE 1.2 Number of Field Testing Permits by APHIS as Pharmaceutical, Industrial, or Novel Traits (1991–2004 Cumulative)

Plant name	Type of products	Total no. of products
Corn	Novel proteins, industrial enzymes, pharma plants	231
Soybeans	Novel proteins, industrial enzymes, pharma plants	30
Alfalfa	Novel proteins, industrial enzymes, pharma plants	4
Barley	Novel proteins, pharma plants	2
Rapeseed	Industrial enzymes, pharma plants	3
Tobacco	Novel proteins, pharma plants	15
Tomato	Pharma plants	1
Rice	Novel proteins, industrial enzymes, pharma plants	11
Safflower	Novel proteins, industrial enzymes	3
Wheat	Novel proteins	2
Sugarcane	Pharma plants	1
Other	Novel proteins, industrial enzymes, pharma plants	22

Source: Information Systems for Biotechnology (2005).

pharmaceuticals, novel proteins, and industrial enzymes. The number of these trials has grown in the past few years, particularly in corn, tobacco, soybeans, and rice (Table 1.2). However, corn is still the crop of choice.

There is immense scope for recombinant protein-based pharmaceuticals, which are manufactured by using plant cell-based systems (Table 1.3). Tobacco was the first plant that was utilized to accumulate a functional murine monoclonal antibody [133–137].

1.3.3 Biotechnology and the Environment

Environmental problems like endangered plants species and large-scale propagation of medicinal plants with elite traits are being resolved by using biotechnology. Several phytoremediation projects are governed by several governments and the private sector to prevent the extinction of certain precious flora. Molecular and heterosis breeding promotes the plant genomics to improve the variety of plants, which may yield better compounds in less time. One more popular achievement of plant biotechnology in environmental sciences was increasing photosynthetic efficiency for biomass production in the plant with the same amount of light and other inputs. There are many uses in environmental biotechnology such as generating microbes and plants for bioremediation.

Plant biotechnology actively participates in the protection of the environment by adopting several new *ex situ* methods. These new *ex situ* conservation methods are necessary for the preservation of lost plant genetic resources. Advancement in biotechnology furnished new methods for plant germplasm conservation and evaluation. Some of the common biotechnological tools like *in vitro* culture, cryopreservation, and molecular markers present a valuable alternative to plant diversity studies, management of genetic resources, and ultimately conservation.

TABLE 1.3   Selected North American and European Biotechnology Companies Specializing in Plant-Made Pharmaceuticals

Biotech company	Vehicle plant	Proprietary technology	Target plant-made pharmaceuticals
Large-scale biology	Tobacco	Viral transfection vector	B-cell non-Hodgkin's lymphoma (Phase III); alpha-galactosidase A (therapy for Fabry's disease); patient-specific cancer vaccines
Crop Tech	Tobacco	Viral vector	Filed for bankruptcy in 2003
Icon genetics	Tobacco	Nuclear and plastid transformation, pro-viral transfection	Antibody and non-Hodgkin's lymphoma vaccine
Chlorogen	Tobacco	Chloroplast-based expression	Cholera vaccine; human serum albumin; interferon (hepatitis C)
Planet biotechnology	Tobacco	Antibody production	CaroRx (targets bacterium that causes tooth decay)
SemBioSys	Safflower	Oil seed-based expression	Anti-obesity peptide; somatotropin; insulin; Apolipoprotein A-1; immunospheres
Medicago	Alfalfa	Expression in forage crop	Hemoglobin
Ventria BioScience	Rice	Seed-based expression	Lactoferrin and lysozyme
Dow/Dow Agro Sciences	Corn/beans of castor plants	Seed-based expression	Phosphinothricin acetyl transferase. Confidential business information – origin: human. RiVax.
Epicyte	Corn	Seed-based expression (contraceptive corn)	Monoclonal antibodies (plantibodies); EPI-19 (bronchiolitis/pneumonia in infants)
Meristem Therapeutics	Corn; tobacco; alfalfa	Seed-based expression	Hemoglobin; gastric lipase (cistic fibrosis, pancreatitis; Phase II); albumin (surgery); cancer therapeutic antibodies
Monsanto Protein Technologies	Corn	Seed-based expression	IgG antiherpes simplex virus. C transcriptional activator.
ProdiGene	Corn	Seed-based expression; October 2002: soybeans accidently mixed with medicine-producing GM corn	Avidin (a diagnostic protein) in GM corn; antibody for traveler's diarrhea. Laccase. Subunit vaccines, recombinant antibodies and further technical enzymes, such as aprotinin and laccase
Syngenta	Corn	Seed-based expression	
Biolex	Corn	Seed-based expression	Duckweed to produce α-interferon and other proteins. Investigational new drug (IND) filing this year

TABLE 1.3 Selected North American and European Biotechnology Companies Specializing in Plant-Made Pharmaceuticals (*cont.*)

Biotech company	Vehicle plant	Proprietary technology	Target plant-made pharmaceuticals
Limagrain	Corn	Phosphinothricin acetyl transferase. Procollagen – origin: human. G glycoprotein serum albumin – origin: human. Alpha-hemoglobin – origin: human. Beta-hemoglobin – origin: human	
Dupoint	Duckweed		
AltaGen (USA)	Potato		Hemoglobin; factor VIII; human growth hormone
Cornell University	Potato		Edible vaccine for hepatitis B
MPB Cologne (appears to be out of business)	Potato; rapeseed		Potatoes
Spanz	Potatoes		Make proteins that will help the body repair itself after heart or circulatory system surgery or nervous diseases
Applied Phytologics	Rice	Seed-based expression	Human-1-antitrypsin Lactoferrin – origin: human. Lysozyme – origin: human. Antithrombin – origin: human. Aminoglycoside 3'-adenylyltransferase – origin: human. Serum albumin – origin: human.
Washington State University	Barley	.	Antithrombin – origin: human. Antitrypsin – origin: human. Lactoferrin – origin: human. Lysozyme – origin: human. Serum albumin – origin: human
Nexgen Biotechnologies	Potato; cucumber; oriental melon; tobacco		Thyroid-stimulating hormone receptor. Hemorrhagic fever virus antigens for diagnosis. Poultry vaccine for avian influenza (H5N1), epidermal growth factor, albumin fusion protein.

Source: Information Systems for Biotechnology (2005).

A list of some of the most common endangered species in India with their type of explant used is revealed in subsequent chapters.

1.3.4 Biotechnology and Agriculture

In agriculture, plant cell, tissue, and organ culture is used for rapid and economic clonal multiplication of fruit and forest trees, for production of virus-free genetic stocks and planting material as well as in the creation of novel genetic variations through somaclonal variation. Genetic engineering techniques are utilized to produce transgenic plants with desirable genes like disease resistance, herbicide resistance, increased shelf-life of fruits, etc. Also, molecular breeding has hastened the process of crop improvement for, for example, molecular markers like RFLP (restriction fragment length polymorphisms) and simple sequence repeats (SSRs) provide powerful tools for indirect selection of both qualitative and quantitative traits and also for studying genotypic diversity (applications are mentioned in Section 5.3.1.9).

In 2002, farmers were expected to plant more than 79 million acres (40 million hectares) of genetically improved corn and soybeans, a 13% increase from the year before. Indian farmers have finally got the official go-ahead for planting insect-resistant cotton. In Brazil it is expected that genetically improved crops will be authorized. In China more than 5 million subsidiary farmers are using insect-resistant plants successfully. Currently, more than 50,000,000 ha of transgenic plants have been used worldwide. In comparison, in Europe farmers had fewer than 15,000 ha of plants. In the last six years, more than 170,000,000 ha of transgenic plants have been used worldwide. Although the Novel Food Regulation has existed since 1997, not a single genetically modified product besides those accepted as substantially equivalent has been authorized under this regulation. And no product was authorized under the Deliberate Release Directive since 1998 due to political opposition to the technology by six member states, including France. Today, some 85 pharmaceuticals made from genetically modified organisms are available on the market and 360 new companies have been set up [138].

1.3.5 Educational Scope

Information technology + Biotechnology = Better tomorrow

Biotechnology graduates are moving into entry-level research positions in the agricultural biotechnology industry, in areas such as tissue culture and transformation, recombinant DNA and molecular biology, protein and nucleic acid biochemistry, genomics, proteomics, and bioinformatics. Biotechnology is a global industry, and a majority companies worldwide have conducted significant research. Students may continue their education in graduate school earning an MS or PhD to enable them to pursue careers in research and/or higher education. Increasingly, professions such as law, technical sales, and business have found students with an education in biotechnology to be strategic hires. There are several large agricultural biotechnology companies in the USA, such as Syngenta at Greensboro and Research Triangle Park (RTP), both in North Carolina; BASF and Bayer also have research facilities at RTP. Monsanto is located in St. Louis, Missouri, Pioneer-Hybred/DuPont in Iowa and Delaware, and Dow AgroSciences is located in Indianapolis. In addition to larger companies, there are many smaller companies and start-ups looking for recent biotechnology graduates.

Currently, Indian plant tissue culture-based industries follow an improved system of quality management system called the National Certification System for Tissue Culture Raised Plants (NCS-TCP), which aims at recognition of commercial tissue culture production facilities, accreditation of test laboratories, and certification of tissue culture raised plants of recognized tissue culture production facilities by the Accredited Test Laboratories. NCS-TCP was established by the Department of Biotechnology (DBT), government of India, which is the first of its kind in the world. Recently lots of plant tissue culture units have flourished in India. Indoor foliage plants dominate the export market. The micropropagation industry in India is providing major support to Indian agriculture in four crop groups: fruits, ornamentals, spices, and forestry/plantation crops. Banana is the largest selling tissue culture fruit crop. Furthermore, tissue culture papaya, rose, anthuriums, sugarcane, vanilla orchids, and gerberas have attained commercial importance.

Skills in tissue culture and transformation, recombinant DNA and molecular biology, protein and nucleic acid biochemistry, genomics, proteomics, and bioinformatics are particularly useful. Moreover, internationally there are various government organizations that are involved in funding research, training, and extension for developing and using biotechnologies for food and agriculture, such as the National Institute of Food and Agriculture, USA, and the Department of Biotechnology, India. Moreover, each year plant biotechnology generates several opportunities for their aspirants so that one can make a career in biotechnology in the following areas:

- Agriculture and environmental biotechnology
- Health sciences and pharmaceutical science
- Plant forensics and reproductive biology
- Food and dairy biotechnology
- Patent attorney
- Clinical research on plant tissue culture-based products
- Drug regulatory affairs
- Good manufacturing practices and good laboratory practices
- Drug designing and new delivery systems of plant tissue culture-based medicines
- Nanobiotechnology and their applications
- Environment protection and conservation through biotechnology
- Regulatory and legal regulations for transgenic and plant tissue culture-based products
- Compounding, dispensing, and packaging of plant tissue culture-based products
- Academics in college and university
- Career as scientist in plant tissue-based research institutes or industries

References

[1] Jha TB, Ghosh B. Plant tissue culture: basic and applied. Hyderabad, India: Universities Press; 2005. p. 1–7.
[2] Bhojwani SS, Razdan MK. Plant tissue culture: theory and practice. 1st ed. Amsterdam, The Netherlands: Elsevier Science; 1996. p. 1–18.
[3] Mishra SP. Plant tissue culture. New Delhi, India: Ane Books Pvt Ltd; 2009. p. 1–20.
[4] Rajdan MK. Introduction to plant tissue culture: plant breeding. 2nd ed. New Delhi: Oxford and IBH Publishing; 2003. p. 1–13.
[5] Chawla HS. Introduction to plant biotechnology. 3rd ed. New Delhi: Oxford and IBH Publishing; 2009. p. 1–13.
[6] Haberlandt G. Culturversuche mit isolierten Pflanzenzellen. Sitz-Ber Mat Nat Kl Kais Akad Wiss Wien 1902;111:69–92.
[7] White PR. A handbook of plant tissue culture. Lancaster, Pa: The Jacques Catlell Press; 1943.

[8] Gautheret RJ. Sur la possibilité de réaliser la culture indéfinie des tissues de tubercules de carotte. C R Soc Biol Paris 1939;208:118–20.

[9] Uspenski EE, Uspenskaja WJ. Reinkultur und ungeschlechtliche Fortpflanzung des Volvox minor und Volvox globator in einer synthetischen Nahrlosung. Z Bot 1925;17:273.

[10] Knop W. Quantitativ Untersuchungen uber den Ernahrungsprozess der Pflanzen. Landw Versuchs-Stat 1865;7:93–107.

[11] Ball. Development in sterile culture of stem tips and adjacent regions of Tropaeolum majus L. and of Lupin albus L. Am J Bot 1946;33:301–18.

[12] Muir WH, Hildebrandt AC, Riker AJ. Plant tissue cultures produced from single isolated plant cells. Science 1954;119:877–8.

[13] Miller CO, Skoog F, Von Saltza MH, Strong F. Kinetin, a cell division factor from deoxyribonucleic acid. J Am Chem Soc 1955;77:1392.

[14] Miller CO, Skoog F, Okumura FS, von Saltza MH, Strong FM. Structure and synthesis of kinetin. J Am Chem Soc 1955;78:2662–3.

[15] Skoog F, Miller CO. Chemical regulation of growth and organ formation in plant tissue cultured in vitro. Symp Soc Exp Biol 1957;XI:118–31.

[16] Cocking EC. A method for the isolation of plant protoplasts and vacuoles. Nature 1960;187:962–3.

[17] Murashige T, Skoog F. A revised medium for rapid growth and bio-assays with tobacco tissue cultures. Physiol Plant 1962;15:473–97.

[18] Mishra SP. Plant tissue culture. New Delhi, India: Ane Books Pvt Ltd; 2009. p. 1–14.

[19] Narayanaswamy S. Plant cell and tissue culture. New Delhi, India: Tata McGraw-Hill Education; 1994. p. 1–7.

[20] Sathyanarayana BN. Plant tissue culture: practices and new experimental protocols. I. K. International Pvt Ltd; 2007. 1–8.

[21] Smith EF, Townsend CO. A plant-tumor of bacterial origin. Science 1907;25:671–3.

[22] Kotte W. Wurzelmeristem in gewebekultur. Ber Deut Ges 1922;40:269–72.

[23] Kotte W. Kulturversuche mit isolierten wurzelspitzen. Beitr Allg Bot 1922;2:413–34.

[24] Robbins WJ. Effect of autolysed yeast and peptone on growth of excised corn root tips in the dark. Bot Gaz (Chicago) 1922;74:59–79.

[25] Robbins WJ. Cultivation of excised root tips and stem tips under sterile conditions. Bot Gaz 1922;73:376–90.

[26] Robbins WJ, Maneval WE. Further experiments on growth of excised root tips under sterile conditions. Bot Gaz 1923;76:274–87.

[27] Went FW. On growth accelerating substances in the coleoptiles of Avina sativa. Proc K Ned Akad Wet Ser 1926;C30:10.

[28] Kögl F, Haagen-Smit AJ, Erxleben H. Über ein neues Auxin ("Hetero-auxin") aus Harn. Z Physiol Chem 1934;228(1-2):90–103.

[29] Gautheret RJ. Sur la culture d extrémités de raciness. New York, NY: Ronald Press; 1932. p. 228.

[30] Gautheret RJ. Recherches sur la culture des tissus végétaux. Essais de culture de quelques tissus méristématiques. Paris: Le François; 1935.

[31] Gautheret RJ. La culture des tissus végétaux. Sonétat actuel, comparaison avec la culture des tissus animaux. Paris: Hermann & Cie; 1937.

[32] Gautheret RJ. Culture du tissue cambial. C R Acad Sci (Paris) 1934;198:2195–6.

[33] White PR. Influence of some environmental conditions on the growth of excised root tips of wheat in liquid media. Plant Physiol 1932;7:613–28.

[34] White PR. Plant tissue cultures. A preliminary report of results obtained in the culturing of certain plant meristems. Archiv für Experimentelle Zellforschung 1932;12:602–20.

[35] White PR. Potentially unlimited growth of excised tomato root tips in a liquid medium. Plant Physiol 1934;9:585–600.

[36] White PR. Potentially unlimited growth of excised plant callus in an artificial nutrient. Am J Bot 1939;26:59–64.

[37] White PR. Controlled differentiation in a plant tissue culture. Bull Torrey Bot Club 1939;66:507–13.

[38] White PR, Braun AC. Crown gall production by bacteria-free tumor tissues. Science 1941;94:239–41.

[39] White PR, Braun AC. A cancerous neoplasm of plants: autonomous bacteria-free crown-gall tissue. Cancer Res 1942;2:597–617.

[40] Loo SW. Cultivation of excised stem tips of asparagus in vitro. Am J Bot 1945;32:13–7.

[41] Steward FC, Caplin SM. A tissue culture from potato tuber: the synergistic action of 2,4-D and coconut milk. Science 1951;113:518–20.

[42] Morel G, Martin C. Guerison de pommes de terre atteintics de maladies a virus. C R Acad Agric Fr 1952;41:471–4.

[43] Muir WH, Hildebrandt AC, Riker AJ. Plant tissue cultures produced from single isolated plant cells. Science 1954;119:877–8.

[44] Steward FC, Shantz EM. The chemical induction of growth in plant tissue cultures. I. Methods of tissue culture and the analysis of growth. II. The chemical nature of the growth promoting substances in coconut milk and similar fluids: the present composition. In: Wain RL, Wightman F, editors. The chemistry and mode of action of plant growth substances. London: Academic Press; 1955. p. 165–86.

[45] Nickell LG. The continuous submerged cultivation of plant tissue as single cells. Proc Nat Acad Sci 1956;42:848.

[46] Steward FC. Growth and development of cultivated cells. III. Interpretations of the growth from free cell to carrot plant. A N J Bot 1958;45:709–13.

[47] Bergmann L. Growth and division of single cells of higher plants cultured in vitro. J Gen Physiol 1960;43:841–51.

[48] Jones LE, Hildebrandt AC, Riker AJ, Wu JH. Growth of somatic tobacco cells in microculture. Am J Bot 1960;47:468–75.

[49] Kanta K, Ranga Swamy F NS, Maheshwari P. Test-tube fertilization in a flowering plant. Nature 1962;194: 1214–7.

[50] Guha S, Maheshwari SC. In vitro production of embryos from anthers of Datura. Nature 1964;204:497.

[51] Power JB, Cummins SE, Cocking EC. Fusion of isolated protoplasts. Nature 1970;225:1016–8.

[52] Carlson PS, Smith HH, Dearing RD. Parasexual interspecific plant hybridization. Proc Natl Acad Sci USA 1972;69:2292–4.

[53] Zenk MH, EI-Shagi H, Schulte U. Anthraquinone production by cell suspension cultures of Morinda citrifolia. Planta Med 1975;Suppl:79–101.

[54] Zenk MH, EI-Shagi E, Arens H, Stockigt J, Weiler EW, Deus B. Formation of the indole alkaloids serpentine and ajmalicine in suspension cultures of Catharanthus roseus. In: Barz W, Reinhard E, Zenk MH, editors. Plant tissue culture and its biotechnological applications. Berlin: Springer-Verlag; 1977. p. 27–43.

[55] Melchers G, Sacristán MD, Holder AA. Somatic hybrid plants of potato and tomato regenerated from fused protoplasts. Carlsberg Res Commun 1978;43:203–18.

[56] Márton L, Wullems GJ, Molendijk L, Schilperoort RA. In vitro transformation of cultured cells from Nicotiana tabacum by Agrobacterium tumefactions. Nature 1979;277:129–31.

[57] Alfermann AW, Schuller I, Reinhard E. Biotransformation of cardiac glycosides by immobilized cell cultures of Digitalis lanata L. Planta Med 1980;40:218–23.

[58] Chilton MD, Saiki R, Yadav N, Gordon M, Quetier F. T-DNA from Ti plasmid is in the nuclear DNA fraction of crown gall tumor cells. Proc Natl Acad Sci USA 1980;77:4060–4.

[59] Willmitzer L, Beuckeleer MD, Lemmers M, Van Montagu M, Schell J. DNA from Ti plasmid present in nucleus and absent from plastids of crown gall plant cells. Nature 1980;287:359–61.

[60] Larkin PJ, Scowcroft WR. Somaclonal variation-a novel source of variability from cell cultures for plant improvement. Theor Appl Genet 1981;60:197–214.

[61] Shuler ML. Production of secondary metabolites from plant tissue culture – problems and prospects. Ann N Y Acad Sci 1981;369:65–79.

[62] Krens FA, Molendijk L, Wullems GJ, Schilperoort RA. In vitro transformation of plant protoplasts with Ti-plasmid DNA. Nature 1982;296:72–4.

[63] Zimmermann U. Electric field-mediated fusion and related electrical phenomena. Biochim Biophys Acta 1982;694(3):227–77.

[64] Zimmermann U, Vienken J. Electric field-induced cell-to-cell fusion. J Membr Biol 1982;67(3):165–82.

[65] Zambryski P, Joos H, Genetello C, Leemans J, Montagu MV, Schell J. Ti plasmid vector for the introduction of DNA into plant cells without alteration of their normal regeneration capacity. EMBO J 1983;2(12):2143–50.

[66] Paszkowski J, Shillito RD, Saul M, Mandák V, Hohn T, Hohn B, et al. Direct gene transfer to plants. EMBO J 1984;3(12):2717–22.

[67] Chen TH, Kartha KK, Leung NL, Kurz WG, Chatson KB, Constabel F. Cryopreservation of alkaloid-producing cell cultures of periwinkle (Catharanthus roseus). Plant Physiol 1984;75(3):726–31.

[68] Block MD, Herrera-Estrella L, Montagu MV, Schell J, Zambryski P. Expression of foreign genes in regenerated plants and in their progeny. EMBO J 1984;3(8):1681–9.

[69] Hernalsteens JP, Thia-Toong L, Schell J, Van Montagu M. An Agrobacterium-transformed cell culture from the monocot Asparagus officinalis. EMBO J 1984;3(13):3039–41.

[70] Tabata M, Fujita Y. Production of shikonin by plant cell cultures. In: Zaitlin M, Day P, Hollaender A, editors. Biotechnology in plant science. Orlando: Academic Press; 1985. p. 207–18.

[71] Horsch RB, Fry JE, Hoffmann N, Eicholz D, Rogers SG, Fraley RT. A simple and general method for transferring genes into plants. Science 1985;227:1229–31.

[72] Fraley RT, Rogers SG, Horsch RB, Eichholtz DA, Flick JS, Fink CL, et al. The SEV system: a new disarmed Ti plasmid vector system for plant transformation. Biotechnology (NY) 1985;3:629–35.

[73] An G. Binary Ti vectors for plant transformation and promoter analysis. Methods Enzymol 1987;153:292–305.

[74] Fromm M, Taylor LP, Walbot V. Expression of genes transferred into monocot and dicot plant cells by electroporation. Proc Natl Acad Sci USA 1985;82(17):5824–8.

[75] Flores HE, Filner P. Metabolic relationships of putrescine, GABA and alkaloids in cell and root cultures of Solanaceae. In: Neuman K-H, Barz W, Reinhard E, editors. Primary and secondary metabolism of plant cell cultures. New York: Springer-Verlag; 1985. p. 174–85.

[76] Mullis K, Faloona F, Scharf S, Saiki R, Horn G, Erlich H. Specific enzymatic amplification of D.N.A. *in vitro*: the polymerase chain reaction. Cold Spring Harb Sym Quant Biol 1986;51:263–73.

[77] Crossway A, Oakes JV, Irvine JM, Ward B, Knauf VC, Shewmaker CK. Integration of foreign DNA following microinjection of tobacco mesophyll protoplasts. Mol Gen Genet 1986;202:179–85.

[78] Sanford JC, Klein TM, Wolf ED, Allen NJ. Delivery of substances in to the cells and tissues using a particle bombardment process. J Part Sci Techn 1987;6:559–63.

[79] Barton KA, Whiteley HR, Yang NS. Bacillus thuringiensis delta-endotoxin expressed in transgenic *Nicotiana tobacum* provides resistance to Lepidoptera insects. Plant Physiol 1987;85:1103–9.

[80] Bytebier B, Deboeck F, Greve HD, Montagu MV, Hernalsteens JP. T-DNA organization in tumor cultures and transgenic plants of the monocotyledon Asparagus officinalis. Proc Natl Acad Sci USA 1987;84(15):5345–9.

[81] Miki BLA, Reich TJ, Iyer VN. Microinjection: an experimental tool for studying and modifying plant cells. In: Hohn T, Schell J (eds.). Plant DNA Infectious Agents. Vienna: Springer 1987;249–65.

[82] Firoozabady E, DeBoer DL, Merlo DJ, Halk EL, Amerson LN, Rashka KE, et al. Transformation of cotton (Gossypium hirsutum L.) by Agrobacterium tumefaciens and regeneration of transgenic plants. Plant Mol Biol 1987;10:105–16.

[83] Klein TM, Frommt M, Weissingert A, Tomest D, Schaaft S, Slettent M, et al. Transfer of foreign genes in to intact maize cells with high-velocity microprojectiles. Proc Natl Acad Sci USA 1988;85:4305–9.

[84] Finer JJ, Nagasawa A. Development of an embryogenic suspension culture of soybean (*Glycine max* Merrill.). Plant Cell, Tiss Org 1988;15:125–36.

[85] Levin R, Gaba V, Tal B, Hirsch S, Denola D, Vasil IK. Automated plant tissue culture for mass propagation. Biotechnology 1988;6:1035–40.

[86] Klein TM, Harpert EC, Svabtt Z, Sanford JC, Fromm ME, Maliga P. Stable genetic transformation of intact Nicotiana cells by the particle bombardment process. Proc Natl Acad Sci USA 1988;85:8502–5.

[87] Crossway A. Microinjection of cells and protoplasts: integration of foreign DNA. Plant Protoplasts and Genetic Engineering II Biotechnology in Agriculture and Forestry 1989;9:228–40.

[88] Miki B, Huang B, Bird S, Kemble R, Simmonds D, Keller W. A procedure for the microinjection of plant cells and protoplasts. J Tiss Cult Meth 1989;12:139–44.

[89] Klein TM, Kornstein L, Sanford J, Fromm ME. Genetic transformation of maize cells by particle bombardment. Plant Physiol 1989;91:440–4.

[90] Williams JG, Kubelik AR, Livak KJ, Rafalski JA, Tingey SV. DNA polymorphisms amplified by arbitrary primers are useful as genetic markers. Nucleic Acids Res 1990;18(22):6531–5. 25.

[91] Finner JJ, McMullen MD. Transformation of soyabean through particle bombardment of embryogenic suspension culture. *In Vitro* Cell Div Biol 1991;27:175–82.

[92] Neuhaus G, Spangenberg G. Plant transformation by microinjection techniques. Physiol Planta 1990;79:213–7.

[93] Dekeyser RA, Claes B, Rycke RD, Habets ME, Montagu MCV, Caplan AB. Transient gene expression in intact and organized rice tissues. Plant Cell 1990;2(7):591–602.

[94] Kaeppler HF, Gu W, Somers DA, Rines HW, Cockburn AF. Silicon carbide fiber-mediated DNA delivery into plant cells. Plant Cell Rep 1990;9(8):415–8.

[95] Huang Y, Diner AM, Karnosky DF. *Agrobacterium rhizogenes*-mediated genetic transformation and regeneration of a conifer: *Larix decidua*. *In Vitro* Cell Dev Biol 1991;27:201–7.

[96] Yun DJ, Hashimoto T, Yamada Y. Metabolic engineering of medicinal plants: transgenic *Atropa belladonna* with an improved alkaloid composition. Proc Natl Acad Sci USA 1992;89(24):11799–803.

[97] Datta SK, Datta K, Soltanifar N, Donn G, Potrykus I. Herbicide-resistant Indica rice plants from IRRI breeding line IR72 after PEG-mediated transformation of protoplasts. Plant Mol Biol 1992;20(4):619–29.

[98] Toivonen L, Laakso S, Rosenqvist H. The effect of temperature on growth, indole alkaloid accumulation and lipid composition of *Catharanthus* roseus cell suspension cultures. Plant Cell Rep 1992;11(8):390–4.

[99] Gundlach H, Müller MJ, Kutchan TM, Zenk MH. Jasmonic acid is a signal transducer in elicitor-induced plant cell cultures. Proc Natl Acad Sci USA 1992;89(6):2389–93.

[100] Kranz E, Lörz H. *In vitro* fertilization with isolated, single gametes results in zygotic embryogenesis and fertile maize plants. Plant Cell 1993;5:739–46.

[101] Flores HE, Dai YR, Cuello JL, Maldonado-Mendoza IE, Loyola-Vargas VM. Green roots: photosynthesis and photoautotrophy in an underground plant organ. Plant Physiol 1993;101:363–71.

[102] Griesbach RJ. An improved method for transforming plants through electrophoresis. Plant Sci 1994;102:81–9.

[103] Xiaojian Y, Brown SK. Genetic transformation of peach tissues by particle bombardment. J Amer Soc Hort Sci 1994;119(2):367–73.

[104] Jaziri M, Shimomura K, Yoshimatsu K, Fauconnier M, Marller M, Homes J. Establishment of normal and transformed root cultures of *Artemisia annua* L. for artemisinin production. J Plant Physiol 1995;145:175–7.

[105] Vos P, Hogers R, Bleeker M, et al. AFLP: a new technique for DNA fingerprinting. Nucleic Acids Res 1995;23:4407–14.

[106] Hansen G, Chilton MD. Agrolistic transformation of plant cells: integration of T-strands generated in planta. Proc Natl Acad Sci USA 1996;93(25):14978–83.

[107] Blattner FR, Plunkett G, Bloch CA, Perna NT, Burland V, Riley M, et al. The complete genome sequence of *Escherichia coli* K-12. Science 1997;277(5331):1453–62. 5.

[108] Fodor SP, Read JL, Pirrung MC, Stryer L, Lu AT, Solas D. Light-directed, spatially addressable parallel chemical synthesis. Science 1991;251:767–73.

[109] Cheng M, Fry JE, Pang S, Zhou H, Hironaka CM, Duncan DR, et al. Genetic transformation of wheat mediated by *Agrobacterium tumefaciens*. Plant Physiol 1997;115:971–80.

[110] Tanaka Y, Tsuda S, Kusumi T. Metabolic Engineering to Modify Flower Color. Plant Cell Physiol 1998;39(11): 1119–26.

[111] Venter JC, et al. The sequence of the human genome. Science 2001;291:1304–51.

[112] Martineau B. First fruit: the creation of the Flavr Savr tomato and the birth of genetically engineered food. New York: McGraw-Hill; 2001.

[113] Yu J, Wang J, Lin W, Li S, Li H, et al. The genomes of *Oryza sativa*: a history of duplications. PLoS Biol 2005;3(2):e38.

[114] James C. Global status of commercialized biotech/GM Crops: 2007. Ithaca, NY: ISAAA Brief; 2007. 37.

[115] Vain P. Thirty years of plant transformation technology development. Plant Biotechnol J 2007;5:221–9.

[116] Thorpe TA. History of plant tissue culture. Mol Biotechnol 2007;37(2):169–80.

[117] Clarke JL, Spetz C, Haugslien S, Xing S, Dees MW, Moe R, et al. *Agrobacterium tumefaciens*-mediated transformation of poinsettia, *Euphorbia pulcherrima*, with virus-derived hairpin RNA constructs confers resistance to poinsettia mosaic virus. Plant Cell Rep 2008;27(6):1027–38.

[118] van Overbeek J, Conklin ME, Blakeslee AF. Factors in coconut milk essential for growth and development of very young Datura embryos. Science 1941;94(2441):350–1.

[119] Skoog F, Tsui C. Growth substances and the formation of buds in plant tissues. In: Skoog F, editor. Plant growth substances. Madison, WI: University of Wisconsin Press; 1951. p. 263–85.

[120] Linsmaier EM, Skoog F. Organic growth factor requirements of tobacco tissue cultures. Physiol Plant 1965;18:100–27.

[121] Gamborg OL, Miller RA, Ojima K. Nutrient requirements of suspension cultures of soybean root cells. Exp Cell Res 1968;50:151–8.

[122] Schenk RU, Hildebrandt AC. Medium and techniques for induction and growth of monocot tyledonous and dicotyledonous plant cell cultures. Can J Bot 1972;50:199–204.

[123] Muir WH, Hilderbrandt AC, Riker AJ. Plant tissue cultures produced from single isolated plant cells. Science 1954;119:877–8.

[124] Muir WH. Cultural conditions favouring the isolation and growth of the single cells from higher plants *in vitro*. PhD thesis, University of Wisconin, USA; 1953.

[125] Reinert J. Uber die kontrolle der morphogenese und die induktion von adventivembryonen an gewebekulturen aus karotten. Planta 1959;53:318–33.

[126] Zaenen I, Van Larebeke N, Teuchy H, Van Montagu M, Schell J. Supercoiled circular DNA in crown-gall inducing Agrobacterium strains. J Mol Biol 1974;86:109–27.

[127] Zambryski P, Holsters M, Kruger K, Depicker A, Schell J, Van Montagu M, et al. Tumor DNA structure in plant cells transformed by *A. tumefaciens*. Science 1980;209:1385–91.

[128] Horsh RB, Fry JE, Hoffman HL, Eicholts D, Rogers SG, Fraley RT. Simple and general method for transferring genes into plants. Science 1985;277:1229–31.

[129] Abel PP, Nelson RS, De B, Hoffmann N, Rogers SG, Fraley RT, et al. Delay of disease development in transgenic plants that express the tobacco mosaic virus coat protein gene. Science 1986;232(4751):738–43.

[130] Nagata T, Takabe I. Plating of isolated tobacco mesophyll protoplasts on agar medium. Planta 1971;99:12–20.

[131] Skoog F. Growth and organ formation in tobacco tissue culture. Am J Bot 1944;31:19–24.

[132] Murashige T, Nakano R. Morphogenetic behavior of tobacco tissue cultures and implication of plant senescence. Am J Bot 1965;52:819–27.

[133] Streber WR, Willmitzer L. Transgenic tobacco plants expressing a bacterial detoxifying enzyme are resistant to 2,4-D. Nat Biotechnol 1989;7:811–6.

[134] Sussex IM. The scientific roots of modern plant biotechnology. Plant Cell 2008;20(5):1189–98.

[135] Altman A. Plant biotechnology in the 21st century: the challenges ahead. EJB Electron J Biotechnol 1999;2(2): 51–5.

[136] Chua NH, Sundaresan V. Plant biotechnology: the ins and outs of a new green revolution. Curr Opin Biotechnol 2000;11:117–9.

[137] Frommer WB, Beachy R. Plant biotechnology A future for plant biotechnology? Naturally! Curr Opin Plant Biol 2003;6:147–9.

[138] Information Systems for Biotechnology. Field test releases in the U.S. Available from: http://www.isb.vt.edu/cfdocs/fieldtests1.cfm.; 2005

[139] Katzek JA. The future of biotechnology. J Comm Biotechnol 2002;9:5–7.

2

Plant Tissue Culture

Saurabh Bhatia

Modern Applications of Plant Biotechnology in Pharmaceutical Sciences. http://dx.doi.org/10.1016/B978-0-12-802221-4.00002-9

2.1 INTRODUCTION

Plant tissue culture is defined as:

The in vitro culture of plant protoplasts, cells, tissues or organs under controlled aseptic conditions which lead to cell multiplication or regeneration of organs or whole plants.

It is one of the best approaches to express the totipotency potential and to induce geno-typical and phenotypical manipulation in plant cells. There are diverse basic and applied applications of plant tissue culture (described in Chapter 5) [1,2]. Several advantages as well as disadvantages of plant tissue culture are mentioned in Table 2.1.

2.2 TYPES OF TISSUE CULTURE

2.2.1 Cultures of Organized Structures

Organized growth contributes toward the creation or maintenance of a defined structure. The growth of higher plants depends on the organized allocation of functions to organs, which in turn become differentiated, modified, and specialized to enable them to undertake their essential roles (Fig. 2.1). Organ cultures are good examples of organized structures. Organ culture is used as a general term for those types of cultures in which an organized form of growth can be continuously maintained [3]. These are the cultures of isolated plant organs including cultures derived from root tips, stem tips, leaf primordia, or immature parts of flowers and fruits [3] (Fig. 2.1). Organ cultures are divided into determinate and indeterminate organs.

2.2.1.1 Culture of Determinate Organs

Kotte and Robins [4,5] established the first organ culture of wheat seedlings. Later on several researchers contributed to this area. Major developments in organ culture are mentioned

TABLE 2.1   Advantages and Disadvantages of Plant Tissue Culture [2]

Advantages	Disadvantages
• Molecular to mass level of work can be performed. The tedious and laborious work such as weeding, spraying, watering, etc. can be skipped in plant tissue culture.	• Requires lot of expensive and specialized procedures, facilities, and advance skills.
• For rejuvenation of plant material and cultures, can be preserved for long time.	• Plants produced are dependent on nutritional sources in contrast to field plants.
• Production is independent on season and can continue throughout the year.	• It is not obligatory to have callus within a short time. Sometimes callus will not appear for months and for some plants callus does not appear.
• It is the best technique for the introduction of temporal characteristics and studying the effects of several mutagens and to attempt immobilizations of cells, for biotransformation or biochemical reactions.	• Plantlets are initially small and have undesirable characteristics.
• It may provide a continuous, reliable source of phytopharmaceuticals and could be used for the large-scale culture of plant cells.	• Plants do not function autotrophically in culture and have to undergo a transitional phase before independent growth.
• Plant tissue culture can produce a large number of clones (with desirable characteristics), draught resistant, flood resistant, disease-free plants, plants of high nutritional values, and high quality plants with improved yields of secondary metabolites (also used to study biogenesis of secondary metabolites).	• Chances of producing genetically aberrant plants may be increased.
• The process offers uniform biomass available all the time, synthesis of medicinal compounds difficult or impossible to synthesize chemically, independent of soil conditions and change in climatic conditions.	• Plantlets are more susceptible to contamination and water loss in the external environment, since they are grown at a high relative humidity.

in Fig. 2.2. A plant with determinate growth stops growing once it reaches its mature phase. Hence, those organs of plants that stop growing at maturity and exhibit determinate growth are called determinate organ cultures. Usually determinate organs cultures have their defined size and shape, e.g., leaves, flowers, and fruits [3]. One of the easiest ways to establish continuous culture of isolated roots *in vitro* is mentioned in Fig. 2.2. There are different types of organ cultures. The types of organ cultures that have limited growth potential are illustrated in Fig. 2.2.

2.2.1.1.1 LEAF CULTURE OR PRIMORDIAL CULTURE

Leaf culture may be described as the culturing of an excised leaf primordial or an immature young leaf of the shoot apex aseptically in a chemically defined medium where they grow and follow the development sequences under controlled conditions. Apical meristem at the tip of the plant stem provides new cells that are needed for stem growth and also acts

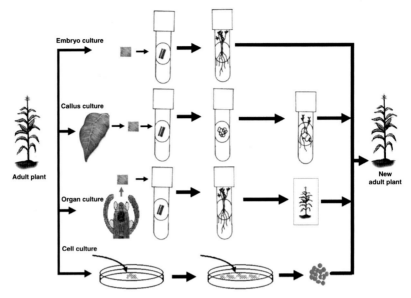

FIGURE 2.1   Types of plant tissue cultures.

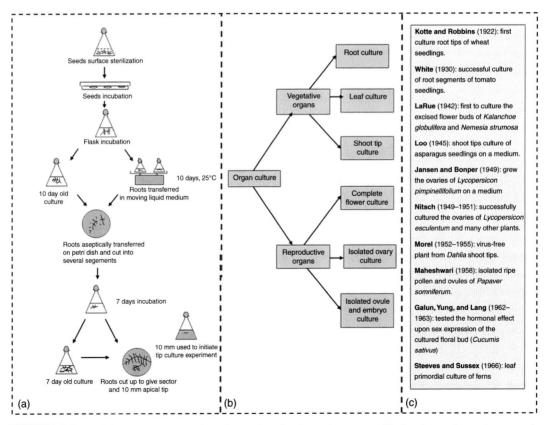

FIGURE 2.2   (a) Schematic representation of procedure for the maintenance of isolated roots in continuous culture; (b) types of organ culture; (c) major developments in organ culture.

as a site of small cellular outgrowths, called leaf primordia that develop into the leaves. Developmental stages of the leaf primordia play an important role in studying phyllotaxy (ordered arrangement of leaf primordia around the circumference of the shoot apical meristem). Auxin and a localized protein called expansin are the key substances that are sufficient to induce a primordium and set into motion all the events needed to produce a mature leaf [6]. A primordium is the simplest set of cells capable of triggering growth of the would-be organ. The most evidenced research on leaf culture to date has been carried out on ferns, particularly cinnamon (*Osmunda cinnamomea*). Padmanabhan reported the leaf culture of *Phoenix sylvestris* [7]. Haight and Kuehnert studied the effect of monochromatic radiations on leaf primordia of the cinnamon fern *O. cinnamomea* L. and later demonstrated the developmental potentialities of leaf primordia of similar plants [8,9]. Orkwiszewsk et al. suggested that leaf identity can be regulated independently of the identity of the shoot apical meristem, which means that vegetative phase change is not initiated by a change in the identity of the shoot apical meristem [10]. The potential of leaf primordia in the development of somatic embryos was successfully established by Almeida et al. He and his coworkers demonstrated the regeneration potential of adult Pejibaye leaf primordia by the development of somatic embryos from it. Leaf primordia also acquire potential in the development of viroid-free plants [11]. Viroid-free multiple-shoot cultures were developed from the *in vitro* culture of grapevine shoot tips from a viroid-infected plant containing one or two leaf primordia [12]. In addition, one recent report suggested that the development of viroid-free *Ipomoea setosa* (sweet potato) from the *in vitro* culture of leaf primordia proved to be a low-cost option toward commercialization [13]. One of the best advantages of leaf primordia culture is the extreme simplicity of the culture medium required for their complete growth and development. Leaf primordium is useful in studying the effects of nutrients, growth factors, and changes in the environmental conditions of the leaf. It is also useful in studying the developmental stages of fern in which they initially become leaves and later sporangia. When nutrient is supplemented with kinetin and devoid of 2,4-dichlorophenoxyacetic acid (2,4-D), it is also useful in the clonal propagation of young leaves to form several buds without the formation of callus [14].

2.2.1.1.2 FRUITS CULTURE

There are various indications of fruit explant cultures that have shown better results. The effect of juice from an "acidless" orange variety on *in vitro* growth of explant (juice vesicle or albedo tissues) cultures from citron (*Citrus medica*), lemon (*Citrus limon*), grapefruit (*Citrus paradisi*), sweet orange (*Citrus sinensis*), and mandarin (*Citrus reticulata*) fruits was studied by Einset. In his study he demonstrated the significant growth stimulation effect of orange juice on various *in vitro* cultured fruits in basal medium containing Murashige and Skoog salts, sucrose, myoinositol, thiamine, 2,4-D, and kinetin. It was also discovered that this stimulation was not due to the presence of citric acid since the addition of "acidless" juice was only responsible for stimulation effects [15]. This report has contradicted the Erner study on growth promoting effects of citric acid as a growth factor from orange juice that affects citrus tissue culture [16]. Yashina et al. reported the successful regeneration of whole, fertile plants of *Silene stenophylla* Ledeb. from immature fruit tissue of the Late Pleistocene age using *in vitro* tissue culture and clonal micropropagation [17]. Oxelman et al. regenerated the 30,000-year-old plant from fruit tissue buried in Siberian permafrost [18]. Protein accumulation in soybeans is highly dependent on the nature of the N (nitrogen) source. Glutamine, asparagines, ureide, and allantoin are equally the most efficient sources of the N. Horta and Sodek showed that the effect of methionine on the storage of protein patterns and free amino acids in the *in vitro* culture of soybean (*Glycine max*) cotyledons using a defined medium containing glutamine and sulfate as sole sources of N and S is a good example of fruit culture [19]. To further study the growth conditions and efficiency of N sources for reserve protein synthesis in *in vitro* culture of soybean fruits, Mosquim and Sodek devised a cultured system consisting of a single fruit attached to a short piece of stem (through which the nutrients were supplied) [20]. This study proved the high metabolic capacity of the fruit tissues for principal N transport compounds of soybean, namely allantoin, asparagine, and glutamine. Gulsen et al. suggested the growth and development of fruit explant culture (pistils and various fruit explants of *C. limon* and *C. sinensis*) in basal medium supplemented with indole-3 acetic acid (IAA), gibberellic acid (GA$_3$), or benzyl-aminopurine, which were successfully cultivated for more than 1 year under *vitro* conditions [21]. Prolonged *in vitro* culture of various citrus fruit explants and especially of juice vesicles and various other studies supported further research in fruit development and physiology.

2.2.1.1.3 STAMENS CULTURE

Stamens are the male reproductive part of a flower. The development of the male reproductive system is a complex biological process, which includes the formation of the stamen with differentiated anther tissues (in which microspores/pollens are generated), then anther dehiscence, and subsequently pollination. Stamen specification and anther development involve a number of extraordinary events such as meristem transition, cell division and differentiation, cell-to-cell communication, etc., which need the cooperative interaction of sporophytic and gametophytic genes [22]. All these stages can be expediently experimented under *in vitro* conditions. Canadian researcher Gary S. Hicks played a major role in the establishment of the stamen culture [23–25]. In his earlier studies he established carpelloids of tobacco stamen primordia under *in vitro* conditions [23]. In 1977 he successfully developed a culture of stamen primordial from a male sterile tobacco [24]. Later on in 1979 he reported the feminized outgrowths on the stamen primordia of tobacco [25]. He has also suggested the strong tendency of some of the young staminal tissues to reorganize into organs of the opposite sex *in vitro* [25]. Similarly, Lu and Enemata have studied the regeneration potential of sepals, stamens, and ovules from perianth explants of *Hyacinthus orientalis* L. in different developmental stages by means of exogenous hormones [26]. In 1988, Rastogi and Sawhney developed a culture of stamen primordia of the normal and male sterile stamenless-2 mutant of tomato (*Lycopersicon esculentum* Mill.) [27]. While establishing stamen cultures from its native explants it was found that growth rates are quite low, e.g., from all explants of *Rosa hybrid* only 14% of plants successfully produced stamen cultures whereas in *Brassica campestris* only 6.5% of regeneration was achieved [28,29]. Among recent studies, Wojciechowicz (2007) compared the regenerative potential of petals, stamens, and pistils of five *Sedum* species *in vitro* [30]. In this study it was demonstrated that petals, stamen, and pistils do not show the capacity for plant regeneration unless they are regenerated through indirect organogenesis [30]. Furthermore, the *Sedum* plant was fully developed by indirect organogenesis using 6-benzylaminopurine (BAP) (cytokinin) and indole butyric acid (IBA) (auxin) as plant growth regulators in contrast to the study conducted by Almann et al. who only succeeded in establishing stamen filament culture out of petal, stamen, and pistil explants [31]. This study also demonstrated that the regenerative potential of stamens and pistils was only half as high as that of petals [30].

2.2.1.1.4 FLOWER CULTURE

Flower culture may be described as the aseptic culture of excised flower buds or a complete flower bud on a chemically defined nutrient medium where it continues developing the full form in a culture vessel. In tissue culture, *in vitro* flowering serves as an important tool for many reasons. One of the most important ones is the ability to shorten the life cycles of plants; other aims include studying flower induction and initiation and floral development. Controlling the environment and media components enables the manipulation of different variables that affect these processes. Flower stamens contain anthers and anthers contain microspores. These microspores then develop an exine around it, called a pollen grain. In other words, when microspores mature they become pollen grains. Under *in vitro* conditions explants such as pollen or anthers are usually utilized for the production of haploid tissues. These pollen grains have the potential to produce both callus and embryos. Anthers (the somatic tissue wall that surrounds and contains the pollen) can be cultured on solid medium (agar should not be used to solidify the medium as it contains inhibitory substances). In anther culture the developing anthers at a particular stage are removed aseptically from the unopened flower bud and are cultured on a nutrient medium. During this process the microspores present in the cultured anther develop into a tissue called callus or embryoid. This tissue further gives rise to haploid plantlets either by organogenesis or embryogenesis.

The flowering process is one of the critical events in the life of a plant. This process involves the switch from the vegetative stage to the reproductive stage of growth and is believed to be regulated by both internal and external factors. A flowering system *in vitro* is considered to be a convenient tool to study specific aspects of flowering, floral initiation, floral organ development, and floral senescence. The application of cytokinins, sucrose concentrations, photoperiod, and subculture time to promote flowering *in vitro* is well documented in many plant species. The aseptic culture of entire flowers, floral parts, and flower initiating explants has been accomplished by several investigators. LaRue maintained the whole flowers and floral parts in a healthy condition for longer periods of time on a synthetic medium. Loo succeeded in the development of flowers from *Cuscuta campestris* despite the development of root and leaves. In his next study he demonstrated the entire life cycle of annual plant *Baeria chrysostoma*, which flowers after 19 days of germination. He postulated that mercuric chloride sterilized explants (*Helianthus annuus*) when cultured on a synthetic medium under the high intensity of fluorescent light, and in the presence of sucrose furnished flowers with greatest regularity in explants bearing small cotyledons. These historical achievements develop further study for future research on flower culture [32].

Flowering is dependent on genes that act to promote flowering (identification of genetic map showing the approximate positions of the genes and quantitative trait loci that affect flowering). In addition photoperiods, vernalization, and the role of carbohydrates and phytohormones also play an important role in promoting flowering [33]. There are several factors that either stimulate or inhibit flowering *in vitro* (Fig. 2.3).

1. *Effect of gene transformation*
   Micropropagation, embryo rescue, mutagenesis, and *in vitro* interspecific hybridization methods have been used by breeders in the floriculture industry for many years. Traditionally, new traits have been introduced into ornamental plants through classical breeding. Genetic modification is an essential tool in the floriculture industry. Genes, for

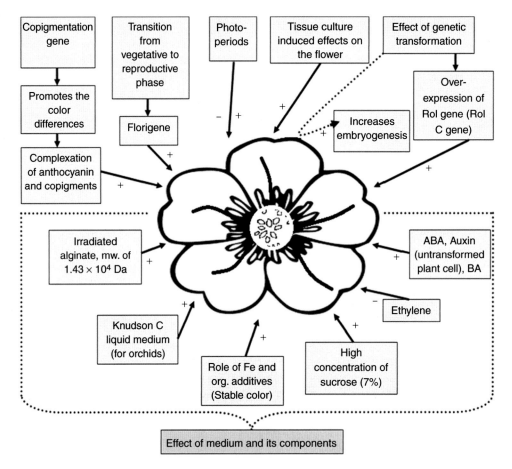

FIGURE 2.3   Factors affecting the *in vitro* flowering of plants.

example rol genes, have potential utility in the floricultural industry. Molecular mechanisms underlying phenotypic expression of these genes are of great importance to the industry. Overexpression of the rol genes of the Ri plasmid of *Agrobacterium rhizogenes* in plants alters the development processes of several plants and affects their architecture. Plants suffering from dwarfed phenotype, reduced apical dominance, smaller, wrinkled leaves, increased rooting, altered flowering, and reduced fertility can be healed by the introduction of rol genes such as rol A, B, C and D, rol C, which forms its major application in improving ornamental and horticultural traits. More specifically, the rol C gene is responsible for inducing smaller flowers and advanced flowering, and therefore offers useful tools for improving ornamental flowers [34].

2. *Regeneration potential of auxin supplementation in transformed explants*

Auxin supplementation is reported to regenerate two to three times more flower buds than explants from untransformed tobacco. Tobacco plant cell pRi 1855 transformation by *Agrobacterium rhizogenes* makes the plant cell insensitive to supplemented ethylene concentration, which inhibits auxin promotion of flower bud formation in its explants, whereas ethylene supplementation in untransformed explants strongly reduces the response to auxin at all concentrations [35].

3. *Gene that promotes copigmentation*
   Color differences in plants can be made by introducing a gene that promotes co-pigmentation. In this process anthocyanins and copigments such as flavones or flavonols (copigmentation) form complexes that lead to the shifting of the visible absorption maximum of the flowers so that it becomes longer and flowers look blue. In 2001, modification of flower color was studied in *Torenia* (*Torenia fournieri* Lind.) by reintroduction of the dihydroflavonol-4-reductase (DFR) gene to produce a bluer trait in flowers [36].

4. *Tissue culture induced stable coloration in flowers*
   The variegated *Saintpaulia* cultivar Thamires (*Saintpaulia* sp.) has pink petals with blue splotches and is generally maintained by leaf cuttings. In contrast, tissue culture-derived progeny of the cultivar showed not only a high percentage of mutants with solid-blue petals but also other solid-color variants, which have not been observed from leaf cuttings. Solid-color phenotypes were inherited stably by their progeny from tissue culture. Tissue culture-induced flower-color changes in *Saintpaulia* are caused by excision of the transposon inserted in the flavonoid 3′,5′-hydroxylase (F3′5′H) promoter [37].

5. *Increased production of embryogenic calli by genetic transformation*
   Parthenocarpy and female sterility made it impossible to improve banana varieties through common hybridization. Genetic transformation for banana improvement is imperative. Recent studies explored that the transformation of tobacco arabinogalactan protein gene significantly increased the production of embryogenic calli from banana immature male flowers when compared with the effect of the control medium, and demonstrated that tobacco arabinogalactan protein can be used to promote banana embryogenesis [38].

6. *Florigen*
   The transition from vegetative to reproductive development is a critical turning point in a plant's life cycle [33]. It is now widely accepted that a leaf-borne signal, florigen, moves via the phloem from leaves to the shoot apical meristem to trigger its reprogramming to produce flowers. In part, the florigenic signal comprises a protein that belongs to the phosphatidylethanolamine-binding protein (PEBP) family that is present in all living organisms but displays diverse functions. Recently, Danilevskaya et al. demonstrated that the maize FT homolog ZCN8 has florigenic function, which plays a pleiotropic role in the regulation of generalized growth of vegetative and reproductive tissues [39].

7. *Effect of hormones*
   Some plants acquire low flowering frequency, e.g., a wild orchid species from China named *Dendrobium candidum* usually requires 3–4 years of cultivation before it can produce flowers. Until 1996 it was widely known that supplementation of spermidine, or benzyladenine (BA), or the combination of 1-naphthylacetic acid (NAA) and BA to the culture medium can induce protocorms or shoots to flower within 3–6 months with a frequency of 31.6–45.8%. But later it was founded that pretreatment of protocorms in an abscisic acid (ABA)-containing medium followed by transfer onto Murashige and Skoog (MS) medium with BA increased flowering frequency by up to 82.8% [40].

Cytokinin benzyladenine plays a key role in flower bud initiation whereas auxin (indoleacetic acid) stimulates in particular the differentiation of flower buds. It was founded that the indoleacetic acid metabolism was not to be influenced by the uptake and metabolism of benzyladenine [41].

The role of different cytokinins on the cultures obtained from flower stalks of *Nicotiana tabacum* was studied by Van der Krieken et al. In this report he has suggested that benzyladenine, benzyladenosine, and dihydrozeatin were the most active compounds for flower bud formation whereas isopentenyladenosine and all active cytokinins bind to the same receptor with different affinities. He has also suggested that the role of isopentenyladenine as a competitive inhibitor of benzyladenine conjugation and therefore simultaneous supplementation of isopentenyladenine with benzyladenine decreased benzyladenine uptake and conjugation [42].

8. *Effect of medium*
Since 2007 it was known that protocorms of an orchid hybrid plant (*Dendrobium madame*) when cultured on Gelrite-solidified medium only produced axillary shoots and roots. Later on it was discovered that transition of vegetative shoot apical meristem to inflorescence meristem occurs when young protocorms were cultured in modified Knudson C liquid medium [43]. Alginate irradiated at 75 kGy with a molecular weight of approx. 1.43×10^4 Da had the highest positive effect in the growth of flower plants, namely *Limonium*, *Lisianthus*, and *Chrysanthemum* [44].

In many plants high levels of iron and organic additives supplementation are required for the development of stable color flowers through many generations *ex vitro*. This was proved by Nhut et al. among two *Torenia* varieties having a white or light purple flower color when developed from the parental variety having violet flowers. In his study he modified MS medium containing half strength of macronutrients, micronutrients, full Fe, and full organic additives. This medium successfully induced early flowering and flower color was found to be stable in two new *Torenia* varieties through three generations *ex vitro* [45].

9. *Role of parthenogenesis and accession-dependent embryo development*
2,4-D supplementation in pollinated flowers stimulates callus development; however, it did not increase the frequency of embryo development from ovules and, thus, was not useful for increasing the frequency of haploid plant recovery. Accession-dependent embryo development increases the efficiency from 0% to 24.29%. It was reported that parthenogenesis and ovules excised from ovaries after pollination with parsley pollen play an important role in the development of carrot haploid and doubled haploid plant production [46].

10. *Photoperiods*
The capacity to form under different photoperiods varies greatly, depending on genotype, source tissue and its developmental stage, and composition of the culture medium, particularly the levels of glucose, auxin, and cytokinin. This capacity in response to different photoperiods was studied in thin-layer explants of flowering plants of several species, cultivars, and lines of *Nicotiana*. Several reports suggested the different capacity of tobacco plant to form flower buds was found to be greatest in the 2 day-neutral plants (*Samsun tobacco* and *Nicotiana rustica*) and least in the two qualitative photoperiodic plants studied (*Nicotiana sylvestris* and *Mammoth tobacco*) [47].

Ohtsubo et al. reported the application of heavy-ion beam irradiation mutation breeding for genetic manipulation, which makes it more convenient to create greater variation in plant phenotypes to produce a large number of mutants with greater variation in floral traits. He and his coworkers succeeded in producing over 200 varieties of transgenic *Torenia* (*Torenia fournieri* Lind.) from over 2400 regenerated plants. Mutant phenotypes were observed mainly in flowers and showed wide variation in color and shape [48].

11. *Effect of sugar*

Sucrose concentration plays an important role in flowering and its absence may also affect the color defect or variation in some plants. Nagira et al. reported that treatment with 7% sucrose elevated endogenous ABA levels (before the induction of anthocyanin synthesis and chlorophyll degradation), whereas 1.5% sucrose medium resulted in a gradual decrease in the ABA level and a failure of induction of anthocyanin synthesis [49].

In vitro flowering overcomes problems associated with flower growth and development as well as fruit and seed production *in vitro* and hence may open up new gates in the field of its conservation and continuous supply of plant material throughout the year by understanding its flowering behavior *in vitro*. *In vitro* flowering of valuable medicinal plants is divided on the basis of its available floral organs as follows.

FLOWER BUDS. Flower cultures have not been a subject of large-scale experimentation. It is evident that there is no transmission of organ determining factors in the meristematic tissue of flowers, e.g., *Nigella damascena* [50]. It has also been reported that application of auxin and cytokinin is required for the formation of flower buds on explants of *Nicotiana tabacum* [51]. Here interaction of auxin and cytokinin with respect to *in vitro* flower bud formation is indirect. A recent *in vitro* flowering report on one of the endangered plants, *Swertia chirayita*, suggested that maximum numbers of flowers buds (12 per culture) can be obtained when shoots were cultured on MS medium containing BAP (1.0 mg/L) and adenine sulfate (70 mg/L) and incubated at 16/8 h light/dark period. Whereas other factors such as optimum temperature, relative humidity, and nature of carbon source also play important roles in the formation of reproductive buds [52].

OVARIES AND OVULES (WHICH DEVELOP AND GROW INTO EMBRYOS). Ovary is the female part of the flower, which consists of either single or many ovules (egg containing part). *Ovary culture may be described as the culture of ovaries isolated from pollinated or unpollinated flowers.* The concept of culturing excised flowers and floral parts *in vitro* originated with Rue (1942, cited by Rangan), who observed rooting from pedicels [53]. Jansen and Bonner grew the ovaries *Lycopersicon pimpinellifolium* on a medium supplemented with casein hydrolysate, IAA, and mixture of vitamins [54]. Later on, Nitsch studied various pollinated and nonpollinated flowers of many plants and also performed similar work on their ovary and ovules [55,56]. Nitsch reported that the production of seedless fruits is possible from the unpollinated ovaries in the case of tomato [55]. He also reported the ovary culture of *Cucumas anguria*, *Nicotiana tabacum*, and *Phaseolus vulgaris* with a reduced fruit size compared to fruit produced in nature [55,56]. In India similar efforts are made to culture ovaries of *Aerva tomentosa*, *Allium cepa*, *Althaea rosea*, *Anethum graveolens*, *Foeniculum vulgare*, *Hyoscyamus niger*, *Iberis amara*, *Linaria maroccana*, and *Tropaeolum majus*, especially at the University of Delhi by using Nitsch's or White's medium supplemented with vitamins, hormones, amino acids, and other growth inducing substances. Maheshwari succeeded in culturing the ovaries from the flowers of *I. amara* 1 day before pollination and found that *in vitro* formed fruits were larger than the natural ones when IAA was supplemented in the nutrient medium [57]. Johri and Sehgal discovered that the supplementation of coconut milk increases the size of naturally formed fruit. From the studies it was discovered that auxins generally act as pollination stimulus [58]. Furthermore, production of viable seeds from cultured ovaries is a big problem. In most of the ovary cultures, nonviable seeds are formed inside the fruits. In 1962, Sachar and Guha produced viable seeds in ovary culture of *Ranunculus sceleratus* [59]. Later on, attempts were made by several researchers to develop ovary culture on different media in various plant species. There are several advantages of ovary culture:

- In certain plants seed development occurs without fertilization by a process called apomixes. In most of the apomictic plants pollination alone stimulates the growth of the ovary and the development of the seeds. In such plants ovary culture may be useful in the study of the stimulus provided by the pollination.
- It is successful in inducing the polyembryony in various parts of the plant.
- It is used in the fundamental and applied aspects of development of fruits and seeds.
- It also provides important information about the role of ancessory floral parts in fruit development.
- It is used to study the effect of hormones on parthogenetic haploid and parthenocarpic development of fruits.
- It is also used to study early development of embryo, fruit development, and various aspects of fruit physiology.
- Test tube fertilization and ovary or pistil culture has been used to circumvent various problems associated with hybridization such as failure of pollen germination on stigmas, insufficient growth of pollen tube, or precocious abscission of flowers and self-incompatibility or sterility.

In addition to ovary culture, ovule or seed culture may also be described as the experimental system by which ovules isolated aseptically from the ovary are grown on chemically defined nutrient medium. The first attempt to isolate ovules and culture them under aseptic conditions was made by White in 1932 in *Antirrhinum majus* (see [53]). However, the technique of ovule culture was successfully performed at the University of Delhi.

Chopra and Sabharwal by using *Gynandropsis gynandra* and *Impatiens balsamina* and Guha and Johri by using *Allium cepa* successfully cultured ovules under *in vitro* conditions [60,61]. In 1961, Maheshwari produced viable seeds from the excised ovules for *Papaver somnifera* [62]. Poddubnaya-Arnoldi studied pollen tube entry into the ovule up to the development of the embryo. She used only 10% of sucrose solution to trace the details [63]. This type of study also indicated that some of the fruit juices such as cucumber, watermelon, parent plant, or ovule extract are known to have beneficial effects on the ovule's development. Environmental conditions exert a profound effect on parent plant *Gossypium* sp. ovules *in vitro*, whose response is multifarious. Since the unsuccessful attempts at the culture of cotton ovules by Joshi, Joshi and Johri made extensive studies on the nutritional and hormonal factors concerned in ovule and fiber development [64,65].

There are several barriers to interspecific hybridization, e.g., late-acting sporophytic self-incompatibility prevents fertilization and silique development following hand pollinations. This technique is useful for raising interspecific hybrids and intergeneric hybrids of plants belonging to the families Cruciferae and Graminae. Pundir successfully produced hybrids by using a cross between *Gossypium arboreum* and *Gossypium hirsutum* [63]. In a normal process these hybrids fail to develop due to early embryo abortion and premature abscission of fruits. Ovule culture can be used to rescue them. Ovule cultures have obvious advantages over whole plants when experimental protocols call for inhibitors, radiolabeled precursors, or controlled environmental conditions to be tested. This technique omits excision of the embryo by culturing the entire ovule, thus greatly facilitating the time and effort involved. Sauer and Friml successfully developed the zygotic Arabidopsis embryos *in vitro* within their ovules [66].

The ovule culture technique for cotton ovules provides significant benefits for using cotton fiber as a model system for plant development. Fiber development is dependent on the addition of phytohormones. Fiber development is also controlled by functional homologs of *Arabidopsis* trichome patterning genes. Wang et al. reported the induction of cotton ovule culture fiber branching by coexpression of cotton BTL, cotton SIM, and *Arabidopsis* STI genes. In this study it was also suggested that the distinctive developmental mechanism of cotton fibers does not depend on endoreduplication. In addition to fiber development, cotton ovule cultures are quite useful for studying early stages of dicot embryogenesis [67]. Unfertilized ovule culture has further advantages than anther culture from the point of view of embryogenesis efficiency, limited influence of donor plant genotype, and a high frequency of haploids and dihaploids production. Doi et al., demonstrated that the unfertilized ovule culture technique of gentians is a powerful tool for obtaining haploids and doubled haploids because of its reproducible and reliable nature and application to a wide range of genotypes [68]. Ramming et al. reported the various *in vitro* conditions for culture of ovules of immature embryos of peach. He also discovered that test tube agar-gelled medium when supplemented with activated charcoal produced significantly larger embryos with a similar conversion rate [69].

ANTHER OR MICROSCOPE CULTURE. This is a technique by which immature pollen is made to divide and grow into tissue (either callus or embryonic tissue), primarily to produce haploids (plants with an N chromosome number) known to be anther culture. Haploid production through anther culture has been referred to as androgenesis. Culturing through anthers or microspores is one of the most popular methods for the production of haploids on artificial culture medium. There are several methods for haploids production but their occurrences are very rare. In this process pollen-containing anthers are isolated from a flower and put into a suitable culture medium. During this process some microspheres survive and develop into tissue. Some yield into embryonic tissue, which when supplemented with favorable medium, is further utilized for shoot and root development. But if callus appears, after hormonal treatment it will differentiate into shoot and root tissue. Datura stramonium was the first haploid plant that was discovered by Bergner in 1921 [70]. Haploids can only be produced in polyploid plants: wheat, tobacco, and clover. Haploids are significant because they carry only one allele of each gene. Thus, any type of mutation is apparent. In haploid plant cells plants with lethal genes are easily eliminated from the gene pool. Through haploid culture homozygous diploid or polyploid plants can be produced, which may be valuable in plant breeding. Production of haploids shortens the time for inbreeding for superior hybrid genotypes. Microspore stage and callus induction from anthers of Kenaf (Hibiscus cannabinus L.) was recently developed by Ibrahim et al. in the optimized semisolid MS medium supplemented with 3.0 mg/L BAP + 3.0 mg/L NAA [71].

2.2.1.1.5 NUCELLUS CULTURE

Nucellus cultures are those cultures in which embryos are derived from the nucellus or integument. Nucellus cultures are taken from pollinated flowers and widely reported in the genus of *Citrus*. It is widely utilized to study the formation of embryos. It is known to be the reliable technique for the production of virus-free citrus plants and can be grown on casein hydrolysate supplemented White's medium giving a callus. The callus may then give rise to pseudobulbils, differentiating into embryos, which can eventually develop into seedlings. The seedlings obtained from the nucellar tissue are of parental type and thus may be important for maintaining purity of horticultural stocks. Weathers and Calavan reported on the importance of using nucellar embryony in polyembryonic citrus to obtain virus-free nucellar plants. Virus particles are generally restricted to the host's vascular tissue, particularly the phloem [72]. Since there is no direct vascular connection between the parent and either the zygotic or nucellar embryos the virus particles can be easily eliminated from the seedling progenies [73]. In 2000, Obukosia and Waithaka reported the nucellar embryo culture of *C. sinensis* L. and *C. limon* L. [74]. In citrus, nucellar seedlings have a tap root and most of the seedlings obtained are virus free. In addition, the vigor that is sometime lost due to repeated propagation by cuttings is restored in nucellar seedlings.

2.2.1.2 *Culture of Indeterminate Organs*

A plant with indeterminate growth can keep growing as long as the environment can support it. Hence, plant organs that grow indefinitely by adding modules exhibit indeterminate growth and are called culture of indeterminate organs.

2.2.1.2.1 MERISTEM CULTURE

Cultivation of shoot apical meristem *in vitro* is known as meristem culture. Meristem culture was developed by Morel and Martin in 1952 for elimination of rivers from *Dahlia*. Morel in 1965 employed meristem culture for micropropagation of orchid cymbidium. Meristem lies in the shoot tip beyond the youngest leaf or first leaf primordium [75]. Culture of the extreme tip of the shoot is used as a technique to free plants from virus infections. Explants are dissected from either apical or lateral buds. They comprise a very small stem apex consisting of just the apical meristem and one or two leaf primordia [76,77]. Meristem lies in the shoot tip and measures up to about 100 mm in diameter and 250 mm in length. Normally shoot tips up to 10 mm are used when the objective is virus elimination (or other pathogenic organism contamination). In such cases it is essential that the apical meristem should be excised with a minimum of the surrounding tissue.

Larger (5–10 mm) explants are required for the rapid clonal propagation of shoot tip culture. Thus, most of the meristem cultures are essentially shoot-tip cultures. If micropropgation is the main objective, the size of shoot tip used for culture is not important. There are two main advantages of working with such small explants. The first is the potential that this apical meristem holds for excluding pathogenic organisms present in the donor plant from the *in vitro* culture, and the second is the stable expression of genetic traits since plantlet production from adventitious organs can be avoided. According to the experimental conditions, if there is no requirement for such benefits, then the related technique of shoot-tip culture may be more expedient for plant propagation [76,77]. Development of shoot directly from the meristem avoids callus tissue formation and adventitious organogenesis, ensuring genetic instability and minimizing somaclonal variation [77]. Meristem culture has become a powerful and successful tool for virus elimination from infected plants and has been successfully applied in many plants such as potato, garlic, etc. [78]. Since the tip meristem is naturally very small (0.1 mm) the percentage of growing meristems is not always satisfactory. To overcome this problem the percentage of tip meristem is increased but this may increases the chances of pathogen penetration. In 1968, Houten et al. demonstrated that heat treatment and meristem culture in combination can be used for the production of virus-free plant material [79]. Later on it was realized that surface sterilization usually by 0.1% $HgCl_2$ for a period of 4 min (in the case of potato) when cultured in MS basal medium furnished the maximum percentage of survived explants [80].

2.2.1.2.2 MERISTEM AND SHOOT CULTURE

The growing points of shoots can be cultured in such a way that they continue uninterrupted and organized growth. As these shoot initials ultimately give rise to small organized shoots, which can then be rooted, their culture has great practical significance for plant propagation. Recently, the meristem culture technique with shoot-tip culture technique was studied for obtaining virus-free (yellow dwarf and leek yellow stripe viruses) plants of two different garlic species (*Allium sativum* and *Allium tuncelianum*). Results of a polymerase chain reaction assay for the detection of viruses proved that more than almost 70% of the obtained cultures are virus free [81].

2.2.1.2.3 SHOOT OR SHOOT TIP CULTURE

The culture of larger stem apices or lateral buds (ranging from 5 to 10 mm in length to undissected buds) is used as a very successful method of propagating plants. The size and relative positions of two kinds of explants in the shoot apex of a typical dicotyledon are considered *in vitro*. Node culture is an adaptation of shoot culture. *In vitro* shoot-tip culture is widely used for clonal progenies that are phenotypically uniform and develop without chromosomal changes or meiotic irregularities. 6-Benzylamino purine and kinetin stimulated shoot development within the range of 0.1–10 μM whereas 6-benzylamino purine at 5 and 10 μM induced shoot multiplication of the apical shoot tip of tomato (*Lycopersicon esculentum* Mill.) [82]. A simple procedure was reported on *Gossypium* meristem shoot-tip culture in which the best shoot development was observed on media containing 0.46 mM kinetin. This simple protocol replaces the existing protocols for meristem tip culture of cotton [83].

2.2.1.2.4 EMBRYO CULTURE

Embryo culture is the culture of isolated immature or mature embryos. Zygotic or seed embryos are often used advantageously as explants in plant tissue culture, for example, to initiate callus cultures. This embryo develops properly when nourishing tissue; endosperm was present in the seed during the development. But crossing between the two distant species resulted in the degeneration of endosperm tissue, which hinders embryo development and in such a case viable plant will not develop. To recover such a hybrid embryo, culturing of the embryo was followed. This culturing of embryo (hybrid) in *in vitro* conditions is known as embryo rescue and is widely used for crop improvement. Hanning in 1904 first cultured isolated mature embryo of a cross between *Cochlearia* × *Raphanus* and successfully obtained the plants [84]. In 1925 and 1929, Laibach isolated zygotic embryos from nonviable seeds of

Linum perenne ×*L. austriacum* [85,86]. These hybrids cannot be developed naturally. In 1941 for the first time Van Overbeek et al. introduced coconut milk for the development of embryo and callus formation in *Datura* [87]. Other research has led to the development of a new area of hybrid embryos through embryo culture, which has given relief to those embryos that are usually aborted (due to various reasons) at early stages and thus cannot be raised naturally. This technique is used for culture where the embryo is incompletely developed (orchids), to overcome seed dormancy, for shortening the breeding cycle, determination of seed viability, microcloning of the source material, for rapid multiplication, and conservation of several medicinally important and endangered plants (e.g., recently embryo culture of medicinally important endangered forest tree species *Strychnos potatorum* with 100% germination rate was conserved by using this technique) [88]. In addition, embryo culture also acts as a rich source of therapeutic secondary metabolites, e.g., an alkaloid (neferine) having the potential for inhibiting human lung cancer has been recently explored from lotus seed embryo [89]. Obtaining contamination-free seeds or embryos without damage or oversterilization is one of the most difficult obstacles in the successful establishment of *in vitro* cultures. Sugii demonstrated the various disinfestation protocols (bleach sterilization, gas sterilization, and ethanol dip and flame) that are successful in establishing *in vitro* cultures of several endangered Hawaiian plant taxa [90].

Applications of embryo culture

Embryo production from sterile seeds (e.g., apricot), viable embryo production (interspecific and intergeneric crosses resulting in nonviable seeds), micropropagation of hard species (*Pinus palustris*), breaking of dormancy, haploid production (*Hordeum vulgare* and *Hordeum bulbosum*), and germination of seeds of obligatory parasites without the host can be achievable with embryo culture.

2.2.1.2.5 SEED CULTURE

Seed culture is an important technique when explants are taken from *in vitro* derived plants and the propagation of orchids. Each explant requires a suitable sterilization procedure, which can otherwise cause contamination and affects the regeneration of plants. In such a case the culture of seeds to raise sterile seedlings is the best method. In addition, there are several plant species in which seed sizes are minute and do not germinate well. Orchid is one of the best examples of this. Orchidaceae is one of the largest families of flowering plants, and many of its species are highly valuable as herbal medicines and to the horticultural industry. To meet commercial requirements and to conserve natural resources, *in vitro* seed germination has been utilized to produce large quantities of uniform seedlings. Limiting factors for the propagation of most of the orchids are: minute size and difficult to use directly in the field, nonendospermous with a low nutrient content, dependent on a specific fungus for germination, early seedling development, and poor germination frequency. Although produced in large numbers (millions per capsule) only a few germinate naturally in the wild. In earlier times, orchids/fungus symbiotic relationship-dependent germination was a major constraint in its *in vitro* culture. Knudson showed that orchid were able to germinate asymbiotically *in vitro* [91]. *In vitro* seed culturing of such plants is dependent on the growth medium supplemented and this is known as asymbiotic germination. However, terrestrial orchid seeds are more difficult to germinate and grow than epiphytic orchids. Terrestrial orchid seeds have a hardened seed coat and more stringent requirements for germination *in vitro*. Lee reported the timing of seed collection and pretreatments for improving *in vitro* germination of some terrestrial Asian orchids [92]. He has also suggested the prominent steps involved *in vitro* germination: (i) the culture of immature seeds (optimal timing of seed harvest is a key to maximizing germination), (ii) the selection of adequate pretreatment conditions (i.e., the duration and concentrations of pretreatment solutions) essential to improve germination, and (iii) subsequent seedling development.

Among various classes of orchids, phalaenopsis orchids have high economic value in the floriculture industry [93]. Hybridization and cross-pollination have proven to be very reliable techniques for the production of a wide range of successful cultivars. *In vitro* propagation makes it possible to clonally mass propagate; however, *in vitro* culture technologies are still a challenge because of the slow growth of plantlets, low multiplication rate, poor rooting, and somaclonal variation. In this regard, micropropagation through protocorm-like bodies obtained from germinating embryos and somatic tissues is an important strategy in obtaining genetically stable plants and the improvement of quality [93]. Seed culture is widely used for large, rapid propagation and large-scale seedling production. For producing large-scale seedlings of *Capparis spinosa* Ma et al. sterilized the seeds with 0.1% $HgCl_2$ (12 min) and utilized optimum MS medium supplemented with activated carbon [94]. Several examples of seed cultures are highlighted in Table 2.2.

2.2.1.2.6 ENDOSPERM CULTURE

The endosperm is a short-lived structure and is consumed during the development of embryo. It is the nourishing tissue in seeds. During the process of fertilization in angiosperms the two male gamete/nuclei fuse separately with two different female nuclei and this process is known as double fertilization. The one male nuclei fuses with egg and forms the zygote (diploid tissue) whereas the other male nuclei fuses with two polar nuclei to form endosperm (triploid tissue) in the embryo sac. This endosperm provides nourishment to the developing embryo in the seed. If the seed's embryo is completely utilized by the embryo then such seeds are called nonendospermous seed whereas if the endosperm is not completely utilized by the embryo such seeds are called endospermous seeds (coconut, coffee). Lamp and Mill in 1933 first cultured the endosperm of maize on the nutrient medium but full success was not obtained [102]. LaRue in 1949 developed callus tissue from the endosperm culture and this made other workers take up the work on endosperm culture for different species of plants [103]. Generally mature endosperm is not a good material for explants, since endosperm undergoes some changes after pollination, which makes it suitable for culturing. Thus, immediately after a few days of pollination endosperm was selected for this purpose. The entire seed or kernel is surface sterilized and endosperm tissue was excised under sterile conditions. For the production of callus, endosperm culture should be placed in the dark and for organ development bright light is required. In addition, for its function of supplying nutrition to the developing embryo it can also be used for the production of triploid plants that are triploid in their chromosomal constitution. Breeding program triploids are produced by crossing tetraploids and diploid plants. But in majority of plants it is not possible and successful, thus endosperm culture was the better and feasible alternative. Triploid plants are useful for the production of seedless fruits (e.g., apple, banana, watermelon, etc.) and for the production of trisomics for cytogenetic studies. Usually these triploids are obtained by crossing colchicine-induced tetraploids with diploids followed by rescuing the triploid embryos. However, there

TABLE 2.2   Past Few Years' Research on Orchids

Plant description	Method	Effective media	Unique features	Growth and survival rates	References
Cephalanthera falcata	Asymbiotic germination (hand pollination and bagging treatment of ovaries)	Kano medium and ND medium	Lignin plays an important role in induction of dormancy	74.5% survived to full maturity	[95]
Malaxis khasiana	Rapid *in vitro* propagation	MS medium 2% sucrose + casein-hydrolysate + BA Second generation medium: MS medium + IAA + BA + Kin	Supported the development of PLBs	Plantlets showed 65% survival under field conditions	[96]
Dendrobium hookerianum	Asymbiotic seed germination	MS medium	The inclusion of plant growth regulators was unnecessary	90% survival of plantlets was achieved	[97]
Coelogyne nervosa	Asymbiotic seed germination	Germination medium: MS medium + 30% coconut water Second generation medium: MS medium + BA (or Kin alone)		Rooted seedlings were successfully transplanted to pots with 91% success	[98]
Juvenile plants of hybrid *Bratonia* orchid	Seed cryopreservation	Liquid morel medium (for protocorm multiplication), liquid ?S medium with half-strength macronutrients (for the development of juvenile plants)	Cryopreservation did not inhibit the germination rate of seeds	Protocorms derived from cryopreserved seeds developed faster than protocorms from control	[99]
Temperate orchid species	Asymbiotic *in vitro* propagation	FAST medium (modified): for both germination and seedling culture	1st phase For sowing, the cultures (dark + 10–12°C) 2nd phase until germination: dark + 25–26°C	After 2 years of aseptic culture they were suitable for transfer *ex vitro*	[100]
Cymbidium mastersii	Mass propagation	MS basal medium 2nd generation medium: MS medium + BAP + NAA (for secondary protocorms)		Survival percentage 88%	[101]

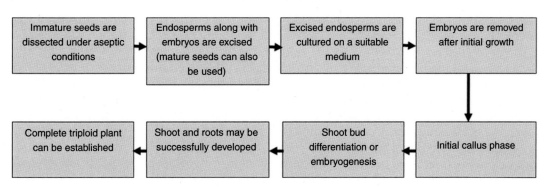

FIGURE 2.4 Steps involved in the endosperm culture technique.

may be a strong crossability barrier making it difficult to produce triploids. A recent report suggested the development of triploid plants of ornamental *Phlox drummondii* from cultures of excised endosperm of immature fruits having zygotic embryo at the early dicotyledonous stage [104]. The sizes of these triploid plants were found to be higher and the plants were more vigorous as compared to naturally occurring diploid plants, whose flowers showed bright color with an enlarged central eye adding to their ornamental value [104]. Similarly, endosperm culture of *Carica papaya* is used to produce 75% of triploid plants having healthy roots and leaves with larger stomata and more chloroplasts in guard cells [105]. High dependence of endosperm efficiency on genotype was studied in *Triticum aestivum*, *Triticum durum*, and *Triticosecale* plants, establishing the relationship between genotype of culture and growth and development of endosperm [106]. Steps involved in the endosperm culture technique are highlighted in Fig. 2.4.

There are two further types of cultures in this class:

- *Mature culture*: Mature culture is derived from the mature endosperm, e.g., mature embryo of *Ricinus communis* on White's medium containing 2,4-D, kinetin, and yeast extract.
- *Immature culture*: Immature culture is derived from the immature endosperm, e.g., maize, wheat, and barley tissue younger than 8 days. This type of culture essentially requires other substances such as yeast extract, vitamins, and casein hydrolysate for its growth and development.

2.2.1.2.7 ISOLATED ROOT CULTURE

Root culture technique was initially experimented by Kotte and Robbins on pea, maize, and cotton root tips [4,5]. These were excised from the plant with minimal trauma and grown aseptically for a few weeks in nutrient media, but ultimately growth ceased. After the breakthrough of White's medium (yeast extract containing inorganic salts and sucrose, which was later replaced by three vitamins) several researchers tried to modify and develop suitable medium for root culture [107]. During this period several researchers were studying the differences in growth parameters between healthy and diseased plants. In 1938, Stanley compared the healthy excised tomato cultured roots with virus infected plant under a similar condition and isolated *Aucuba* mosaic virus protein from diseased excised tomato roots grown *in vitro* [108]. Later on several investigations were conducted to retain the regenerative ability of isolated roots over a longer period. By modification in White's medium Miguel Raggio and Nora Raggio in 1956 developed a novel method for the cultivation of isolated roots [109]. Most of the studies were based on modification in White'smedium [107,110]. In 1984 isolated root cultures of *Brassica* species by serial subculture were established by using modified White's medium [111]. It was demonstrated that the regenerative ability of isolated roots was retained over a period of 5 months in culture [111]. Therefore, it is possible to regenerate shoots from segments of cultured roots by incubation on agar-solidified media containing cytokinin and auxin.

Root tip cultures are generally maintained in an agitated liquid medium with an appropriate auxin. Roots of the solanaceous species contain tropane alkaloids in higher amounts. Regeneration of such roots from the undifferentiated calli increases the production of alkaloids drastically. Therefore, root culture of *Datura, Hyoscyamus,* and *Atropa* are cultured to produce the high amount of alkaloids. However, owing to the slow growth rate and growth related culturing resistance offered by the many species, interest in them as a source of secondary products has been limited.

Isolated root cultures have been utilized for a number of different research purposes (e.g., study of nematode infections, used to grow beneficial mycorrhizal fungi, to study the process of nodulation with nitrogen-fixing *Rhizobium* bacteria in leguminous plants, and for the production of various proteins and secondary metabolites). Root culture methods have several advantages: the nutrition of excised roots grown *in vitro* can be controlled, substances normally contributed by the shoot can be excluded, and substances whose effects are to be tested can be added to the medium in known amounts [112]. In addition to these advantages isolated root cultures have the potential to develop "super roots": these are roots from regenerated plants and roots formed directly on protoplast-derived calli that were once established in new root cultures for longer periods. These newly initiated cultures expressed all the super root qualities again, including prolific shoot regeneration upon transfer to light, indicating that the super-growing character is not lost through protoplast isolation and regeneration. The super root pathway of regeneration, from protoplasts to callus, roots, root culture, and plants, allows the virtually unlimited mass regeneration of plants from root protoplasts. Regenerating super root protoplasts adds an important component to tissue culture systems for legume/rhizobium research. In 2001, for the first time Akashi et al. developed a long-term root culture (super root) of *Lotus corniculatus* [113]. Furthermore, root cultures exhibit a higher degree of genetic stability than other tissue cultures. Hence, it is suitable and widely used for storing the germplasm of certain species. Auxins or gibberellins are known for inhibiting the growth of root culture. Naturally adventitious shoots raised from roots indicate the concept that roots have the power to differentiate into shoots. This can be done by supplementation of shoot inducing hormones (cytokinin to the medium). Tomato is the most widely known example of a plant regenerated from root-derived culture.

2.2.2 Culture of Unorganized Cells

2.2.2.1 Callus Cultures

A callus consists of an amorphous mass of loosely arranged thin-walled parenchymatous cells arising from the proliferating cells of the parent tissue. More often callus is confused by the term callose, which is a polysaccharide secreted by the plants (sieve elements) during any stress or microbial, insect, or any other pathogen attack. Calli can be obtained from almost any part of the plant. Frequently, as a result of wounding, a callus is formed at the cut end of the stem or root. It is more or less nonorganized tissue that contains differentiated (starting material for callus induction, e.g., leaves, root, shoot, etc.) as well as undifferentiated cells. It is also known that different types of callus in *Arabidopsis thaliana* have distinct gene expression profiles [114]. Therefore, the term callus includes cells with various degrees of differentiation. The cellular mass of callus is composed of unspecialized parenchyma cells. Parenchymatous cells present in the explants usually undergo this differentiation. Hence, in principle, callus can be defined as an unorganized and less differentiated parenchymatous tissue. This amorphous tissue is generally formed when plant cells proliferate in an unsystematic way. Thus, callus cultures are basically clumps of cells raised due to disorganized proliferation of cells from the segment of plant organs. In this technique plant cells propagate on suitable media to form clumps of undifferentiated cells called callus. When callus contains differentiated cells present in isolated explants then dedifferentiation (i.e., cells undergo changes to become meristematic) must take place before cell division can occur. If explants only contain meristematic tissue when isolated, then cell division takes place without dedifferentiation. During the dedifferentiation process, mature adult cells are temporarily able to revert from adult to the juvenile state. The rejuvenated cells have a greater growth and division potentiality. These cells under special circumstances are able to regenerate organs and/or embryos. Therefore, dedifferentiation is a prominent step to consider during *in vitro* propagation of plants. Callus initiation is usually accompanied by supplementation of suitable callus induction hormones. Growth-supporting medium and sterile conditions are obligatory for its growth and development. Exogenously supplied growth regulators present in the nutrient medium influence callus formation from the explants. Hormone supplementation for callus development can be categorized in three ways (auxin alone, cytokinin alone, both auxin and cytokinin).

Major developments in callus culture are illustrated in Table 2.3. After the major discoveries, callus has been widely used in both basic research and industrial applications. Apart from auxin and cytokine other hormones, such as brassinosteroids or abscisic acid, also induce callus and in some species may substitute auxin or cytokinin in callus formation. Factors that contribute in callus formation and their different possible mechanisms are highlighted in Fig. 2.5. Major factors (auxin, cytokinin, wound, egg cell, and embryonic and meristematic fate) that are responsible for callus induction are highlighted in dark gray circles and their respective transcription factors are highlighted in light boxes. In *Arabidopsis*, shoot or root explants incubated on auxin- and cytokinin-containing callus-inducing medium (CIM) form callus from pericycle cells adjacent to the xylem poles. This report has proved that callus is an organized mass and depending upon environmental conditions (in nature and in *in vitro* conditions) they acquire different morphology. Depending upon their potential in organ regeneration there are different types of callus (Fig. 2.6). In addition callus-inducing medium grown callus and wound-induced callus show different morphology. In nature, calli are formed by wounds, tumor causing bacteria (Ti gene), and genetic tumors (Fig. 2.6).

2.2.2.1.1 MORPHOLOGICAL FEATURES OF CALLUS

Callus varies significantly in form and texture, ranging from hard nodular cell masses to friable soft ones. It may be white or creamish, green either in whole or in part of the chloroplast development, or purple due to anthocyanin accumulation in the vacuoles. The shape of the individual cells within the callus mass ranges from near spherical to markedly elongated. The nondividing cells within the cell mass are thin walled with a large central vacuole whereas the cells in the region of active cell division, the meristematic region, are smaller with reduced

TABLE 2.3   Major Contributions of Classical and Modern Era in Callus Culture Development

Year	Contributor	Contribution	References
Classical era for callus culture development			
1939	Gautheret, Nobécourt, White	Successful establishment of continuously growing callus cultures	[115–117]
1941	Overbeek	Coconut milk as a new component of nutrient media for callus cultures	[87]
1950	Ball	Studied the differentiation in a callus culture of *Sequoia sempervirens*	[118]
1953	Tulecke	Production of haploid callus of the gymnosperm *Ginkgo biloba* pollen	[119]
1954	Jablonski and Skoog	Developed a technique for the generation and culture of wound tumor tissue from isolated shoot parts of tobacco (*Nicotiana tabacum*)	[120]
1955	Miller et al.	Discovery of kinetin, a cell division hormone	[121,122]
1957	Skoog and Miller	Discovery of the regulation of organ formation by changing the ratio of auxin: cytokinin	[123]
1958	Steward and Reinert	Regeneration of somatic embryos from callus clumps and cell suspension of *Dacus carota*. Differentiation has been demonstrated in callus tissues of carrot	[124,125]
1963	Kato and Takeuchi	Plants were obtained from callus culture tissue, from single carrot cell in suspension and differentiation has been demonstrated in callus tissues of carrot	[126]
1965	Gibbs	Reported the growth of single cells from *Nicotiana tabacum* callus tissue in nutrient medium containing agar	[127]
1965	Murakishi	Survival of dissociated tomato callus cells inoculated with tobacco mosaic virus	[128]
1966	Furuya	Nicotine and anatabine in tobacco callus tissue	[129]
1966	Hansen and Hildebrandt	The distribution of tobacco mosaic virus in plant callus cultures	[130]
1966	Vasil and Hildebrandt	Differentiation has been demonstrated in callus tissues of endive and parsley	[131]
1967	Chandra and Hildebrandt; Vasil and Hildebrandt	Plants can be obtained in single isolated cell of tobacco	[132]
1968	Wilmar and Hellendoorn	Differentiation has been demonstrated in callus tissues of asparagus	[133]
1968	Heble et al.	First evidence for the production of steroid alkaloids (solasonine) by callus tissue of *S. xanthocarpum*	[134]
1969	Kaul et al.	Reported the factors that influence the production of diosgenin from callus and suspension cultures of by *Dioscorea deltoidea*	[135]

TABLE 2.3 Major Contributions of Classical and Modern Era in Callus Culture Development *(cont.)*

Year	Contributor	Contribution	References
1988	O'Hara and Street	Established wheat callus culture derived from various explants and proved that the presence of the auxin was essential for continued proliferation of the wheat callus tissue	[136]
1988	Chen et al.	Explored three morphologically distinct types of callus from sugarcane cultures: a white compact callus capable of plant regeneration, a friable nonmorphogenic callus and a mucilaginous nodular callus that could revert to these other two types depending on the concentration of 2,4-D in the culture medium.	[137]

New era for callus culture development

Year	Contributor	Contribution	References
1979	Goren et al.	Reported the potential of abscisic acid in inducing callus	[138]
1983, 1984	Akiyoshi et al.	Reported the expression of bacterial genes (isopentenyl transferase) encoding biosynthetic enzymes of cytokinin forces infected plants to produce galls	[139,140]
2001	Bourgaud et al.	Described that callus has been widely used in both basic research and industrial applications (secondary metabolites production)	[141]
2000	Hu et al.	Explored role of brassinosteroids in inducing callus	[142]
2002	Stobbe et al.	Discovered that wound-induced calli regenerate new organs or new tissues, suggesting that they are highly pluripotent	[143]
2002	Iwai et al.	Systematic deposition of structural cell wall polysaccharide, such is significant for establishing and/or maintaining the cellular differentiation status. Loss-of-function mutations in cell wall production often lead to callus formation. Iwai has reported nonorganogenic callus of *Nicotiana plumbaginifolia*, having loosely attached cells and develop callus on the shoot apex	[144]
2003	Dewitte et al.	Reported that the activation of a single core cell cycle regulator, such as cyclins or cyclin-dependent kinases, alone is usually not sufficient to induce callus	[145]
2004	Udagawa et al.	Explored the genetic tumors induced by interspecific crosses between *Nicotiana glauca* and *Nicotiana langsdorffii*	[146]
2004	Udagawa et al.	Described that senescence and wounding further enhance tumorization within the hybrid plants	[146]
2005	Ohtani and Sugiyama	Examined the RNA processing and protein translation during callus formation	[147]
2006	Eckardt	Explored the tumor-induced callus by bacterial infection	[148]

(Continued)

TABLE 2.3   Major Contributions of Classical and Modern Era in Callus Culture Development *(cont.)*

Year	Contributor	Contribution	References
New era for callus culture development			
2007	Umehara et al.	Reported the callus induction by the reacquisition of embryonic or meristematic fate	[149]
2008	Tooker et al.	Reported that gall formation caused by other pathogenic organisms has also been well documented (gall formation by insects)	[150]
2009	Atta et al.	Suggested that *Arabidopsis* calli are not a mass of unorganized cells; instead, they have organized structures resembling the primordia of lateral roots	[151]
2006/2009	Chiappetta et al.	Found that some genetic tumors are accompanied by misexpression of key regulators in embryogenesis or meristem development	[152,153]
2010	Sugimoto et al.	Explored gene expression profiles of *Arabidopsis* calli, which are highly similar to that of root meristems	[154]
2011	Iwase et al.	Reported the distinct gene expression in different types of callus in *Arabidopsis thaliana*, which proved that callus has various degrees of differentiation	[114]
2012	Hwang et al.	Reported that cytokinins induced transcription factor activation and induced the expression of many target genes	[155]
2013	Stroud et al.	Reported the stable epigenome changes (loss of methylation) in rice. These epigenome changes are stable across generations in regenerated plants compared to nonregenerated plants	[156]
2014	Xu and Huang	Callus formation actually represents a form of *de novo* organogenesis	[157]

vacuole size and densely staining cytoplasm. In some instances, there may be some differentiation within the cell mass with phloem cells and lignified xylem cells becoming apparent.

2.2.2.1.2 INDUCTION OF CALLUS

Stems, leaves, roots, flowers, seeds, and many other parts (preferably young plants) of plant species can be used to induce the callus tissue; however, successful callus production is dependent on the plant species and conditions provided. Dicot plants are rather amenable for callus induction, as compared to monocot, whereas in woody plants growth of callus is generally slow. In culture this dedifferentiated mass can be preserved indefinitely provided the callus is subcultured on the fresh medium.

2.2.2.1.3 MAINTAINACE OF CALLUS

The callus formed on the original explants is called primary callus. Secondary callus cultures are initiated from pieces of tissue dissected from the primary callus. Such a culture

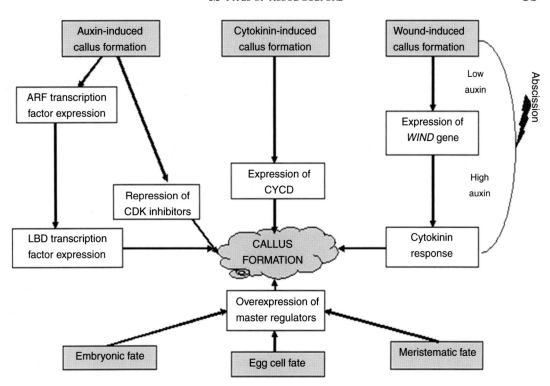

FIGURE 2.5 **Mechanism involved in callus formation.**

can be kept for indefinite periods by successive subculturing. During subculturing, callus cultures are divided to provide new inoculums for culture initiation on a fresh medium. The period from initiation of culture or a subculture to the time of its transfer is called passage. Further callus cultures are not cell cultures since whole tissue associations are cultivated. During long-term cultures, genetic and epigenetic changes occur. The callus can then be said to be composed of a population of cells with slightly different genotypes resulting in differences between one strain of callus and another.

In cases where the callus is difficult to induce, or if young callus is needed, then immature embryos or seedlings or parts of these are used. Callus growth within a plant species may depend on the type of starting material (juvenile or old), original position of the explants, the plant, age of the plant, physiology of the plant, and the growth conditions. Once the callus tissue is formed from the explants the callus is further transferred on to a new medium. This process of transfer is called subculturing. When subcultured regularly on agar medium callus culture will exhibit an S-phase or sigmoid pattern of growth during each passage. There are five phases of callus growth: *lag phase* (where calls prepare to divide), *exponential phase* (where the rate of cell division is highest), *linear phase* (cell division slows down but the rate of cell expansion continues to increase), *deceleration phase* (where the rate of cell division and elongation continues to decrease), *stationary phase* (where the number and size of cells remain constant).

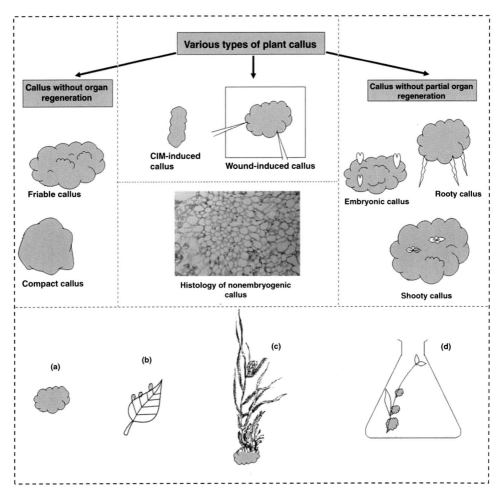

FIGURE 2.6 **Illustration representing types, histology, and various forms of callus (derived from *in vitro* and Nature).** (a) Callus formed under *in vitro* conditions; (b) callus induced at wound site; (c) tumor induced by bacterial infection; (d) genetic tumors caused by interspecific cross between two *Nicotiana* sp.

2.2.2.1.4 APPLICATIONS OF CALLUS CULTURE

Callus culture provides information on the regeneration potentiality of the plant and acts as a good source material for protoplast isolation. Callus can be used as inoculums for the initiation of suspension cultures, serve as a better source of cells for the genetic manipulation of plant genomes, and be maintained indefinitely in the *in vitro* condition for longer periods of time.

2.2.2.2 Cell Suspension Cultures

Haberlandt made the first attempt to isolate single cells from leaves of flowering plants [158]. Muir in 1958 clearly showed that plant cells can be grown in liquid (suspension) cultures similar to microorganisms [159]. However, plant cells individually in a population of cultured cells invariably show cytogenetical and metabolic variations depending upon the stage of the growth cycle and culture conditions. This type of variability is called spatial heterogeneity [160]. Suspension culture is the culturing of isolated cells in liquid media. Cells can be isolated from *in vivo* plant material, either by mechanical means or through enzymatic digestion, and form callus induced from any explants. Cell suspension cultures can be initiated from virtually any part of the plant, just as callus culture. It is the most common way to initiate suspension cultures from callus already growing in culture. Broadly callus cultures are divided into two different categories: friable and compact. Cells are densely aggregated in compact callus whereas cells are loosely associated in friable callus. Based on the type of callus (friable callus or soft callus requires less force to break apart easily than compact callus) suspension cultures are produced. These types of callus offer the inoculums to form cell suspension cultures. For initiating cell suspensions relatively large inoculums should be used so that the released concentration increases quickly. Such types of cells represent a lower level of organization than tissue or callus culture and are often called cell cultures. This liquid medium is typically similar in composition to the one on which the callus is grown. However, adjustments may have to be made in the concentration of hormone and inorganic salts. Agitation is required for suspension cultures for three purposes: it serves to break up the cell aggregates; it maintains a uniform distribution of cells of various sizes and shapes; and cell clumps in the medium provide gaseous exchange for the cells to sustain cell respiration in the liquid medium. As cell division proceeds, the inoculums break up and shed new cell clusters, which fracture again to give individual cells and other small groups. Due to the natural tendency of plant cells to adhere together, it is not always possible to grow a suspension of single cells only. Different types of suspension cultures are highlighted in Fig. 2.7.

2.2.2.2.1 BATCH CULTURES

Batch culture is a closed culture system that contains limited amounts of nutrients. In batch culture cells grow in a finite volume of liquid medium and are usually maintained in conical flasks on orbital shakers at a speed of 80–120 rpm. There are many types of batch culture: slowly rotating culture, shake culture, spinning culture, and stirred culture.

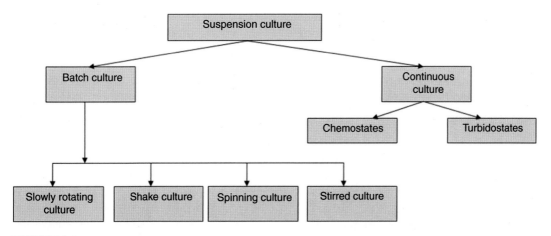

FIGURE 2.7 Types of suspension culture.

2.2.2.2.2 CONTINUOUS CULTURES

Cultures that require a continuous supply of the cell suspension or the product in the medium are known as continuous cultures. This system is maintained in a steady state for prolonged periods by draining out the used liquid medium and adding fresh medium to stabilize the physiological state of growing cells. The growth medium is designed in such a way that one of the nutrients is in limited quantity therefore during exponential growth as the nutrient is exhausted the growth will stop. However, before the nutrient is exhausted the fresh medium with limited nutrient is added. Due to the continuous flow of the nutrients and steady state of the cells' nutrients depletion does not occur. A wide range of bioreactor configurations and sizes have been designed for continuous cultures depending on the variety of plant cells [161,162]. There are two types of continuous cultures: (i) *closed continuous culture* – in this system cells are separated from the drained medium and added back to suspension culture and (ii) *open continuous culture* – in this system addition of the medium is accompanied by harvest of an equal volume of suspension culture.

2.2.2.2.3 SUSPENSION CULTURE TECHNIQUES

Suspension cultures of higher plant cells in synthetic media were demonstrated by Torrey [163]. In 1965, Earle and Torrey suggested the defined media for the cells isolated from *Convolvulus*. Well colonies were formed on his suggested media. Later on several researchers defined different media for different plant cell cultures [164]. For initiating cell cultures at low inoculum density a conditioned medium is used. Culture medium for cell suspension and its conditioning was demonstrated by Torres (Fig. 2.8) [165]. This involves the separation of high-density cell culture from a low-density culture medium by a barrier that permits the diffusion of solutes and air. There are so many techniques used for the culturing of cell culture. Among them the oldest and most frequently utilized technique is Bergmann's cell plating technique (Fig. 2.8). In this technique free cells are suspended in liquid medium (if cell aggregates are present, the culture is filtered), and a culture medium with agar (0.6–1%) is cooled and maintained at 35°C in a water bath [166]. An equal volume of these liquid and agar media are mixed and rapidly spread in a Petri dish, so that cells are evenly distributed in a thin layer, after solidification. The Petri dishes are sealed with parafilm and examined with an inverted microscope to mark single cells (marking is done on the outer surface of the dish). The plates are incubated in the dark at 25°C and cell colonies developing from marked single cells are used to obtain single cell cultures. Various other methods (e.g., filter paper raft-nurse technique; microchamber technique, bioreactors, etc.) have also been developed to grow individual cells. The microchamber technique was first attempted by De Ropp, then successfully accomplished by Jones et al. In this technique a drop of medium containing a single cell is placed over a microscopic slide and covered with three different cover slips in such a fashion that a microchamber is formed [167,168]. Before placing each cover slip, mineral oil is poured on each occasion aseptically. The formed microchamber protects the plant cell from water loss but permits the gaseous exchange (Fig. 2.8). These cultured cells can be preserved by cryopreservation. Mustafa et al. demonstrated the two-step (controlled rate) freezing technique, also known as the slow (equilibrium) freezing method for long-term storage, which has been applied successfully to a wide range of plant cell suspension cultures [169].

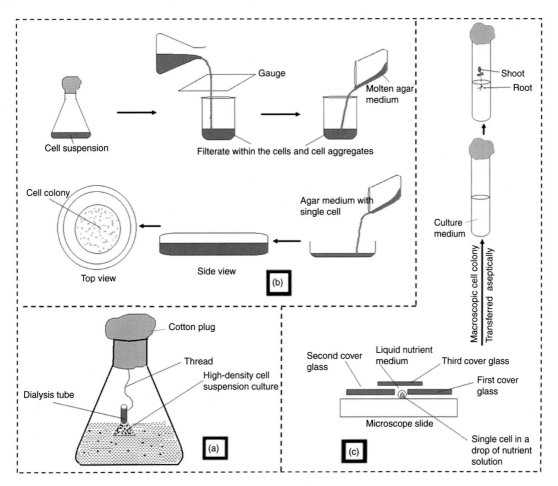

FIGURE 2.8 (a) Conditioning apparatus for low-density cell culture medium [163]; (b) Bergmann's cell plating technique for culturing single cells [166]; (c) microchamber technique for cell plating [168].

2.2.2.2.4 PATTERN OF GROWTH

Cells in suspension can exhibit much higher rates of cell division than those in callus culture. Suspension cultures when maintained under controlled conditions of light, temperature, and aeration follow a predictable pattern of growth curve (Fig. 2.9)

- *Lag phase*: The culture first passes through a lag phase in which there is little growth. The lag phase is the period when the cells adjust to the replenished supplies of nutrients and undertake all the necessary synthesis prior to cell division.
- *Log phase*: The cultures then pass through the logarithm phase or exponential phase of growth in which cells divide very rapidly, causing a logarithmic increase in cell number. Under optimum conditions, cell numbers double every 20–50 h, depending upon their species.
- The culture passes through a further period of rapid cell division that results in a linear increase in number, slowing at the phase as some nutrients become limiting.

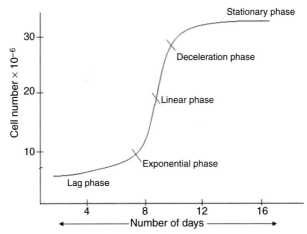

FIGURE 2.9   Growth curve showing different phases of growth.

- *Stationary phase*: The cultures then reach a stationary phase, when the rate of cell division within the culture decreases, and the cell number is stabilized and growth finally halts. As nutrients are depleted, some of the cells of the culture begin to show senescent characteristics and a low level of cell division will maintain cell numbers. If the cells are left in the stationary phase too long, they will die.

2.2.2.2.5 APPLICATION OF CELL CULTURE

For production of secondary metabolites (discussed in Chapter 7), mutant selection (discussed in Chapter 11), biotransformation (discussed in Chapter 7), somatic embryogenesis (discussed in Chapter 6), immobilization (discussed in Chapter 7), commercial production of cell mass and induction of mutation and genetic manipulation of plant cells, studying the effect of different chemicals, for obtaining individual isolated cells used for protoplast production, commercial production of cell mass, single cell protein hybrids or cybrids, to develop the single cell line or cell clone and easily preserved by using cryopreservation technique than other tissues or organ of the plant.

2.2.2.3 *Protoplast Culture*

A cell without a cell wall is called a protoplast. An earlier definition of protoplast (cells with their walls stripped off and removed from the proximity of their neighbouring cells) was modified by Vasil:

> The protoplast is a part of plant cell which lies within the cell wall and can be plasmolysed and isolated by removing the cell wall by mechanical or enzymatic procedure [170].

Major developments in protoplast culture are highlighted in Table 2.4. Somatic hybridization involves isolation, fusion, selection, and culture of the hybrid cells for the regeneration of hybrid plants from them.

2.2.2.3.1 METHODS FOR ISOLATION OF PROTOPLAST

The isolated protoplast is highly fragile and the outer plasma membrane is fully exposed. The plasma membrane is the only barrier between the interior of the living plant cell and the

TABLE 2.4   Prominent Research Finding Related to Protoplast Culture

Year	Contributor	Findings	References
1880	Hanstein	The word protoplast was coined for the living matter surrounded by the cell membrane	[171]
1892	Klercker	Klercker was the first to isolate protoplasts from plasmolyzed cells of *Stratiotes aloides* by microsurgery on plasmolyzed cells by mechanical method; however, the yields were extremely low and this method is not useful	[172,173]
1927	Küster	Demonstrated that the cell wall was hydrolyzed during fruit ripening process so that free protoplasts and protoplasmic units are left. He preferred such physiological method for isolating protoplasts	[174]
1931	Chambers	Protoplast isolation from tissues of onion bulb (onion scales immersed in 1 M sucrose until the protoplast shrunk and then plasmolyzed)	[175]
1960	Cocking	Cocking was the first to use enzymes to release protoplasts	[176]
1971	Nagata and Takebe	Developed a technique to derive cell and plant clones from isolated mesophyll protoplasts of tobacco	[177]
1972	Carlson and others	Carlson was the first to produce somatic hybrids by using two different species of *Nicotiana* (*N. glauca* × *N. langsdorfii*). He has also demonstrated the use of protoplast culture technique in genetic research	[178,179]
1972	Potrykus and Durand	Reported the callus formation from single protoplasts of *Petunia*	[180]
1973	Frearson et al.	Reported the isolation, culture, and regeneration of *Petunia* leaf protoplasts	[181]
1974	Vasil and Vasil	Reported the regeneration of tobacco and *Petunia* plants from protoplasts and culture of corn protoplasts	[182]
1975	Shepard and Roger	Described a method for the isolation of large numbers of tobacco mesophyll cell protoplasts under relatively low external osmotic conditions	[183]
1977	Potrykus et al.	Reported the callus formation from stem protoplasts of corn	[184]
1979	Potrykus et al.	Reported the callus formation from cell culture protoplasts of corn	[185]
1980	Veronica	Isolated protoplast from *Aspergillus fumigatus* using a lytic enzyme mixture from *Trichoderma harzianum*	[186]
1984	Glimelius	Isolated protoplasts from *Brassica*-produced callus with high efficiency in media containing casein hydrolysate and high concentrations of the auxin	[187]
1986	Firoozabady and Deboer	Isolated protoplasts of cotton (from cotyledons and foliage leaves). Protoplast yield and viability, cell wall regeneration, and cell division were influenced by several factors, e.g., genotype, age, tissue, and growth condition of donor plant, enzyme mixture and concentration, preplasmolysis period, incubation period, and culture medium	[188]
1986	Yamada et al.	Reported that protoplast derived calli from Fujiminori (*Oryza sativa* L.) produced whole plants in the regeneration medium	[189]

(Continued)

TABLE 2.4   Prominent Research Finding Related to Protoplast Culture (*cont.*)

Year	Contributor	Findings	References
1988	Wei and Xu	Protoplasts were isolated from immature cotyledons of six cultivars of *Glycine max* L. and cultured in the KP8 liquid medium supplemented with 0.2 mg/L 2,4-D, 1 mg/L NAA, and 0.5 mg/L ZT. Eighty-seven plants have been regenerated from four cultivars, and normal seeds were obtained from them after transplanting into pots	[190]
1988	Lührs and Lörz	Protoplast isolated from morphogenic suspension cultures of barley was studied for its regenerative potential	[191]
1988	Harris et al.	Protoplasts were isolated from anther-derived suspension cultures of commercial wheat (*Triticum aestivum* L. cv. Chris)	[192]
1990	Li and Murai	Established an efficient and reproducible procedure for protoplast propagation and fertile plant regeneration of rice (*O. sativa* L.) cultivars Nipponbare and Taipei 309	[193]
1990	Hayashimoto et al.	Protoplast transformation and regeneration of fertile transgenic plants of rice (*O. sativa* L.) cultivars Nipponbare and Taipei 309	[194]
1991	Arya et al.	Somatic embryos were formed from protoplast-derived embryogenic callus, which regenerated into plantlets	[195]
1992	Hayakawa et al.	The coat protein gene of rice stripe virus was introduced into two *Japonica* varieties of rice by electroporation of protoplasts	[196]
1995	Jain et al.	An improved procedure for plant regeneration from *Indica* and *Japonica* rice protoplasts was introduced by plating embryogenic cell suspension-derived protoplasts on the surface of filter membranes overlying agarose-embedded feeder cells of *Lolium multiflorum* and *O. ridleyi*, combined with the use of a maltose-containing shoot regeneration medium	[197]
2004	Rosenbluh et al.	Nonendocytic penetration of core histones into *Petunia* protoplasts and cultured cells: a novel mechanism for the introduction of macromolecules into plant cells	[198]
2007	Yoo et al.	Arabidopsis mesophyll protoplasts: a versatile cell system for transient gene expression analysis	[199]
2008	Yang et al.	Expression profile analysis of genes involved in cell wall regeneration during protoplast culture in cotton by suppression subtractive hybridization and microarray	[200]

external environment. Mechanical or enzymatic isolation are the most common approaches to remove the cell wall without damaging the protoplast. Mechanical isolation, although possible, often results in low yields, poor quality, and poor performance in culture due to substances released from damaged cells. Enzymatic isolation is a safe method that is usually carried out in a simple solution with a high osmoticum (substance that acts to supplement osmotic pressure in a plant or a culture of a plant cell, e.g., sucrose), along with cell wall degrading enzymes. A high quality mixture of *cellulase* and *pectinase* enzymes must be used for this purpose. The general protocol for the isolation, culture, and regeneration of plantlets from leaf protoplasts is mentioned in Fig. 2.10. Isolation of protoplast can be done by three methods:

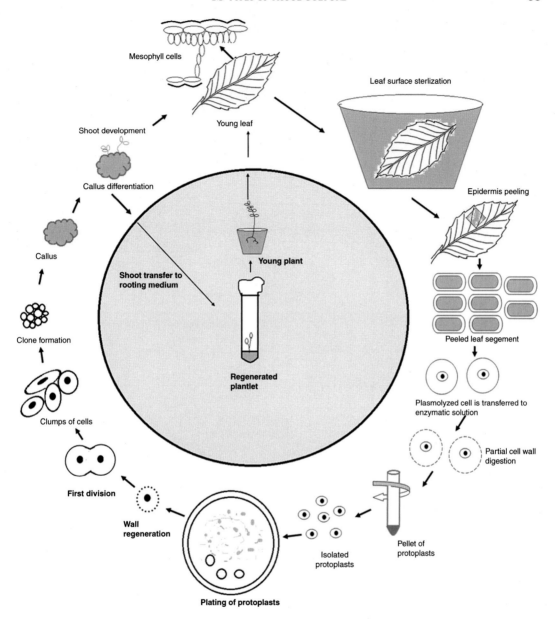

FIGURE 2.10 Diagrammatic representation of the technique used for isolation, culture, and regeneration of plantlets from leaf protoplasts.

- *Mechanical method*: Mechanical method of protoplast isolation was first done by Klercker [170] (Fig. 2.11).
- *Sequential enzymatic method*: The sequential enzymatic method was first used by Takebe and others in 1968, wherein they used commercially available enzymes (Table 2.5) in two steps [177] (Fig. 2.11).

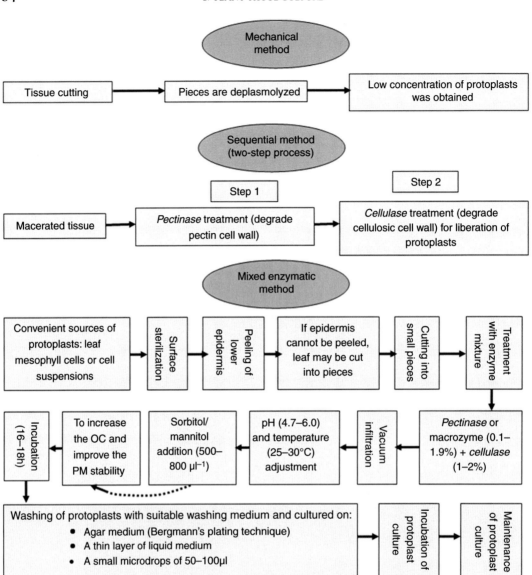

FIGURE 2.11 **Methods for the isolation of the protoplasts (mechanical, sequential, mixed enzymatic methods).** OC: Osmotic concentration; PM: Plasma membrane.

- *Mixed enzymatic method*: Nagata and Takebe reported the first plant regeneration from isolated protoplasts in 1971 and since then this has been achieved in 330 species of higher plants (gymnosperm 10, monocots 32, dicots 288) [177]. In the mixed enzymatic method both the enzymes were used together to reduce time and chances of contamination. Power and Cocking used this method for the isolation of protoplasts from a number of plant sciences and it gives very good yields, as high as 2.5×10^6 protoplasts/gram of leaf tissue [201] (Fig. 2.11).

TABLE 2.5 Various Commercially Available Enzymes Commonly Used for the Isolation of Protoplast

Enzyme	Source organism
1. Zymolyase	*Arthrobacter luteus*
2. Cellulose onozuka	*Trichoderma viride*
3. Rhozyme	*Aspergillus niger*
4. Macrozyme	*Rhizopus arrhizus*
5. Hemicellulase	*Aspergillus niger*
6. Macerase	*Rhizopus arrhizus*
7. Helicase	*Helix pomatia*
8. Pectolyase	*Aspergillus japonica*
9. Drisclease	*Irpex lacteus*
10. Cellulysin	*Trichoderma viride*

2.2.2.3.2 PROTOPLAST FUSION AND SOMATIC HYBRIDIZATION

Protoplast fusion or somatic hybridization is one of the most important uses of protoplast culture. This is particularly significant for hybridization between species or genera, which cannot be made to cross by conventional methods of sexual hybridization. Although somatic hybridization was achieved first in animals and only later in plants, its significance has been realized fully in plants because the hybrid cell can be induced to regenerate into whole plants. Various examples of somatic hybridization of interspecific, intergeneric, and intertribal plants are highlighted in Table 2.6.

2.2.2.3.3 TECHNIQUES OF PROTOPLAST FUSION

(a) *Chemical fusogen*

High molecular weight water-soluble polymer, polyethylene glycol (PEG), has been identified as a potent fusogen. The polymer binds with the lipid membrane of cells and thus induces fusion (Fig 2.12). Various fusogens are highlighted in Fig. 2.13. The most effective chemical fusion of protoplast is obtained by combining PEG and calcium. $NaNO_3$ is not preferred due to low frequency of fusion, particularly when highly vacuolated mesophyll protoplasts are used.

(b) *Electric fusion*

In electric fusion protoplasts are placed into a small culture vessel containing electrodes and a potential difference is applied, then the protoplast will line up between the electrodes. Alternate generation of AC and DC pulse are two steps required for electric fusion. This method is more reproducible and less damaging but requires expensive equipment.

2.2.2.3.4 APPLICATIONS

- *To overcome sexual incompatibility*: Production of novel interspecific and intergeneric crosses between plants that are difficult or impossible to hybridize conventionally. Therefore, sexual incompatibility may be overcome. Melchers and Labib used albino mutants for the complementation selection of green intraspecific hybrids of tobacco [202].

TABLE 2.6   Examples of Somatic Hybridization in Different Plants

Genus	Parent species and their chromosome number	Chromosome number of hybrid
Interspecific hybrids		
Brassica	*B. oleracea* (2n = 18) + *B. campestris* (2n = 20) *B. napus* (2n = 38) + *B. oleracea* (2n = 18) *B. napus* (2n = 38) + *B. nigra* (2n = 16) *B. napus* (2n = 38) + *B. carinata* (2n = 34)	Wide variation
Nicotiana	*N. tabacum* (2n = 48) + *N. alata* (2n = 18)	66–71
	N. tabacum (2n = 48) + *N. glauca* (2n = 14)	72
	N. tabacum (2n = 48) + *N. rustica* (2n = 48)	60–91
	N. tabacum (2n = 48) + *N. octophora* (2n = 24)	48
	N. tabacum (2n = 48) + *N. mesophila* (2n = 48)	96
	N. tabacum (2n = 48) + *N. glutinosa* (2n = 24)	50–88
Intergeneric hybrids		
Raphanus × *Brassica*	*Raphanus sativus* + *B. oleracea*	Raphanobrassica
Moricandia × *Brassica*	*Moricandia arvensis* + *B. oleracea*	Moricandiobrassica
Eruca × *Brassica*	*Eruca sativa* + *B. napus*	Erucobrassica
Nicotiana × *Lycopersicon* *Nicotiana* × *Petunia*	*Nicotiana tabacum* + *Lycopersicon esculentum* *Nicotiana tabacum* + *Petunia inflorata*	Nicotiopersicon Nicotiopetunia
Solanum × *Lycopersicon*	*Solanum tuberosum* + *Lycopersicon esculentum*	Solanopersicon
Datura × *Atropa*	*Datura inoxia* + *Atropa belladonna*	Daturotropa
Intertribal hybrids		
Arabidopsis × *Brassica*	*Arabidopsis thaliana* + *B. campestris*	Arabidobrassica
Thlaspi × *Brassica*	*Thlaspi perfoliatum* + *B. napus*	Thlaspobrassica

Interspecific somatic hybrid plants from sexually incompatible species have been raised in *Nicotiana, Petunia, Daucus,* and *Datura.*

- *Production of cybrids*: Cybrids are cells or plants containing the nucleus of one species and cytoplasm of both parenteral species. These are generally produced during protoplast fusion in variable frequencies. Cybrid formation may result by fusion of normal protoplasts of one species with enucleated protoplasts (cytoplasm), elimination of the nucleus of one species from a normal heterokaryon, or gradual elimination of the chromosomes of one species from a hybrid cell during further mitotic division (Fig. 2.12). The cybrids can be produced in high frequencies by irradiation of one parenteral protoplast before fusion in order to inactivate the nuclei or by preparing enucleate protoplasts of one species and fusing them with normal protoplasts of another species.
- *Uptake of foreign materials*: Being naked in nature, isolated protoplasts are considered to be very suitable for genetic and cytoplasmic modifications. It has been reported that plant protoplast has a unique property in uptaking isolated nuclei, DNA, chromosomes, chloroplasts, cyanobacteria, nitrogen fixing bacteria, and virus particles.

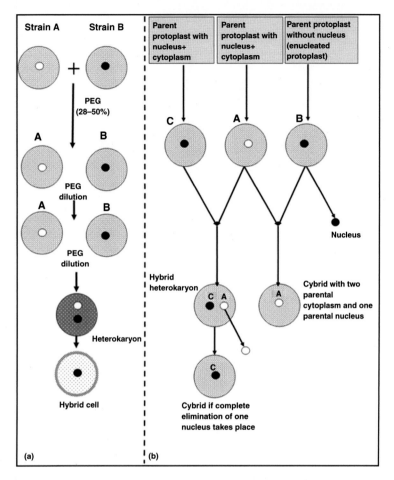

FIGURE 2.12 Protocol for the polyethylene glycol induced protoplast fusion (a) and production of cybrids through protoplast fusion (b).

- *Gene transfer with use of protoplast*: Direct gene transfer by using isolated protoplasts is an alternative to the use of *Agrobacterium*. In 1974, Jeff Schell and coworkers revealed that the engineering ability of the *Agrobacterium* cell lies in its plasmids, not in the bacterial chromosomes. *Agrobacterium*-mediated transformation of the tobacco protoplast led to an extraordinary breakthrough in recovering the first transgenic plant [203].

2.2.2.4 Immobilized Cell Cultures (Described in Chapter 7)

Plant cells can be encapsulated or entrapped in a gel or any suitable polymeric matrix that is afterwards solidified. Earlier, this technique was limited to micropropagation, but now it is employed widely in plant tissue culture practices that are focusing on producing secondary products or for the biotransformation of chemical compounds through plant cells.

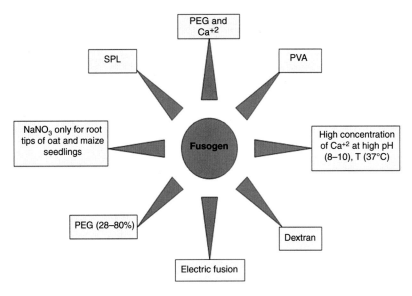

FIGURE 2.13   **Techniques of protoplast fusion.**

2.3 PLANT TISSUE CULTURE MEDIA

Culturing of microorganisms on simply agar medium or many other complex or defined media is a common practice that has been practiced from very earlier times. After exploring the regeneration or differentiation or totipotent potential of plant cells, the *in vitro* propagation technique introduced the same concept in plant science, which provides the foundation for further plant tissue culture studies. In nature, soil nourishes plants and provides the basic nutrients for their further growth and development. Apart from carbon, hydrogen, and oxygen, plants require large amounts of elements denoted as major elements [nitrogen (N), potassium (K), calcium (Ca), phosphorus (P), magnesium (Mg), and sulfur (S)] with small quantities of minor elements [iron (Fe), nickel (Ni), chlorine (Cl), manganese (Mn), zinc (Zn), boron (B), copper (Cu), and molybdenum (Mo)]. These 17 elements are known to be the essential elements for healthy and vigorous growth of intact plants, therefore they are the essential part of most of the plant culture media. However, certain others, such as cobalt (Co), aluminum (Al), sodium (Na), and iodine (I), are also essential for some species [204]. Thus, soil and plant mineral analysis (elementary composition) can give a better idea regarding the basic requirements of plants. Otherwise development and optimization of new media becomes tedious. In 2008 George et al. compared the elementary composition of healthy plants against the most commonly used Murashige and Skoog medium [204,205]. Each plant strain has its different requirement. Some plant strains easily grow on simple media (inorganic nutrients, carbon sources, growth regulators, and gelling agents) and some essentially require the supplementation of vitamins, growth, and certain selective substances. During the *in vitro* culturing process plant tissue absorbs the inorganic nutrients (ions) from media in a similar fashion to that from soil. In nutrient medium (weak aqueous solution) these inorganic salts

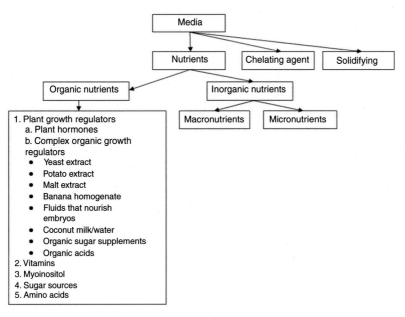

FIGURE 2.14 Outline describing the main components of media.

dissociate and are subsequently absorbed by the plant cells in the form of cations and anions. Uptake of each ion is generally proportional to its respective salt concentration in the medium [204]. But this not true since concentration of other salts may also affect the uptake of ions, e.g., under conditions of high K^+ or Ca^{2+} concentrations, Mg deficiency can result, and vice versa. Therefore, in plants nutrients are either taken up passively or through active mechanisms that are generally less dependent on ionic concentration than passive uptake [204]. The composition of media is described in Fig. 2.14. Tables 2.7, 2.8, 2.9, and 2.10 describe the different types of media along with the different roles of the elements required for plant growth and development.

2.3.1 Types of Media

Different types of media and their basic features are highlighted in Table 2.11.

2.3.2 Functions of Plant Tissue Culture Media

Plant tissue culture media provide water, minerals, vitamins, hormones, growth regulators, organic compounds, and other desirable nutrients for the further growth and development of cell or tissue into the undifferentiated mass of the callus, as well as provide desirable pH to substrate and act as a dumping ground for secondary metabolites. They also provide access to the atmosphere for gaseous exchange. Different types of media, their composition, and different roles of their prominent elements are described in Tables 2.7, 2.8, 2.9, and 2.10.

TABLE 2.7 Different Types of Media and Their Special Features

Medium	Special feature	References
Hoagland and Arnon, 1938	• This is a hydroponic nutrient solution and is one of the most popular solution compositions for growing plants. • This solution provides every nutrient necessary for plant growth and is appropriate for the growth of a large variety of plant species. • It has been modified several times, mainly to add iron chelates.	[206,207]
Gautheret, 1939	• Reported potentially unlimited growth of cultures derived from carrot tip root tissue when the growth substance indole-3-acetic acid (IAA) was incorporated in the culture medium. • Gautheret's medium was based on Knop's salt solution.	[115]
Knudson (K), 1946	• Knudson C orchid medium was the first medium specially formulated for *in vitro* orchid cultures.	[208]
Vacin and Went (VW), 1949	• This medium is used for orchid culture.	[209]
Burkholder and Nickell, 1949	• Modified the White's medium by adding extra phosphate and vitamin B_1.	[210]
Hellers, 1953	• This is a low salt, reduced-growth medium, which is similar to White's medium and allows explants to develop and grow at a slower rate. • Hellers has experimented with root culture of certain orchids and later on started clonal propagation of orchids on a large scale.	[211]
Reinert and White, 1956	• Reinert and White have used a variety of vitamins for the culture of callus tissue of *Picea glauca*.	[212]
Murashige and Skoog (MS), 1962	• MS medium was initially developed for tobacco and was formulated on the basis of mineral analysis of tobacco tissue. • The significant feature of the MS medium is its very high concentration of nitrate, potassium, and ammonia. • MS medium is economical as compared to other media like White's medium. • It promotes organogenesis and regeneration of plants. • MS medium is used for micropropagation, organ culture, callus culture, and cell suspension culture.	[205]
White (W), 1963	• This is one of the earliest media in plant tissue culture. • First developed for root culture medium of tomato root. • White's medium was based on Uspenski and Uspenska's medium for algae.	[213]
Linsmaier and Skoog (LS), 1965	• This is a version of MS medium with modified organic constituents.	[214]
Eriksson, 1965	• Eriksson medium was developed for cell suspension cultures of *Haplopappus gracilis*.	[215]
Gamborgs (B5), 1968	• This medium was first developed for soybean callus culture. Contains much greater content of nitrate as compared to ammonium ions. • Designed for callus and cell suspension culture and protoplast culture. • Used for regeneration of protoplast-derived plants.	[216,217]
Nitsch and Nitsch (N and N), 1969	• This medium is utilized for anther callus culture, supports embryogenesis, and promotes the growth of protoplast culture. • Contains lower salt solution than MS medium but not as low that of White.	[218]

TABLE 2.7   Different Types of Media and Their Special Features (*cont.*)

Medium	Special feature	References
Schenk and Hildebrandt medium (SH), 1972	• This medium is used for growth of both monocyte and dicotyle cell suspensions. • It is also used for callus and cell suspension culture.	[219]
Gresshoff and Doy, 1974	• This medium has been specially formulated for plant cell, tissue, and organ cultures. • Potassium nitrate and ammonium nitrate serve as the sources of nitrate. • Glycine serves as the amino acid source. • Medium does not contain sucrose and agar; hence, these components have to be added to the medium before use.	[220]
Chu (N6), 1975	• Establishment of an efficient medium for anther culture of rice, through comparative experiments on the nitrogen sources. • This medium is used to promote organ culture and cell suspension culture.	[221]
Kao and Michayluk, 1975	• This medium was developed according to the nutritional requirements for growth of *Vicia hajastana* cells and protoplasts at a very low population density in liquid media.	[222]
Mitras (M), 1976	• Mitras medium is used for orchid culture.	[223]
Lloyd and McCown (LM), 1981	• This medium is a woody plant medium and was first utilized for *Kalmia latifolia*.	[224]
Lichter, 1982	• The production of haploid plants from isolated microspores of *Brassica napus* (L.) was first reported by Lichter in 1982. • This medium was derived from that described by Nitsch and Nitsch and was developed to support the initiation and growth of haploid plants from anther and pollen cultures of *Brassica napus*. • This medium contains the equivalent of 500 mg/L calcium nitrate tetrahydrate as described in the original formulation.	[225]
Driver and Kuniyuki, 1984 and McGranahan, et al. 1987	• This medium was developed specifically for walnut. • It was also developed for the multiplication of shoots from nodal explants. • The medium was supplemented with 4.5 µM BA and 5 nM IBA. • Larger diameter and more homogeneous microshoots were obtained from this medium.	[226,227]
Hickok et al., 1995	• This medium is suitable for spore germination and gametophyte cultures.	[228]
Quoirin and Lepoivre, 1977	• Quoirin and Lepoivre medium has been specially formulated for plant cell, tissue, and organ cultures. • Ammonium nitrate and potassium nitrate serve as nitrate sources. • Medium does not contain sucrose and agar; hence, these components have to be added to the medium before use.	[229]
Quoirin et al. 1977 and Coke, 1996	• Coke has been elaborated for *in vitro* culturing of loblolly pine whereas Quoirin et al. showed that dilution of macronutrients improved the rooting of several *Prunus* species.	[230,231]
Vuylsteke, 1998	• IBA has been used in this medium to induce rooting.	[232]
Maliro, 2004	• Tissue culture medium gelled with cassava flour to support shoot proliferation of stem nodal sections of *Uapaca kirkiana* and *Faidherbia albida*.	[233]

TABLE 2.8   Some of the Elements Important for Plant Nutrition and Their Physiological Function

Elements	Function	Deficiency	Source salts
Nitrogen	Component of proteins, nucleic acids, and some coenzymes. This element is required in greatest amount	Inhibition of protein synthesis	KNO_3, NH_4NO_3, $Ca(NO_3)_2$
Potassium	Regulates osmotic potential, principal inorganic cation	Inactivation of enzymes and osmotic pressure imbalance	KNO_3
Calcium	Cell wall synthesis, membrane function, cell signaling	Membrane and shoot-tip necrosis	$CaCl_2$, $Ca(NO_3)_2$
Magnesium	Enzyme cofactor, component of chlorophyll	Enzymatic reaction and ATP synthesis will be affected	$MgSO_4$
Phosphorus	Component of nucleic acids, energy transfer, component of intermediates in respiration and photosynthesis	Delayed growth and dark green color of the leaves	KH_2PO_4
Sulfur	Component of some amino acids (methionine, cysteine) and some cofactors	Inhibits protein synthesis and decreases chlorophyll in leaves	$MgSO_4$, K_2SO_4
Chlorine	Required for photosynthesis	Decrease in photosynthesis	$COCl_2$
Iron	Electron transfer as a component of cytochromes	Severe effects on growth and development	Na_2Fe EDTA
Manganese	Enzyme cofactor	Various enzymatic activities will be affected	$MNSO_4$
Cobalt	Component of some vitamins	Vitamin synthesis will be decreased	$COCl_2$
Copper	Enzyme cofactor, electron-transfer reactions	Decrease in photosynthesis	Cu_2SO_4
Zinc	Enzyme cofactor, chlorophyll biosynthesis	Decrease in the synthesis of tryptophan	$ZnSO_4$
Molybdenum	Enzyme cofactor, component of nitrate reductase (participates in the conversion of nitrate to ammonium)	Inhibition of nitrate to ammonium conversion	Na_2MoO_4
Boron	Involved in different enzymatic activity	Various enzymatic activities will be affected	H_3BO_3

These elements have to be supplied by the culture medium in order to support the growth of healthy cultures *in vitro*.

2.3.3 Components of Tissue Culture Medium

2.3.3.1 Inorganic Nutrients

In vitro growth of plants also requires a combination of macro- and micronutrients as for *in vivo* growth. Their concentration is presented in the form of millimolar quantities. The role of different elements with their respective source salts is shown in Table 2.8.

TABLE 2.9 The Concentrations of Major and Minor Compounds and Vitamins in Different Types of Media

Constituents	Concentration in culture medium (mg/mL)					
	MS	W	SH	B5	H	LS
MAJOR SALTS						
$Ca(NO_3)_2 \cdot 4H_2O$	–	142	–	–	–	–
KNO_3	1900	81	2500	3000	–	1900
$NaNO_3$	–	–	–	–	600	–
NH_4NO_3	1650	–	–	–	–	1650
$NH_4H_2PO_4$	–	–	300	–	–	–
$(NH_4)_2SO_4$	–	–		134	–	–
$MgSO_4 \cdot 7H_2O$	370	74	400	500	250	370
$CaCl_2 \cdot 2H_2O$	440		200	150	75	440
KCL		65	–	–	750	–
KH_2PO_4	170	12	–	–		170
$NaH_2PO_4 \cdot H_2O$	–	–	–	150	125	–
MINOR SALTS						
$MnSO_4 \cdot H_2O$	22.3	–	10	10	–	–
$MnSO_4 \cdot 4H_2O$	–	–	–	–	0.1	22.3
KI	0.83	–	1	0.75	0.01	0.8
H_3BO_3	6.2	–	5	3	1	6.2
$ZnSO_4 \cdot 7H_2O$	8.6	–	1	2	1	8.6
$CuSO_4$	–	–	0.2	0.025	–	–
$CuSO_4 \cdot 5H_2O$	0.025	–	–	–	0.03	0.02
$NaMoO_4 \cdot 2H_2O$	0.25	–	0.1	0.25	–	0.25
$CoCl_2 \cdot 6H_2O$	0.25	–	0.1	0.025	–	0.02
$AlCl_3$	–	–	–	–	0.03	–
$NiCl_2 \cdot 6H_2O$	–	–	–	–	0.03	–
CHELATING AGENTS						
$FeCl_3 \cdot 6H_2O$	–	–	–	–	1	–
$FeSO_4 \cdot 7H_2O$	27.95	–	15	–	–	27.86
$Fe(SO_4)_3$	–	2.46	–	–	–	–
Sequestrene 330 Fe	–	–	–	28	–	–
Na_2EDTA	37.23	–	20	–	–	37.20
VITAMINS						
Myoinositol	100	–	1000	100	–	100
Thiamine–HCl	0.10	–	5	10	–	0.4

(Continued)

TABLE 2.9   The Concentrations of Major and Minor Compounds and Vitamins in Different Types of Media *(cont.)*

	Concentration in culture medium (mg/mL)					
Constituents	**MS**	**W**	**SH**	**B5**	**H**	**LS**
Nicotinic acid	0.50	–	5	1	–	–
Pyridoxine–HCl	0.50	–	0.5	1	–	–
COMPLEX ADDITIONS						
Yeast extract	–	100	–	–	–	–
SUGAR						
Sucrose	30,000	20,000	30,000	20,000	–	30,000
pH						
pH	5.8	–	5.9	5.5	–	5.8

MS, Murashige and Skoog, 1962; W, White's, 1953; SH, Schenk and Heldebrandt, 1972; B5, Gamborg, 1968; H, Heller's, 1953; LS, Lismaier and Skoog, 1965. Complex additions (e.g., coconut milk, malt extract, potato extract, banana homogenate, casein hydrolysate, algal compounds used in the conjugation) are not listed. Compositions are as in the original formulations. Sucrose (20–30 g/L) should be added to Heller's salt medium.

TABLE 2.10   Concentrations of Major and Minor Compounds and Vitamins in Different Types of Media

	Concentration in culture medium (mg/mL)							
Constituents	**K**	**M**	**KM**	**VW**	**LM**	**N-6**	**GT**	**N and N**
MAJOR SALTS								
$Ca_3(PO_4)_2$	–	200	–	200	–	–	–	–
$Ca(NO_3)_2$	1000	–	–	–	556	–	500	–
KNO_3	250	180	1900	525	–	2830	125	2000
$NaNO_3$	–	–	–	–	–	–	–	–
$NH_4 NO_3$	–	–	1650	–	400	–	–	–
$NH_4H_2PO_4$	–	–	–	–	–	–	–	–
$(NH_4)_2SO_4$	–	100	–	500	–	–	–	–
$MgSO_4 7H_2O$	250	250	370	250	370	185	–	250
$CaCl_2 2H_2O$	–	–	440	–	96	166	–	–
$CaCl_2$	–	–	–	–	–	–	–	25
KCL	–	–	–	–	–	–	–	1500
KH_2PO_4	250	150	170	250	170	400	125	–
$NaH_2PO_4H_2O$			–	–	–	–	–	250
K_2SO_4			–	–	990	–	–	–

TABLE 2.10 Concentrations of Major and Minor Compounds and Vitamins in Different Types of Media (*cont.*)

Constituents	Concentration in culture medium (mg/mL)							
	K	M	KM	VW	LM	N-6	GT	N and N
MINOR SALTS								
$MnSO_4H_2O$	–	–	–	–	–	–	–	–
$MnSO_44H_2O$	–	–	22.30	–	29.43	3.3	3	3
KI	–	0.03	0.83	–		0.8	0.5	–
H_3BO_3	–	0.6	6.20	–	6.2	1.6	0.05	0.5
$ZnSO_47H_2O$	–	0.05	8.6	–	8.6	1.5	0.18	0.5
$CuSO_4$	–	–	–	–	–	–	–	–
$CuSO_45H_2O$	–	–	0.025	–	0.25	–	0.5	0.025
$NaMoO_42H_2O$	–	0.05	0.25	–	0.25	–	–	0.025
$CoCl_26H_2O$	–	–	0.025	–	–	–	–	–
$AlCl_3$	–	–	–	–	–	–	–	–
$NiSO_4$	–	–	–	–	–	–	0.05	–
$Ti(SO_4)_3$	–	–	–	–	–	–	0.20	–
$BeSO_4$	–	–	–	–	–	–	0.1	–
H_2SO_4	–	–	–	–	–	–	1	–
$Fe(C_4H_4O_6)_3 \cdot 2H_2O$	–	–	–	28	–	–	–	–
$MnCl_2$	0.4							
CHELATING AGENTS								
$FeCl_36H_2O$	–	–	–	–	–	–	–	–
$FeSO_47H_2O$	27.8	27.8	–	27.8	27.8	0.05	–	
$Fe(SO_4)_3$	–	–	–	–	–	–	–	
Na_2EDTA	37.3	37.3	–	37.3	37.3	–	–	
VITAMINS								
Myoinositol	–	100	–	100	–	–	–	
Thiamine–HCl	0.3	1	–	1	1	0.1	–	
Nicotinic acid	1.25	0.5	–	0.5	0.5	0.5	–	
Pyridoxine–HCl	0.3	0.5	–	0.5	0.5	0.1	–	
COMPLEX ADDITIONS								
Yeast extract	–	–	100	–	–	–	–	
SUGAR								
Sucrose	–	30,000	20,000	30,000	30,000	30,000	34,000	
AMINO ACIDS								
Glycine	–	2	–	2	–	3	–	
pH								
pH		5.8	–	5.9	5.5	–	5.8	

K, Knoop; M, Mitra, 1976; KM, Kudson modified, 1946; VW, Vacin and Went, 1949; LM, Lloyd and McCown, 1980; N-6, Chu, 1978; GT, Gautheret, 1939; N and N, Nitsch and Nitsch, 1969 media.

TABLE 2.11 Different Types of Media

Types of media	Features
Basal medium	• Contains macro- and micronutrients, but no vitamins, carbohydrates, or growth regulators.
Normal medium	• Typically it is complete and requires no additional components (except gelling agent, if desired).
Modified basal salt medium	• Indicates that one or more of the components varies in concentration or from that originally published.
Natural media	• Media that contain only natural substances supplemented by organic acids, e.g., potato extract.
Defined media/ synthetic media	• Synthetic media are the chemically defined media that are devoid of the biological component such as yeast, animal, or plant tissue.
Prepared media	• It is not obligatory to use synthetic media (marketed by different companies such as Sigma, Flow, Gibco) as such. • Founder of each medium has successfully designed a formula of different components that is suitable for either broad or sometimes limited class of plants. • No stock solution is needed for such media; each packet may be dissolved directly in a specified amount of distilled water. Otherwise preparation of stock solutions for media preparation is really time consuming.
Growth medium	• On the basis of growth and development process plant medium is divided into four parts: • *Roots induction medium*: high concentrations of auxin relative to cytokinin produced roots • *Shoot induction medium*: high concentrations of cytokinin relative to auxin produced shoots • *Callus induction medium*: auxin- and cytokinin-containing callus-inducing medium • *Precallus induction medium*: Preincubation is essential to permit the dedifferentiation of tissues that will ultimately redifferentiate into organs [234–236]. Treatment of explants with preincubation medium is a two-step process, explants are preincubated on an auxin-rich (CIM) and then are transferred to a cytokinin-rich shoot induction medium (SIM). During CIM preincubation, root explants acquire competence to respond to shoot induction signals during subsequent incubation on SIM.
Selective media	• Media that are used for the growth of only selected cultures, e.g., a selective tissue culture medium for growth of compact (dwarf) mutants of apple. • A selective reagent may also be included in a culture medium to either promote or restrict the growth of certain cultures.
Minimal media	• Media that contain the minimum nutrients possible for tissue growth, generally without the presence of amino acids to grow "wild type" of plant stains, e.g., Murashige and Skoog basal salts with minimal organics medium.
Universal media	• Universal media are those media that, once designed, can be used for a group of the plants present in a class, species, or genus. • No media of such type have so far been developed. • Each medium requires optimization for the proper growth and development of the cell or tissue. • Murashige and Skoog medium is known for the development of callus for many plants but it also requires optimization in tissue culture experimentation.

- *Macronutrients* are required at a concentration greater than 0.5 mM/L. These include salts of nitrogen, potassium, phosphorus, calcium, magnesium, and sulfur. These all have different roles in development such as protein synthesis (N, S), nucleotide synthesis (S, N, P), membrane integrity (Mg), cell wall synthesis (Ca), and enzyme cofactor (Mg). Nitrogen is supplemented in the form of organic (amino acids, casein hydrolysate, and other organic acids) and inorganic form. Inorganic nitrogen is usually supplied in the form of ammonium (NH^{4+}) and nitrate (NO^{3-}) ions. Nitrate is superior to ammonium as the sole N source but use of NH^{4+} checks the increase of pH toward alkalinity. Nitrates and sulfates have to be reduced before they can participate in the synthesis of amino acids, protein, and enzymes. Culture media should contain 25 mM/L nitrogen and potassium. Other major elements are adequate in the concentration range of 1–3 mM/L.
- *Micronutrients* are required at a concentration less than 0.05 mM/L. These include iron, manganese, zinc, boron, copper, and molybdenum. These inorganic elements although required in small quantity are essential for plant growth, most critical of them being iron, which is not available at low pH. Free iron is very low in plants. Iron is mainly bound to chelator ethylenediaminetetraacetic acid (EDTA) that helps iron to be available in the culture. Therefore, it is provided as iron EDTA complex to make it available at a wide range of pH.

2.3.3.2 *Carbon Source*

During plant tissue culture growth sucrose acts as a fuel source for sustaining photomixotrophic metabolism (organisms can use different sources of energy and carbon), ensuring optimal development, although other important roles such as carbon precursor or signaling metabolite have more recently been highlighted. Sucrose is a very important part of nutrient medium as an energy source, since most plant cultures are unable to photosynthesize effectively owing to poorly developed cellular and tissue development, lack of chlorophyll, inadequate gas exchange and carbon dioxide in tissue culture vessels, etc. Hence, they lack auxotrophic ability and need external carbon for energy. Sugar uptake in plant tissue cultures appears to be partially through passive permeation and partially through active transport. Sucrose also supports the maintenance of osmotic potential (osmoticum) and the conservation of water in cells. Hence, in anther culture a higher concentration of sucrose (6–12%) is used. It has been also proven that plant tissue cultures do not fix enough CO_2 to sustain growth in the absence of sucrose, mainly due to limited CO_2 inside the vessel. However, high sucrose concentration in the media restricts the photosynthetic efficiency of cultured plants by reducing the key enzymes for photosynthesis, levels of chlorophyll, and epicuticular waxes promoting the formation of structurally and physiologically abnormal stomata. The most preferred carbon or energy source is sucrose at a concentration of 20–60 g/L. But the levels of sucrose that are normally used to support the growth of tissue cultures are often inhibitory to chlorophyll synthesis. During autoclaving the medium sucrose is hydrolyzed to glucose and fructose, which are then used by the plant material for their growth. Fructose, if autoclaved is toxic. It has been found that a plant tissue culture medium containing glucose or fructose sterilized by autoclaving inhibits the growth of carrot root tissue cultures. More growth inhibition occurs when sugar and culture medium is autoclaved together [237]. Other mono- or disaccharide and sugar alcohols like glucose, sorbitol, raffinose, etc., may be used depending upon plant species. Sucrose is still the best source of carbon followed by glucose, maltose, and raffinose; fructose was less effective and mannose and lactose were the least suitable. Carbohydrate sucrose is generally required to be present in addition to IAA before tracheid elements are differentiated in tissue cultures. Different types of sugars and their different roles in growth and development of plant cell are mentioned Table 2.12.

2.3.3.3 Organic Supplements

2.3.3.3.1 VITAMINS

Vitamins are organic substances required for metabolic processes as cofactors or parts of enzymes. Hence, for optimum growth, medium should be supplemented with vitamins. Thiamine (B1), nicotinic acid (B3), pyridoxine (B6), pantothenic acid (B5), and myoinositol are commonly used vitamins of which thiamine (0.1 to 5 mg/L) is essentially added to medium as it is involved in carbohydrate metabolism. Four vitamins (myoinositol, thiamine, nicotinic acid, and pyridoxine) are the ingredients of MS medium. They have been used in different ratios for the culture of tissues and their requirement may vary according to the nature of the plant and the type of culture. It has been proven that only myoinositol and thiamine are required for the optimum growth of tobacco callus tissue on MS salts. In 1965, Linsmaier and Skoog modified the medium by increasing the level of thiamine up to fourfold over that of Murashige and Skoog, but other vitamins such as nicotinic acid, pyridoxine, and glycine (amino acid) were unnecessary [214]. Different roles of vitamins in growth and development of plant cells are found in Table 2.13.

2.3.3.3.2 AMINO ACIDS

These nitrogenous substances are not essential but addition of amino acids augments the nitrogen supply to media, which is important for stimulating cell growth in protoplast cultures and also in inducing and maintaining somatic embryogenesis. This reduced organic nitrogen is more readily taken up by plants than the inorganic nitrogen. L-Glutamine, L-asparagine, L-cysteine, and L-glycine are commonly used amino acids that are being added to the culture medium in form of mixtures as individually they inhibit cell growth.

2.3.3.3.3 COMPLEX ORGANICS

Complex organics are also called natural supplements or undefined supplements. They are the group of undefined supplements such as casein hydrolysate, coconut water, yeast extract, orange juice, tomato juice, etc. When the completely defined plant culture media did not give the desired results, employing natural supplements have beneficial effects on *in vitro* plant cell and tissue cultures. The first successful cultures of plant tissue involved the use of yeast extract [5,107]. Recently, casein hydrolysate has given significant success in tissue culture and potato extract also has been found useful for anther culture. However, these natural extracts are avoided as their composition is unknown and varies from batch to batch, affecting the reproducibility of results. Organic supplementation is essential for proper growth and regeneration of plants. These organic substances are the active source of several amino acids, hormones, vitamins, fatty acids, carbohydrates, and several other plant growth substances. Their required quantity varies with plant and species. Inclusion of natural complexes is not essential or may not be critical but is often beneficial. Some of the most common organic supplements of plant tissue culture media from natural sources are highlighted in Table 2.14.

TABLE 2.12 Different Types of Carbohydrates Used in Plant Tissue Culture Medium with Their Uses

Nature of sugar	Name	Uses
Reducing sugar	Glucose	• Autoclaved glucose sometimes supports the growth of callus. • In some cases supports cell division and tracheid formation. • Acts as an osmolyte during protoplast isolation. • Its stimulatory effect on morphogenesis is due to its action as a respiratory substrate.
	Fructose	• Effective in preventing hyperhydricity. • Best sugar for the production of adventitious shoots for some plants. • Filter sterilized fructose supports the growth of callus cultures in some plants. • Autoclaved fructose was proved to be toxic in some plants.
	Galactose	• Galactose is said to be toxic to most plant tissues. • Induces early somatic embryo maturation. • Reduces or overcomes hyperhydricity in shoot cultures. • In some cases cells can become adapted and grown on galactose (due to induction of the enzyme galactose kinase).
	Mannose	• Broken down to glucose and fructose, can also sometimes be used as partial replacement for sucrose.
	Maltose	• Callus induction in some plants. • Shows slow intra- and extracellular hydrolysis in plants. • Acts as carbon source and as an osmoticum. • Supports embryogenesis in some cases.
	Cellobiose	• Broken down to glucose fructose, can also sometimes be used as a partial replacement for sucrose
	Lactose	• Induces the activity of β-galactosidase enzyme. • Plant cells have been shown to become adapted.
Nonreducing sugar	Sucrose	• Inhibits chlorophyll formation and photosynthesis. • Supports cell division and tracheid formation. • Acts as an osmolyte during protoplast isolation. • Differentiation of floral buds. • Effective translocation of sucrose to apical meristems from isolated roots.
	Raffinose	• Some plant cells have been shown to become adapted.
	Trehalose	• Broken down to glucose fructose, can also sometimes be used as a partial replacement for sucrose
Slow reducing sugar	Arabinose	• Broken down to glucose fructose, can also sometimes be used as a partial replacement for sucrose
	Ribose	• Broken down to glucose fructose, can also sometimes be used as a partial replacement for sucrose
	Xylose	• Broken down to glucose fructose, can also sometimes be used as a partial replacement for sucrose

Aforementioned uses are collected from different reports [281]. They are not universal; each sugar utilization varies according to varieties, genus, species, and environment of the plant.

TABLE 2.13 Different Roles of Vitamins in Growth and Development of Plant Cell

Name	Role of vitamins in growth of plant cell
Myoinositol	<ul><li>This is a plant vitamin, but sometimes related to supplementary carbohydrate as it does not have actions like carbohydrate (energy source or as an osmoticum). Presence of six hydroxyl group makes it more reactive against various acids to form esters.</li><li>Effect of myoinositol was first shown by Jacquiot in bud formation [238].</li><li>Pollard et al. reported that growth promoting property of coconut milk is due to presence of *myo*inositol content. He also founded that it contains an additional vitamin called *scyllo*-inositol [239].</li><li>In media when it is supplemented against inositol it can promote tissue growth [240].</li><li>It acts by being involved in biosynthetic pathways to form pectin, and hemicellulose is essentially required in cell walls and hence promotes growth [241].</li><li>Plays an important role in the uptake and utilization of ions [242]. It has the capability to promote cell division alone and sometimes with other hormones [243].</li></ul>
Thiamine	<ul><li>This is one of the most frequently utilized vitamins, which are supplemented to media in the form of thiamine pyrophosphate.</li><li>It is an essential cofactor in carbohydrate metabolism and is directly involved in the biosynthesis of some amino acids.</li><li>MS medium contains a low concentration 0.3 μM thiamine. This concentration may not be sufficient to obtain the desirable results [244].</li><li>There can be an interaction between thiamine and cytokinin growth regulators, which may affect the growth of the plant.</li><li>More often its supplementation (post-, pre-, or during the different development stages) finally decides its action against growth of plant cell [245].</li></ul>
Vitamin C	<ul><li>This is also used during explant isolation and to prevent blackening.</li><li>Powerful antioxidant.</li><li>Induces cell division and elongation [246].</li><li>Enhances shoot formations and reverses the inhibition of shoot formation by gibberellic acid in young callus (less effective in old callus).</li></ul>
Vitamin E	<ul><li>α-Tocopherol has a strong antioxidant activity potential and plays a vital role in plant cell growth and development.</li></ul>
Adenine	<ul><li>Adenine sulfate is widely used in tissue culture media, but its effects are quite similar to those produced by cytokinins, which hinders its utilization.</li></ul>
Riboflavin	<ul><li>This inhibits the callus formation but may improve the growth and quality of shoots [247].</li></ul>
Pantothenic acid	<ul><li>Drastic variation in its potential in influencing plant growth has been seen. In some plants it shows growth whereas in others it does not induce any effect.</li></ul>

2.3.3.4 *Plant Growth Regulators (PGRs)*

Plant growth regulators stimulate cell division and hence regulate the growth and differentiation of shoots and roots on explants and embryos in semisolid or in liquid medium cultures. In 1957, Skoog and Miller showed that the developmental fate of regenerating tobacco pith tissue in culture could be directed by the plant hormones cytokinin and auxin. High concentrations of cytokinin relative to auxin-produced shoots while roots were formed when the ratios were reversed. Callus formed at hormone concentrations that were optimal

TABLE 2.14   Organic Supplements of Plant Tissue Culture Media from Natural Sources

Type	Features
COMPLEX ORGANICS	
Coconut water	• This is a colorless liquid endosperm of green coconut (*Cocos nucifera*), whereas coconut milk is the extract of white, solid endosperm of matured coconut. Both are used in tissue culture media, but coconut water is a more complex combination of various compounds.
	• It was first used in tissue cultures by Van Overbeek et al. [248] He found that the addition of coconut milk to a culture medium was necessary for the development of very young embryos of *Datura stramonium*.
	• This complex water mixture is an active source of several amino acids, organic acids, plant growth regulators (cytokinins and auxins), vitamins, sugar, minerals, nucleic acids, and unidentified growth substances, which are collectively responsible for growth and development of the tissue *in vitro* conditions.
	• This liquid has been found to be beneficial for inducing growth of callus and suspension culture and for the induction of morphogenesis.
	• It is commonly used in orchid tissue culture.
	• Unlike others it is very difficult to replace by fully defined media. It covers the action of both auxin and cytokinins.
	• It was reported that its auxin-like activity is increased by autoclaving, because any such growth substances exist in a complex form and are released by hydrolysis.
	• In comparison to auxin, GAs, and ABA it contains large amounts of natural cytokinins.
Yeast extract	• Used less as an ingredient in plant tissue culture media than previously. In earlier times it was treated as an active source of amino acids and vitamins [249,250].
	• It was only used where vitamins and amino acids are in either low concentration or absent.
	• White established the first culture medium containing yeast extract and only macro- and micronutrients [107]. It was later discovered that amino acids such as glycine, lysine, and arginine, and vitamins such as thiamine and nicotinic acid, could serve as replacements for yeast extract [251].
	• Yeast extract has been recently introduced under biotic elicitor classification since it has the ability to stimulate the defense mechanism, which leads to increased secondary metabolite production [252].
	• But yeast extract has shown to have some serious unusual effects such as accumulation of phytoalexins in media and induced direct formation of adventitious embryo. This may be due to the concentration and composition of amino acids present in yeast extract.
Malt extract	• Acts as a source of carbohydrates but no longer commonly used except for certain species of citrus [253,254].
	• Shown to induce embryogenesis in citrus plants [255].
	• Some plant hormones such as auxins and gibberellins have been identified in malt extract [256].
	• Malt extract also promoted the germination of early cotyledonary stage embryos arising from the *in vitro* rescue of zygotic embryos of sour orange [257].
Potato extract	• Contains carbohydrates, vitamins (C, B_1, B_6), amino acids, and mineral elements (potassium, iron, magnesium).
	• Useful medium for anther culture of wheat and some other cereal plants.
	• Potato extract alone or combined with components of conventional culture media has since been found to provide a useful medium for the anther culture of wheat and some other cereal plants [258].
	• In some reports its utilization for orchid propagation is also promoted.

(Continued)

TABLE 2.14 Organic Supplements of Plant Tissue Culture Media from Natural Sources *(cont.)*

Type	Features
Banana homogenate	• Contains cytokinins and several other substances as found in other natural sources. • The reason for its stimulatory effect is unknown, but some reports consider its pH stabilizing property as a cause behind its stimulatory effect. • It is widely used for orchid cultures. • It has been also found that utilization of banana homogenate manifests cytokinin compounds in media [259].
Casein hydrolysate	• It is a complex mixture of 18 amino acids, vitamins, calcium, phosphate, and several microelements [260]. • The proportion of amino acid depends on the source protein composition from which it is prepared. • More effective for plant tissue culture than the addition of major amino acids. • The best quality of casein hydrolysate can be examined by content of reduced glutamine in extract.
Algal extract	• Micro- and macroalgae are found to be an active source of phytohormones [261,262]. • Widely used in *in vitro* cultivation of higher plants such as pea, tobacco, and beet. • Gives brown, hard, and compact calli, when supplemented without any exogenous plant growth regulators. But when supplemented with exogenous substances gives white–green calli with small shoots, especially seen in pea micropropagation.
Embryo-nourishing fluids	• There are various extracts, e.g., liquid present in the embryo sac of immature fruits of *Aesculus* (e.g., *A. woerlitzensis*), that have been found to have a strong growth-promoting and nourishing effect on embryo but coconut is still acquires more significant activity than others [263].

ACTIVATED CHARCOAL

Type	Features
Activated charcoal	• Use in the promotion and inhibition of culture growth. • Stimulates growth and differentiation in orchids, carrot, ivy, and tomato, whereas it inhibits growth in tobacco, soybean, etc. • Adsorbs brown–black pigments and oxidized phenolics produced during culture and thus reduces toxicity. • Adsorbs other organic compounds like PGRs, vitamins, etc., which may cause the inhibition of culture growth. • Causes darkening of culture medium and helps root induction and growth.

for callus growth, but not for shoot or root formation. Supplementation of PGRs in various cultures leads to the expression of different genes (transcription factors) that further regulates the different development phases (regeneration of shoots, roots, or calli from root explants) in plants. This can be better explained on the basis of identifying groups of genes that serve as molecular signatures of the different developmental processes, i.e., genes that were specifically up- or downregulated on one developmental pathway. The role of cytokinin and auxin signaling to direct the course of development is still unclear in several plants. As mentioned in above (Fig. 2.5), cytokinin signal transduction involves a multicomponent phosphorelay signaling system in which sensory His kinase serves as a cytokinin receptor. The cytokinin signal is transduced to the nucleus via His phosphotransfer proteins. This signal is further transmitted to two types of gene expression regulators that finally regulate the various development processes of the plant. Therefore, once a group of such genes have been identified, vigorous efforts during optimization for different hormonal concentrations will be hopefully reduced and hence promote the specified hormones with their effective concentration to regulate the expression of genes in the development process. In 2006, Che et al. identified a transcription factor gene (RAP2.6L) that appears to be part of a network involved in regulating the expression of many other genes in shoot regeneration [234]. The four major PGRs used are auxins, cytokinins, gibberellins, and abscisic acid, and their addition is essential to the culture medium. Ethylene is also among these.

Various types of hormones and their roles are highlighted in Tables 2.15 and 2.16.

- *Auxins* induce cell division, cell elongation, apical dominance, adventitious root formation, and somatic embryogenesis. Went discovered auxin more than 70 years ago [264]. When used in low concentration, auxins induce root initiation and in high concentration act as a selective herbicide/weedkiller and in some cases callus formation may also occur. Commonly used synthetic auxins are NAA, 2,4-D, IAA, IBA, etc. Both IBA and IAA are photosensitive so the stock solutions must be stored in the dark. 2,4-D is used to induce and regulate somatic embryogenesis as well as callusing. Also 2-methoxy-3,6-dichlorobenzoic acid (Dicamba), 2,4,5-trichlorophenoxyacetic acid (2,4,5-T), 2-methyl-4-chlorophenoxyacetic acid (MCPA), 2-naphthyloxyacetic acid (NOA), and 4-amino-2,5,6-trichloropicolinic acid (Picloram) are used as auxins. Auxins are easily dissolved in either absolute alcohol or ethanol and diluted NaOH or KOH. Both natural and synthetic auxins are thermostable.
- *Cytokinins* are the derivatives of adenine, promote cell division, and stimulate initiation and growth of shoots *in vitro*. These are 4-hydroxy-3-methyl-trans-2-butenylaminopurine (Zeatin), 6-furfurylaminopurine (kinetin), 6-benzylaminopurine (BAP), N^6-(2-isopentenyl) adenine (2iP(IPA)), and 1-phenyl-3-(1,2,3-thiadiazol-5-yl) urea (thidiazuron), frequently used cytokinins. They modify apical dominance by promoting axillary shoot formation. A higher concentration of cytokinin causes inhibition of root formation and promotes adventitious shoot formation. The ratio of auxin/cytokinin plays an important role in morphogenesis. A high ratio leads to embryogenesis and root initiation whereas a low ratio leads to axillary bud and shoot proliferation, though an intermediate ratio is required for the formation of callus. Cytokinins are subdivided into two major classes: natural (*trans*-zeatin, *cis*-zeatin, iP, dihydrozeatin, and zeatin riboside) and synthetic cytokinins. Organic supplements such as yeast extract or coconut milk are the rich source of natural cytokinin. Kinetin is not acknowledged under a natural cytokinin since it is present in nature by structural rearrangement [266], therefore many natural cytokinins that are structurally related to kinetin have been identified [265,266]. Synthetic cytokinins are again subdivided into two classes: purines (N^6-substituted adenine derivatives and some other less structurally related compounds such as 4-alkylaminopteridines and 6-benzyloxypurines) and phenylureas analogs (1,3-diphenylurea and thidiazuron). Some of these purine analogs are more active than kinetin or benzyladenine (BA), and are particularly effective in promoting morphogenesis.
- *Gibberellins*: Gibberellins are numerous, naturally occurring, structurally related compounds that are normally used in plant regeneration. Only a few gibberellins are used in the plant tissue culture media. Water soluble and thermo-unstable gibberellic acid (GA$_3$) is mostly used for internode elongation and meristem growth, and usually inhibits

TABLE 2.15   List of Plant Growth Hormones and Their Functions

PGR	Product name	Function in plant tissue culture

Ax	Indole-3-acetic acid
	Indole-3-butyric acid
	Indole-3-butyric acid, potassium salt
	α-Naphthaleneacetic acid
	2,4-Dichlorophenoxyacetic acid
	p-Chlorophenoxyacetic acid
	  • Picloram
	  • Dicamba
		• Adventitious root formation (high conc.)
		• Adventitious shoot formation (low conc.)
		• Induction of somatic embryos
		• Cell division
		• Callus formation and growth
		• Inhibition of axillary buds
		• Inhibition of root elongation

Cy	6-Benzylaminopurine
	6-γ,γ-Dimethylallylaminopurine (2iP)
	Kinetin
	Thidiazuron (TDZ)
	N-(2-chloro-4-pyridyl)-N′phenylurea
	  • Zeatin
	  • Zeatin riboside
		• Adventitious shoot formation
		• Inhibition of root formation
		• Promotes cell division
		• Modulates callus initiation and growth
		• Stimulation of axillary bud breaking and growth
		• Inhibition of shoot elongation
		• Inhibition of leaf senescence

GA	• Gibberellic acid	• Stimulates shoot elongation • Releases seeds, embryos, and apical buds from dormancy • Inhibits adventitious root formation • Paclobutrazol and ancymidol inhibit gibberellin synthesis, thus resulting in shorter shoots, and promoting tuber, corm, and bulb formation.
AA	• Abscisic acid	• Stimulates bulb and tuber formation • Stimulates the maturation of embryos • Promotes the start of dormancy
PA	• Putrescine • Spermidine • Spermine	• Promotes adventitious root formation • Promotes somatic embryogenesis • Promotes shoot formation
Et	• Ethylene	• Leaves senescence • Induction of adventitious roots and root hairs • Breaking of seed and bud dormancy in some species • Promotion or inhibition of adventitious regeneration
JA	• Jasmonic acid	• Promotion of tuber and bulb formation • Enhancement of meristem formation (tissue differentiation) • Stimulation of root formation • Promotion of pigment formation • Promotion of tissue differentiation
SA	• Salicylic acid	• Inhibition of seed germination • Induction of flowering • Promotion of bud formation • Blocking of wound response
BA	• Brassinosteriods	• Promotion of germination • Inhibition of root growth and development • Promotion of shoot elongation • Inhibition of root growth and development • Enhancement of xylem differentiation

Ax, auxins; Cy, cytokinin; GA, gibberellic acid; AA, abscisic acid; PA, polyamines; Et, ethylene; JA, jasmonic acid; SA, salicylic acid; BA, brassinosteroids.

TABLE 2.16 Recent List of Plant Growth Stimulators and Inhibitors

Plant growth regulators	
Auxins	4-CPA, 2,4-D, 2,4-DB, 2,4-DEP, dichlorpropfenoprop, IAA, IBA, naphthaleneacetamide, α-naphthaleneacetic acids, 1-naphthol, naphthoxyacetic acids, potassium naphthenate, sodium naphthenate, 2,4,5-T
Antiauxins	Clofibric acid, 2,3,5-tri-odobenzoic acid
Cytokinins	2iP, benzyladenine, 4-hydroxyphenethyl alcohol, kinetin, zeatin
Gibberellins	Gibberellin derivatives
Defoliants	Calcium cyanamide, dimethipin, endothal, ethephon, merphos, metoxuron pentachlorophenol, thidiazuron, tribufos
Gametocides	Fenridazon, maleic hydrazide
Ethylene inhibitors	aviglycine, 1-methyl-cyclopropene
Ethylene releasers	ACC, etacelasil, ethephon, glyoxime
Gametocides	Fenridazon, maleic hydrazide
Growth inhibitors	Abscisic acid, ancymidol, butralin, carbaryl, chlorphonium, chlorpropham dikegulac, flumetralin, fluoridamid, fosamine, glyphosine, isopyrimol, jasmonic acid, maleic hydrazide, mepiquat, piproctanyl, prohydrojasmon, propham, tiaojiean, 2,3,5-tri-iodobenzoic acid, morphactins (chlorfluren, chlorflurenol, dichlorflurenol, flurenol)
Growth retardants	Chlormequat, daminozide, flurprimidol, mefluidide, paclobutrazol, tetcyclacis, uniconazole
Growth stimulators	Brassinolide, brassinolide-ethyl, DCPTA, forchlorfenuron, hymexazol, prosuler, pyripropanol, triacontanol
Unclassified plant growth regulators	Bachmedesh, benzofluor, buminafos, carvone, choline chloride, ciobutide, clofencet, cloxyfonac, cyanamide, cyclanilide, cycloheximide, cyprosulfamide, epocholeone, ethychlozate, ethylene, fuphenthiourea, furalane, heptopargil, holosulf, inabenfide, karetazan, lead arsenate, methasulfocarb, prohexadione, pydanon, sintofen, triapenthenol, trinexapac

adventitious shoot formation. Their inhibitory action is found during organogenesis and dedifferentiation of tissue.

• *Abscisic acid* (ABA) is used only for somatic embryogenesis and for culturing woody species. It inhibits cell division and has a favorable effect on abscission. ABA is soluble in water and thermostable in nature but sensitivity against light often limits its application.

• *Ethylene* is a naturally occurring PGR, which occurs in a gaseous state and is most commonly associated with controlling fruit ripening in climacteric fruits. Its production in some plant cell cultures often inhibits the growth and development of the culture. For its utilization in the gaseous state, 2-chloroethane phosphoric acid powder is added in the medium to liberate ethylene.

2.3.3.5 Solidifying Agents

Solidifying agents are used for preparing semisolid tissue culture media to enable explant to be placed on culture media (slightly embedded) to provide sufficient aeration. Agar is a high molecular weight polysaccharide obtained from seaweeds and can easily bind with water. Its binding with water increases with concentration. However, *in vitro* growth may be adversely affected if the agar concentration is too high. At higher concentrations agar medium becomes hard and does not allow the diffusion of nutrients into the tissues. It is added to the medium in concentrations ranging from 0.5%–1% (6–8 g/L). Agar is preferred over other gelling agents such as agarose and phytagel because it is inert; it neither reacts with media constituents nor is digested by plant enzymes. Difco Bacto agar is often used by plant tissue culturists at a concentration of 0.6–1.0% (w/v). A purified extract of agar called agarose is used for protoplast culture. Other gelling products such as Gelrite at 0.2% (in the presence of divalent cations) form clear gels (unlike agar which is translucent) and hence it is easier to detect contamination, which might develop during culture growth. At higher concentrations (10%), gelatin was also experimented with, but has limited use since it melts at low temperature (25°C). Without using any gelling agent mechanical support for cell or tissue growth can also be provided by glass beads, a filter paper bridge, perforated cellophane, polyurethane foam, sponge underneath filter paper, etc.

2.3.3.6 *pH*

It is the negative logarithm of hydrogen ion activity that affects the absorption of ions and solidification of culture media. Optimum pH for culture media is 5.6–5.8 before sterilization. The values of pH lower than 4.5 or higher than 7.0 greatly inhibit growth and development of tissue *in vitro*. The pH of culture media generally drops by 0.3–0.5 units after autoclaving and keeps changing through the incubation of culture due to oxidation as well as differential uptake and secretion of substances by the cultured tissue. If the pH drops appreciably during plant tissue culture (pH below 5.0 it does not allow gelling of the agar and the medium becomes liquid), then a fresh medium should be prepared, whereas a pH greater than 6.0 gives hard medium (interferes with the absorption of nutrients). It is well established that pH of the medium affects the gelling efficiency of agar, uptake of ingredients, solubility of different salts, and chemical reactions (especially those catalyzed by enzymes) in the medium.

2.4 SELECTION OF A SUITABLE NEW MEDIUM

Selection of the new or already established medium for new explants (new species or varieties) requires a great deal of optimization to establish its *in vitro* cell line. Not all cells in explants contribute to the formation of callus and not all plants easily form cell lines *in vitro*. Therefore, media optimization is essential for those plants that are difficult to grow under *in-situ* and *ex-situ* conditions. Since there is no ideal approach that benefits the media easily for unexplored explants (of new genotypes), a lot of strategies can be employed to evaluate the nutritional requirement of newly found plant, which can be later manipulated for further research (Fig. 2.15).

2.5 PREPARATION OF MEDIA

Plant tissue culture chemicals used for preparing media should be free from impurities and all are of research grade (analytical grade). Media preparation is a very crucial step to induce desirable features or to check the growth and development of the selected tissue. Stock solution preparation is the initial step, which is followed by media preparation as mentioned in Fig. 2.16. According to the nature of cells or tissues, standard composition of media should

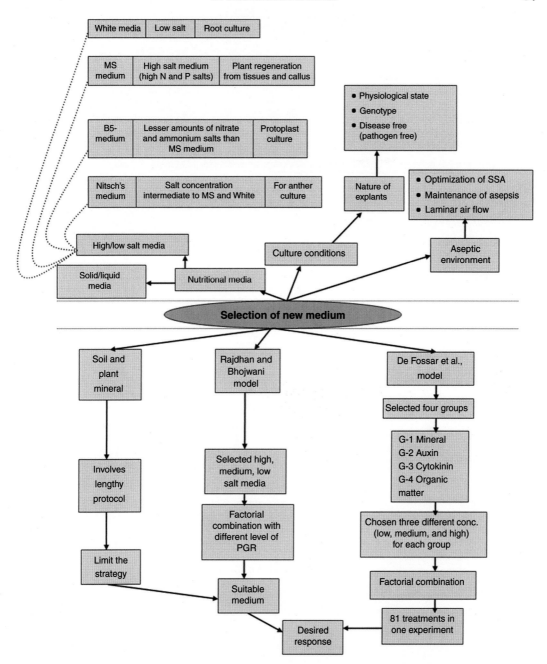

FIGURE 2.15 Strategies for the selection of the medium. These are based on the complete soil or plant organic and inorganic components analysis, which is limited now days. Other approaches suggested by Bhojwani and Razdan and De Fossard et al. can prove to be a solution [267]. Nature of explants, medium, and aseptic conditions also assist in selection of suitable media.

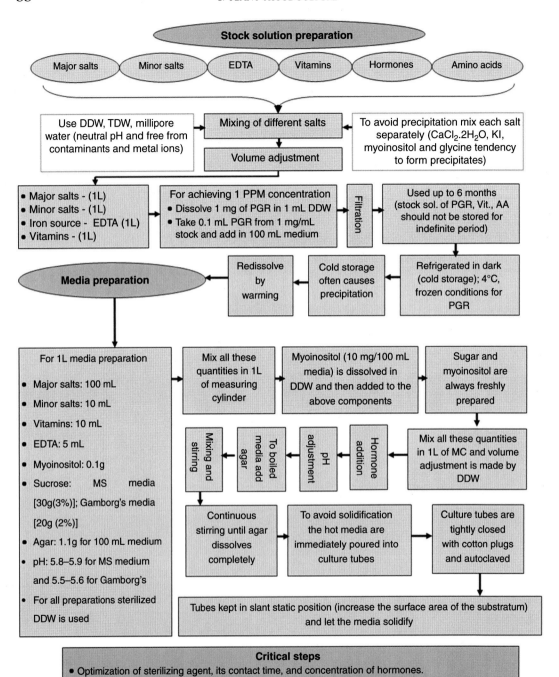

FIGURE 2.16 Steps involved in media preparation. First step involved is stock solution preparation and second is media preparation.

be used for their desirable growth and development, which can be further optimized for obtaining better results.

2.6 CALLUS INDUCTION, SUBCULTURE, AND MAINTENANCE

Different steps involved in callus growth and development are highlighted in Fig. 2.14.

2.6.1 Selection of Plant Material

Cultivar is selected and explant is separated. A tip of the shoot meristem is normally taken as explant.

2.6.2 Surface Sterilization of Explants

In surface sterilization all explants are treated with an appropriate agent to kill contaminating microbes present on their surface. The surface sterilization procedure will depend mainly on the source and type of the explants, which will determine the contamination load and tolerance to the sterilizing agent. The common sterilizing agents used for surface sterilization are found in Table 2.17. Among these, calcium or sodium hypochlorite and mercuric chloride are the most commonly used reagents showing satisfactory results. The period of treatment varies from 5 to 30 min. As these agents are also toxic to plant tissues, the time and concentration used should be such that it causes minimum tissue damage. The basic protocol generally used for surface sterilization is shown in Fig 2.17.

2.6.3 Preparation of Explants

For initiation of callus, disinfected explants were prepared as illustrated in Fig. 2.17.

TABLE 2.17 Chemicals Used for the Surface Sterilization of Explants

Disinfectant	Concentration	Exposure period
Benzalkonium chloride	0.01–0.1%	5–20 min
Sodium hypochlorite	0.5–5%	5–30 min
Silver nitrate	1%	5–30 min
Mercuric chloride	0.1–1.0%	2–10 min
Hydrogen peroxide	3–12%	5–15 min
Ethyl alcohol	75–95%	30–60 s
Calcium hypochlorite	9–10%	3–30 min
Bromine water	1–2%	2–10 min

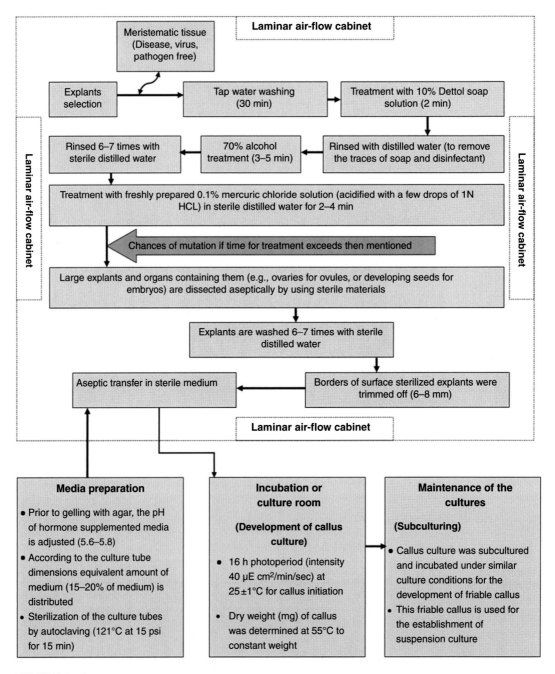

FIGURE 2.17   Protocol for surface sterilization of explants.

2.6.4 Media Preparation and its Inoculation

This was mentioned in Section 2.6.3 (Figs 2.16 and 2.17).

2.6.5 Incubation of Cultures

The inoculated cultures are transferred to another room called the culture room, where light and temperature are strictly controlled.

2.6.6 Subculture

For maintenance, the developed callus can be cut into segments and subcultured (Fig. 2.17).

2.7 OPTIMIZATION OF MEDIA

Most of the potential applications of plant tissue culture are dependent on its growth, which can be regulated and controlled by the composition of culture media. The plant tissue culture medium can be easily manipulated by changing the type and quantity of ingredients used. However, this is not particularly easy as this process involves manipulation of various chemical and physical factors. Optimization strategies usually vary according to the type of culture and growth levels. It can be different for basal medium first generation, second generation, callus induction, suspension culture, organogenesis, embryogenesis, and nature of explants, and different according to other objective set during experimentation. One of the primary objectives of optimization is to increase the accumulation of secondary metabolites and other products at higher levels than those in native plants. This is achieved by manipulation of physical factors and nutritional elements in a culture medium. Rosmarinic acid by *Coleus blumei*, ubiquinone-10 by *Nicotiana tabacum*, ginsenosides by *Panax ginseng*, berberin by *Coptis japonica*, and shikonin by *Lithospermum erythrorhizon* are the most cited examples where accumulation of these products in cultured cells was found to be higher than in intact plants. Development of optimized media for various species and applications requires a number of different laborious and time-consuming approaches. Identification of those factors that may directly or indirectly influence the growth and development of cultured tissue is a very complex task. The following approaches are designed to reduce the workload during this process.

2.7.1 Soil and Plant Mineral Analysis for Evaluating the Essential Minerals in Inert Growth Medium [268–270]

Soil and plant analysis gives a brief idea regarding the primary and secondary nutritional requirements of plant tissue cultures, which further helps in determining the uptake as well as the optimum concentration. The study related to plant requirements for macro- and micronutrients is based on two basic principles. First, evaluation of those parameters that affect the uptake process of nutrients and their optimum concentration in the soil helps in deciding the basic needs of the respective plant. Atomic absorption spectroscopy is widely used for this purpose. Media can be easily designed after the confirmation of macro and micronutrients in plants. The second aspect is the variation in soil conditions even in the same cultivation area, which causes changes in nutrient absorption capacity and further affects optimal soil concentration, causing a problem in evaluating the essential minerals of the plants. Disturbances in pH, temperature, porosity of the soil, and other factors sometimes causes imbalance between the nutrients and their uptake rate. Some plants adapt to this variation but some do not survive. Thus, it is difficult to identify those factors that lead to change in soil mineral composition. Furthermore, interaction between the nutrients causes a great problem in evaluating the optimized concentration of each component. Therefore, designing of new inert material (quartz sand) that shows no reactions with nutrients at controlled optimal environmental conditions (moisture, temperature, light) can be a good approach.

2.7.2 Interactions Among Mineral Nutrients [270–274]

Under the influence of several biotic and abiotic stresses, minerals show interaction in the growth medium as well as within plant tissues, which can lead to synergism and antagonism. These effects sometime cause deficiency or toxicity of particular minerals, resulting in decrease in plant growth and crop yield. Replacement of the toxic concentration of minerals or any complexes with nontoxic elements is known to be a better approach. Normally, there are three steps for grading the concentration in plants: (i) at optimal level; (ii) at drastic deficiency; and (iii) at high toxicity. After evaluation of these concentrations, toxic concentrations can be easily be displaced with optimized concentration to eliminate the negative effect of toxic contents of nutrients in substrate on plant biomass production. The negative effect of higher levels of P, Cu, Zn, and Mn could be considerably diminished by increasing the levels of Ca, Mg, and Fe, as well as N, P, K, Zn, Co, Mo, and B in substrate.

2.7.3 Effect of Physical and Chemical Properties of Soil on Nutrient Accumulation in Plants [269,270]

The physical and chemical properties of soil significantly affect the availability of nutrients. It was found that soil texture, pH level, organic matter, carbonate, and oxides of iron and aluminum are important parameters that should be considered during the optimization of nutrient medium for plants (e.g., increased organic matter content in the substrate clearly reduced nutrient availability to plants).

2.7.4 Complex Method for Optimization of Mineral Nutrition [270,272,274]

Development of optimized mineral composition for plants is a very tedious and time-consuming task, though some preliminary exercise reduces the efforts in optimizing suitable culture medium for elite and extinct species. For the development of any nutritional medium, two important facts should be considered. First is a stable and balanced mineral nutrition regimen and second is maintaining the conditions necessary for optimal plant mineral nutrition. To achieve this set of objectives Rinkis et al. (1989) developed a scheme of a complex method for optimization of plant mineral nutrition (Fig. 2.18).

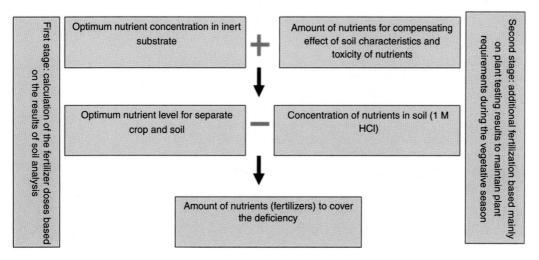

FIGURE 2.18   Illustration of complex method for optimization of plant mineral nutrition [273,274].

2.7.5 Neurofuzzy Logic Technology

Neurofuzzy logic is a hybrid technology and combines the adaptive learning capabilities from artificial neural networks with the generality of representation from fuzzy logic through simple rules. Hildebrandt et al., 1946 [275]

The nonlinear and time variant nature of all biological processes increases their complexity, which can be understood by the evaluation of external factors that influence its elemental composition. Evaluation of one external factor is not sufficient to provide entire knowledge of the whole process, such as growth parameters at whole plant level. In plant tissue culture, practice, media designing, optimization, and development are the most laborious and time consuming. This can be explained on the basis of earlier suggestions, for example:

- More than 16,000 cultures of tobacco were required to design Hildebrandt's medium [275].
- A broad spectrum of 43 factorial designs with 81 combinations for tobacco was employed by De Fossard et al. [267].
- To finish their design of MS medium, Murashige and Skoog spent 5 years [205].
- In last 70–80 years thousands of articles have described over 2000 different culture media in plant tissue culture [276].

Optimization of *in vitro* conditions provides the best survival conditions to the transferred healthy explants. However, in some cases the best *in vitro* conditions do not provide optimal *ex vitro* results. Therefore, a better understanding can be established by optimizing variables that are involved during *in vitro* growth and linking them with *ex vitro* acclimatization results, which may result in improvement of the process (Fig. 2.19). Recently, large and complex factorial designs have been employed in plant tissue culture. Several studies have also demonstrated the effectiveness of computational techniques like artificial neural networks (ANNs) and neurofuzzy logic in studying different plant tissue culture processes [277,278]. Gago et al. in 2011 introduced neurofuzzy logic technology to reduce different laborious and time-consuming approaches in development of optimized media in plant tissue culture science [278]. Neurofuzzy

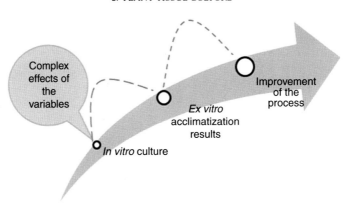

FIGURE 2.19   Strategy used in neurofuzzy logic technology to draw the relationship between different variables in growth phase with *ex vitro* acclimatization results in plant tissue culture.

logic technology draws a perfect connection between various factors affecting plant growth and soil mineral composition. This is achieved by extracting biologically useful information from each database and then combining them to create significant models. It is promoted nowadays to evaluate the effect and importance of plant tissue media composition in plant growth. Neurofuzzy logic alone is not sufficient for analyzing complex multivariate datasets in biological processes, therefore its combination with an additional soft-computing technique (artificial neural networks) appears to be quite fruitful in addressing complex analyses in biological studies. Artificial neural networks (ANNs) are mathematical tools useful for modeling nonlinear relationships between variables. Compared to old statistics, ANNs have shown higher accuracy in prediction, as pointed out in several plant science papers [279]. A combination of ANNs and fuzzy logic technology (neurofuzzy logic) can be applied to model complex multivariate datasets in order to find the best combination of factors, which allows the handling of large databases and increases knowledge about the factors that potentially affect any responses in data mining. This has recently been reported for apricot [277] and the *in vitro* culture of grapevine [280]. Neurofuzzy logic generates understandable and reusable knowledge that helps in understanding the cause/effect relationships and present results in the form of linguistic terms [278].

2.8 MAINTENANCE OF CULTURES CELL LINES

Explant selection and sterilization, medium selection, and optimization and callus induction are the most important steps used for establishing the callus culture. Maintenance of callus culture is required for attaining successful growth of the plant cell. During the maintenance phase the obtained callus is subcultured and maintained for short and long periods. As mentioned in Fig. 2.20, the subculturing period depends on various factors. It is widely known that callus acquires unexpected growth patterns, i.e., certain cultures are maintained for a short period (having poor regeneration power) whereas some cultures can be maintained for several decades (retaining their regeneration power for longer periods). The future of these cultures can be defined by their regeneration potential, genotype variation, and chances of occurrence of various technical problems (hyperhydricity). In addition, growth factors like cell count, cell density, cell viability, and pack cell volume evaluation ensure the future life of transferred explants. The scope of regeneration is mainly examined by evaluating cell viability. Primary culture is required to be subcultured when cell density increases and large amounts of medium are consumed. These types of heterogeneous primary cultures contain many types of cells (derived from the original tissue) that form homogeneous cell lines during subculturing. Such homogeneous cells are now called cell line and can be propagated, characterized, and stored for their further usage. If most of the cells of the cell line exhibit a specific property or function then they are called cell strain. A cell line or cell strain may be finite or continuous. Finite cell lines grow up to 20–80 population doublings before extinction. After maintaining the cell line, hormones are supplemented to direct further growth. These steps are also demonstrated in Fig. 2.20.

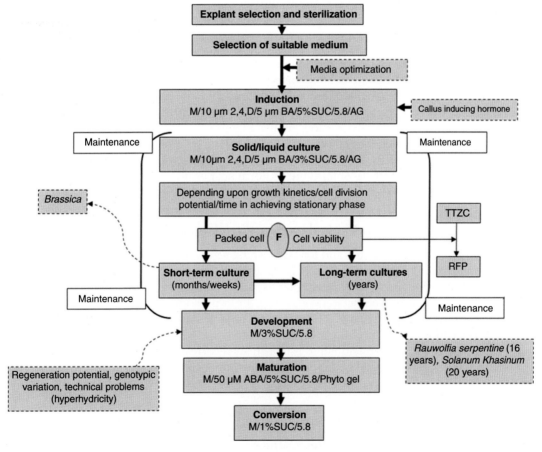

FIGURE 2.20 **Representation of sequential protocols (induction, maintenance, development, maturation, conversion) carried out in plant tissue culture.** M, medium; BA, N6-benzyladenine; 2,4-D, 2,4-dichlorophenoxyacetic acid; ABA, abscisic acid; PDT, partial drying treatment; RFP, red formazin precipitate; TTZC, 2,3,5-triphenyltetrazolium chloride; SUC, sucrose; AG, agar; F, growth parameters factors.

2.9 ASSESSMENT OF THEIR GROWTH PARAMETERS

Assessment of growth parameters in the different types of cultures plays an important role in evaluating the growth kinetics of plant cell and tissue culture. The growth measurements of most common *in vitro* systems, i.e., callus and cell suspension cultures, are focused on in this section.

2.9.1 Callus Cultures

Callus culture is the most essential step to initiate an *in vitro* culture and requires optimum supply of nutrients for their sufficient growth. However, slow growth rate and high biochemical variability hinder its utilization in plant tissue culture. Therefore, media optimization is an essential parameter to evaluate the effect of different media components on the growth rate of the tissue. Parameters like growth index, fresh weight, and dry weight are frequently used to determine the growth of the callus cultures.

2.9.2 Suspension Cultures

Free cell adhesion (large clumps formation) and failure of the cell to separate after division are the most common problems seen in suspension culture. However, accessibility of friable callus tissue (easily disaggregated into single cells and small clusters) can successfully assist in establishing the cell suspension cultures. Fast growth of segregated cells is due to the availability of the nutrition from all directions, which makes it more suitable for biochemical studies. Adhesiveness between the cells can also be overcome by modification in culture medium at late lag phase of growth. Furthermore, enzymatic degradation and sieving are the most frequently utilized methods to obtain fine uniform suspensions of free cells. However, once established it has the propensity to revert to a clumped state condition again.

2.9.3 Growth Evaluation Methods for *In Vitro* Cultures

For evaluating growth kinetics and for establishing a good linear correlation with dry weight data, several parameters (mentioned later in the chapter) are assessed at different stages for the different cultures derived from different plant species. During the growth cycle these cultures usually go through a marked heterogeneity in cell morphology or high degree of aggregation or cell lysis at the stationary phase, which causes a great disturbance in this correlation. Parameters like cell counting and turbidity give a good correlation with the dry-cell weight parameter, whereas DNA, RNA, and protein fail to establish such correlation with the dry weight, which results in wide variations. Cell counting is the most time-consuming, complicated, and long-standing method but still represents the best way to assess culture growth in suspension cultures.

2.9.4 Measurement of Growth in Callus and Suspension Culture

2.9.4.1 Measuring Growth in Callus Cultures

The growth index of the callus culture is measured by fresh and dry weight measurement. For the fresh weight measurements harvested tissue is carefully weighed on the balance to avoid tissue desiccation. Whereas for dry weight measurement tissue is either lyophilized or dried (microwave oven drying, 60°C) until the constant weight is not achieved.

2.9.4.2 *Measuring Growth in Cell Suspension Cultures*

- *Fresh cell weight and dry cell weight*: This is a more precise measurement of cell growth than the sole culture volume; however, both require the manipulation of samples in nonsterile conditions.
- *Settled cell volume (SCV) and packed cell volume (PCV)*: SCV is the percentage of the total volume of suspension occupied by the cell mass, whereas in PCV total volume of suspension occupied by the cell mass after compacting the suspension by centrifugation.
- *Cell number/mL of media*: Cell counting is done by pipetting 1 mL of the suspension culture and counting the total number of cells under the microscope (cell counting chamber).
- *Culture cell density*: This is estimated after the complete disaggregation of the cell, which can be achieved by incubating them with an 8% chromium trioxide solution, or with hydrolytic enzymes, such as cellulase and pectinase. Chromium trioxide hinders the estimation of cell viability; however, careful use of enzymes maintains cell viability.
- *Protein and/or DNA content*: Ethidium bromide or propidium cell staining is used for such determination. Stained cells in excited state cells emit reddish orange fluorescence.
- *Medium conductivity*: This represents the ionic concentration (uptake of ions by the cells) of the culture medium and decreases inversely to biomass gain. By application of an electromagnetic field an electroporator is used to determine medium conductivity.
- *Oxygen and mass transfers*: Factors like viscosity, density, cell buoyancy, and aggregation directly affect the solubility of oxygen and mass transfers.
- *Cell viability*: A staining reagent, fluorescein diacetate, is widely used to check cell viability.
- *Osmolarity*: Osmotic pressure and ionic strength of culture medium influence the membrane transport pH, extracellular enzymes, and secondary metabolite production.

2.9.4.3 *Evaluation of Growth Efficiency*

2.9.4.3.1 GROWTH INDEX (GI)

Growth index is calculated by the ratio of the total mass transferred and final volume accumulated during propagation of the culture. In more actual terms growth index is the measurement of the final and the initial masses at sampling time, which is represented as follows:

$$GI = \frac{F_m - I_m}{F_m}$$

where GI is growth index, and F_m and I_m represent the final and initial masses, respectively (either as fresh or dry weight).

2.9.4.3.2 SPECIFIC GROWTH RATE (S_G)

The specific growth rate period is defined as the rate of increase of biomass of a cell population per unit of biomass concentration. In the sigmoid curve it occurs between the lag and stationary phases where cell growth follows a straight-line equation as follows:

$$\ln F_m = S_g t + \ln I_m$$

$$S_g = \ln F_m - \ln I_m / t$$

where S_g is the specific growth rate, F_m is the biomass (or cell density) at time t, and I_m is the initial biomass (or cell density).

2.9.4.3.3 DOUBLING TIME (T_D)

This is the time consumed by the particular concentration of the cells to double from their initial concentration, e.g., T_D of microorganism (hours) > plant cell (days). Among all the plant tissue cultures the fastest doubling time is reported for tobacco cells (15 h). T_D is represented as follows: $T_D = \ln 2 / S_g$, where S_g represents the specific growth rate.

References

[1] Smith MK, Drew RA. Current applications of tissue culture in plant propagation and improvement. Aust J Plant Physiol 1990;17(3):267–89.
[2] Jha TB, Ghosh B. Plant tissue culture: basic and applied. Hyderabad, India: Universities Press; 2005.
[3] Chawla HS. Introduction to plant biotechnology. 3rd ed. New Delhi: Oxford & IBH Publishing Company Pvt Ltd; 2011.
[4] Kotte W. Kulturversuch isolierten Wurzelespitzen. Beitr Allg Bot 1922;2:413–34.
[5] Robbins WJ. Cultivation of excised root tips and stem tips under sterile conditions. Bot Gaz 1922;73:376–90.
[6] Cleland RE. Unlocking the mysteries of leaf primordia formation. Proc Natl Acad Sci USA 2001;98(20):10981–2.
[7] Padmanabhan D. *In vitro* culture of leaf primordia of *Phoenix silvestris* L. Naturwissenschaften 1966;53(18):483.
[8] Haight TH, Kuehnert CC. Photomorphogenesis of *Osmunda cinnamomea* cultured leaf primordial. Can J Bot 1970;48(5):911–21.
[9] Haight TH, Kuehnert CC. Developmental potentialities of leaf primordia of *Osmunda cinnamomea*. VI. The expression of P1. Can J Bot 1971;49(11):1941–5.
[10] Orkwiszewski JAJ, Poethig RS. Phase identity of the maize leaf is determined after leaf initiation. Proc Natl Acad Sci USA 2000;97(19):10631–6.
[11] Almeida MD, Almeida CVD. Somatic embryogenesis and *in vitro* plant regeneration from Pejibaye adult plant leaf primordial. Pesq Agropec Bras 2006;41(9):1449–52.
[12] Duran-Vila N, Juárez J, Arregui JM. Production of viroid-free grapevines by shoot tip culture. Am J Enol Vitic 1988;39(3):217–20.
[13] Alam I, Sharmin SA, Naher MK, Alam MJ, Anisuzzaman M, Alam MF. Elimination and detection of viruses in meristem-derived plantlets of sweetpotato as a low-cost option toward commercialization. Biotechnology 2013;3(2):153–64.
[14] Mishra SP. Plant tissue culture. New Delhi: Ane Books Pvt Ltd, 2009. p. 68–75.
[15] Einset JW. Citrus tissue culture: stimulation of fruit explant cultures with orange juice. Plant Physiol 1978;62(6):885–8.
[16] Erner Y. Partial purification of a growth factor from orange juice which affects citrus tissue culture and its replacement by citric acid. Plant Physiol 1975;56(2):279–82.
[17] Yashina S, Gubin S, Maksimovich S, Yashina A, Gakhova E, Gilichinsky D. Regeneration of whole fertile plants from 30,000-y-old fruit tissue buried in Siberian permafrost. Proc Natl Acad Sci USA 2012;109(10):4008–13.
[18] Oxelman B, Petri A, Elven R, Lazkov G. The taxonomic identity of the 30,000-y-old plant regenerated from fruit tissue buried in Siberian permafrost. Proc Natl Acad Sci USA 2012;109(41):E2735.
[19] Horta ACG, Sodek L. Free amino acid and storage protein composition of soybean fruit explants and isolated cotyledons cultured with and without methionine. Ann Bot 1997;79(5):547–52.
[20] Mosquim PR, Sodek L. Culture of soybean fruit explants: growth conditions and efficiency of nitrogen sources for reserve protein synthesis. Plant Cell Tissue Organ Cult 1991;27(1):71–6.
[21] Gülsen Y, Altman A, Goren R. Growth and development of citrus pistils and fruit explants *in vitro*. Physiol Planta 1981;53(3):295–300.
[22] Zhang DB, Wilson ZA. Stamen specification and anther development in rice. Chin Sci Bull 2009;54:2342.
[23] Hicks GS. Carpelloids on tobacco stamen primordia *in vitro*. Can J Bot 1975;53(1):77–81.
[24] Hicks GS. *In vitro* culture of stamen primordial from a male sterile tobacco. Plant Sci Lett 1977;10:257–63.
[25] Hicks GS. Feminised outgrowths of the stamen primordia of tobacco *in vitro*. Plant Sci Lett 1979;17:81–9.

[26] Lu W, Enomoto K, Fukunaga Y, Kuo C. Regeneration of tepals, stamens and ovules in explants from perianth of *Hyacinthus orientalis* L. importance of explant age and exogenous hormones. Planta 1988;175(4):478–84.

[27] Rastogi R, Sawhney VK. *In vitro* culture of stamen primordia of the normal and a male sterile stamenless-2 mutant of tomato (*Lycopersicon esculentum* Mill.). J Plant Physiol 1988;133:349–52.

[28] Noriega C, Söndahl MR. Somatic embryogenesis in hybrid tea roses. Nat Biotechnol 1991;9:991–3.

[29] Choi PS, Soh WY, Liu JR. Somatic embryogenesis and plant regeneration in cotyledonary explant cultures of Chinese cabbage. Plant Cell Tissue Organ Cult 1996;44(3):253–6.

[30] Wojciechowicz MK. Comparison of regenerative potential of petals, stamens and pistils of five Sedum species *in vitro*. Biodivers Res Conserv 2007;5(8):87–94.

[31] Alemanno L, Berthouly M, Michaux-Ferrière N. Histology of somatic embryogenesis from floral tissues cocoa. Plant Cell Tissue Organ Cult 1996;46(3):187–94.

[32] Henrickson CE. The flowering of sunflower explants in aseptic culture. Plant Physiol 1954;29(6):536–8.

[33] Levy YY, Dean C. The transition to flowering. Plant Cell 1998;10(12):1973–89.

[34] Casanova E, Trillas MI, Moysset L, Vainstein A. Influence of rol genes in floriculture. Biotechnol Adv 2005;23(1):3–39.

[35] Smulders MJM, Croes AF, Kemp A, Hese KM, Harren F, Wullems GJ. Inhibition by ethylene of auxin-promotion of flower bud formation in tobacco explants is absent in plants transformed by *Agrobacterium rhizogenes*. Plant Physiol 1991;96(4):1131–5.

[36] Aida R, Yoshida K, Kondo T, Kishimoto S, Shibata M. Copigmentation gives bluer flowers on transgenic torenia plants with the antisense dihydroflavonol-4-reductase gene. Plant Sci 2000;160(1):49–56.

[37] Sato M, Kawabe T, Hosokawa M, Tatsuzawa F, Doi M. Tissue culture-induced flower-color changes in Saintpaulia caused by excision of the transposon inserted in the flavonoid 3′5′ hydroxylase (F3′5′H) promoter. Plant Cell Rep 2011;30(5):929–39.

[38] Shu H, Xu L, Li Z, Li J, Jin Z, Chang S. Tobacco arabinogalactan protein NtEPc can promote banana (Musa AAA) somatic embryogenesis. Appl Biochem Biotechnol 2014;174:2818–26.

[39] Danilevskaya ON, Meng X, McGonigle B, Muszynski MG. Beyond flowering time: pleiotropic function of the maize flowering hormone florigen. Plant Signal Behav 2011;6(9):1267–70.

[40] Wang G, Xu Z, Chia TF, Chua NH. *In vitro* flowering of *Dendrobium candidum*. Sci China C Life Sci 1997;40(1):35–42.

[41] Peeters AJM, Gerards W, Barendse GWM, Wullems GJ. *In vitro* flower bud formation in tobacco: interaction of hormones. Plant Physiol 1991;97(1):402–8.

[42] Van der Krieken WM, Croes AF, Smulders MJ, Wullems GJ. Cytokinins and flower bud formation *in vitro* in tobacco: role of the metabolites. Plant Physiol 1990;92(3):565–9.

[43] Sim GE, Goh CJ, Loh CS. Induction of *in vitro* flowering in *Dendrobium madame* Thong-In (Orchidaceae) seedlings is associated with increase in endogenous N(6)-(Delta (2)-isopentenyl)-adenine (iP) and N (6)-(Delta (2)-isopentenyl)-adenosine (iPA) levels. Plant Cell Rep 2008;27(8):1281–9.

[44] Le QL, Nguyen QH, Nagasawa N, Kume T, Yoshii F, Nakanishi TM. Biological effect of radiation-degraded alginate on flower plants in tissue culture. Biotechnol Appl Biochem 2003;38:283–8.

[45] Nhut DT, Hai NT, Thu PT, Thi NN, Hien TT, Tuan TT, et al. Protocol for inducing flower color somaclonal variation in Torenia (*Torenia fournieri* Lind.). Methods Mol Biol 2013;11013:455–62.

[46] Kiełkowska A, Adamus A, Baranski R. An improved protocol for carrot haploid and doubled haploid plant production using induced parthenogenesis and ovule excision *in vitro*. In Vitro Cell Dev Biol Plant 2014;50:376–83.

[47] Rajeevan MS, Lang A. Flower-bud formation in explants of photoperiodic and day-neutral Nicotiana biotypes and its bearing on the regulation of flower formation. Proc Natl Acad Sci USA 1993;90(10):4636–40.

[48] Ohtsubo N, Sasaki K, Aida R, Ryuto H, Ichida H, Hayashi Y, et al. Efficient modification of floral traits by heavy-ion beam irradiation on transgenic Torenia. Methods Mol Biol 2012;847:275–89.

[49] Nagira Y, Ikegami K, Koshiba T, Ozeki Y. Effect of ABA upon anthocyanin synthesis in regenerated Torenia shoots. J Plant Res 2006;119(2):137–44.

[50] Raman K, Greyson RI. Changes during development in the compartmentalization patterns of extractable gibberellin-like substances in "single" and "double" genotypes of *Nigella damascene*. Can J Bot 1977;55(15):2115–21.

[51] Tran TVM, Dien NT, Chlyah A. Regulation of organogenesis in small explants of superficial tissue of *Nicotiana tabacum* L. Planta 1974;119(2):149–59.

[52] Sharma V, Kamal B, Srivastava N, Dobriyal AK, Jadon VS. *In vitro* flower induction from shoots regenerated from cultured axillary buds of endangered medicinal herb *Swertia chirayita* H. Karst. Biotechnol Res Int 2014; 2014 (Article ID 264690). DOI: http://dx.doi.org/10.1155/2014/264690.

[53] Rangan TS. Ovary, ovule and nucellus culture. In: Johri BM, editor. Experimental embryology of vascular plants. Heidelberg: Springer-Verlag; 1982. 105–129.

[54] Jenson LL, Bonner J. Development of fruits from excised flowers in sterile culture. Abstr Am J Bot 1949;36:826.

[55] Nitsch JP. Growth and development *in vitro* of excised ovaries. Am J Bot 1951;38:566–77.

[56] Nitsch JP. The *in* vitro culture of flowers, fruits. In: Maheshwari, P, Ranga Swamy, NS, editors. Plant tissue, organ culture: a symposium. Delhi, India: International Society of Plant Morphologists; 1963. p. 198–214.

[57] Maheshwari N, Lal M. *In vitro* culture of ovaries of *Iberis amara* L. Nature 1958;181:631–2.

[58] Johri BM, Sehgal CB. Growth responses of ovaries of *Anethum, Foeniculum* and *Trachyspermum*. Phytomorphology 1966;16:364–78.

[59] Narayanaswamy S. Plant cell and tissue culture. New Delhi: Tata McGraw-Hill Education; 1994. 167.

[60] Chopra RN, Sabharwal PS. *In vitro* culture of ovules of *Gynandropsis* gynandra and *Impatiens* balsamina. In: Maheshwari P, Rangaswamy NS, editors. Plant tissue and organ culture:– a symposium. Delhi: International Society of Plant Morphologists; 1963. p. 255–64.

[61] Guha S, Johri BM. *In vitro* development of ovary and ovule of *Allium cepa* L. Phytomorphology 1966;16: 353–64.

[62] Maheshwari N. *In vitro* culture of excised ovules of *Papaver somniferum*. Science 1958;127(3294):342.

[63] Poddubnaya-Arnoldi VA. Study of fertilization in the living material of some angiosperms. Phytomorphology 1960;10:185–98.

[64] Joshi PC, Johri BM. *In vitro* growth of ovules of (*Gossypium hirsutum* L). Phytomorphology 1972;22:195–209.

[65] Pundir NS. Experimental embryology of *G. arboreum* L. × *G. hirsutum* L. and their reciprocal crosses. Bot Gaz 1972;133:7–26.

[66] Sauer M, Friml J. *In vitro* culture of Arabidopsis embryos within their ovules. Plant J 2004;40(5):835–43.

[67] Wang G, Feng H, Sun J, Du X. Induction of cotton ovule culture fibre branching by co-expression of cotton BTL, cotton SIM, and Arabidopsis STI genes. J Exp Bot 2013;64(14):4157–68.

[68] Doi H, Hoshi N, Yamada E, Yokoi S, Nishihara M, Hikage T, et al. Efficient haploid and doubled haploid production from unfertilized ovule culture of gentians (Gentiana spp.). Breed Sci 2013;63(4):400–6.

[69] Ramming DW, Emershad RL, Foster C. *In vitro* factors during ovule culture affect development and conversion of immature peach and nectarine embryos. HortScience 2003;38(3):424–8.

[70] Guha S, Maheshwari SC. Development of embryoids from pollen grains of Datura *in vitro*. Phytomorphology 1967;17:454–61.

[71] Ibrahim AM, Kayat FB, Hussin ZESM, Susanto D, Ariffulah M. Determination of suitable microspore stage and callus induction from anthers of Kenaf (*Hibiscus cannabinus* L.). Sci World J 2014; 2014 (Article ID 284342). DOI: http://dx.doi.org/10.1155/2014/284342.

[72] Weathers LG, Calavan EC. Nucellar embryony – a means of freeing citrus from viruses. In: Wallace JM, editor. Citrus virus diseases. Berkeley: Univeristy of California, Agricultural Science Division; 1959. p. 197–202.

[73] Button J, Kochba J. Tissue culture in the citrus industry. In: Reinert J, Bajaj YPS, editors. Applied and fundamental aspects of plant cell, tissue and organ culture. New York: Springer-Verlag; 1977.

[74] Obukosia SD, Waithaka K. Nucellar embryo culture of *Citrus sinensis* L. and *Citrus limon* L. Afr Crop Sci J 2000;8(2):109–16.

[75] Morel G, Martin C. Guerison de dahlias atteints d'ume maladie a virus. C R Acad Sci, Paris 1952;235:1324–5.

[76] Grout BW. Meristem-tip culture. Methods Mol Biol 1990;6:81–91.

[77] Grout BWW. Meristem-tip culture for propagation and virus elimination. Plant Cell Cult Prot: Methods Mol Biol 1999;111:115–25.

[78] Al-Taleb MM, Hassawi DS, Abu-Romman SM. Production of virus free potato plants using meristem culture from cultivars grown under Jordanian environment. Am Eurasian J Agric Environ Sci 2011;11(4):467–72.

[79] ten Houten JG, Quak F, van der Meer FA. Heat treatment and meristem culture for the production of virus-free plant material. Neth J Plant Pathol 1968;74(1):17–24.

[80] Bhuiyan FR. *In vitro* meristem culture and regeneration of three potato varieties of Bangladesh. Res Biotechnol 2013;4(3):29–37.

[81] Tas̗kın H, Baktemur G, Kurul M, Büyükalaca S. Use of tissue culture techniques for producing virus-free plant in garlic and their identification through real-time PCR. Sci World J 2013; 2013 (Article ID 781282). DOI: http://dx.doi.org/10.1155/2013/781282.

[82] Novák FJ, Mašková I. Apical shoot tip culture of tomato. Sci Horticult 1979;10(4):337–44.

[83] Saeed NA, Zafar Y, Malik KA. A simple procedure of Gossypium meristem shoot tip culture. Plant Cell Tissue Organ Cult 1997;51(3):201–7.

[84] Hanning E. Zur Physiologie pflanzenlicher Embryonem, I Uberdie Kultur von Cruciferen-Embryonen ausserhalb des Embryosacks. Z Bot 1904;62:45–80.

[85] Laibach F, Das. Taubwerden von Bastardsmen und die Kunstliche Aufzucht fruh absterbender Bastardembryonen. Z Bot 1925;17:417–59.

[86] Laibach F. Ectogenesis in plants. Methods and genetic possibilities of propagating embryos otherwise dying in the seed. J Hered 1929;20:201–8.

[87] Van Overbeek J, Conklin ME, Blakslee AF. Factors in coconut essential for growth and development of very young Datura embryos. Science 1941;94:350–1.

[88] Kagithoju S, Godishala V, Kairamkonda M, Nanna RS. Embryo culture is an efficient way to conserve a medicinally important endangered forest tree species *Strychnos potatorum*. J Forest Res 2013;24(2):279–83.

[89] Paramasivan P, Ching FW, Padma VV. Neferine, an alkaloid from lotus seed embryo, inhibits human lung cancer. BioFactors 2014;40(1):121–31.

[90] Sugii NC. The establishment of axenic seed and embryo cultures of endangered Hawaiian plant species: special review of disinfestation protocols. *In Vitro* Cell Dev Biol 2011;47(1):157–69.

[91] Knudson L. Nonsymbiotic germination of orchid seeds. Bot Gaz 1922;73(1):1–25.

[92] Lee YI. *In vitro* culture and germination of terrestrial Asian orchid seeds. Methods Mol Biol 2011;710:53–62.

[93] Paek KY, Hahn EJ, Park SY. Micropropagation of Phalaenopsis orchids via protocorms and protocorm-like bodies. Methods Mol Biol 2011;710:293–306.

[94] Ma SJ, Lu T, Zhang AQ, Wang Y, Zhou L. Tissue culture and rapid propogation of seeds of Uyghur traditional herbal *Capparis spinosa*. Zhong Yao Cai 2010;33(12):1833–6.

[95] Yamazaki JUN, Miyoshi K. *In vitro* asymbiotic germination of immature seed and formation of protocorm by *Cephalanthera falcata* (Orchidaceae). Ann Bot 2006;98(6):1197–206.

[96] Deb CR. Temjensangba. *In vitro* propagation of threatened terrestrial orchid, Malaxis khasiana Soland ex. Swartz through immature seed culture. Indian J Exp Biol 2006;44(9):762–6.

[97] Paul S, Kumaria S, Tandon P. An effective nutrient medium for asymbiotic seed germination and large-scale *in vitro* regeneration of *Dendrobium hookerianum*, a threatened orchid of northeast India. AoB Plants 2012; 2012:22. DOI: 10.1093/aobpla/plr032

[98] Abraham S, Augustine J, Thomas TD. Asymbiotic seed germination and *in vitro* conservation of *Coelogyne nervosa* A. Rich. An endemic orchid to Western Ghats. Physiol Mol Biol Plants 2012;18(3):245–51.

[99] Popov AS, Popova EV, Nikishina TV, Kolomeytseva GL. The development of juvenile plants of the hybrid orchid Bratonia after seed cryopreservation. Cryo Lett 2004;25(3):205–12.

[100] Szendrák E, Read PE. Asymbiotic *in vitro* propagation of temperate terrestrial orchids (orchidaceae). HortScience 1996;31(4):588.

[101] Mohanty P, Paul S, Das MC, Kumaria S, Tandon P. A simple and efficient protocol for the mass propagation of *Cymbidium mastersii*: an ornamental orchid of Northeast India. AoB Plants 2012; 2012:pls023.

[102] Lampe and Mills, 1933. Cited by LaRue CD. The growth of plant embryos in culture. Bull Torrey Bot Club 1936; 63:365–382.

[103] LaRue CD. Cultures of the endosperm of maize. Am J Bot 1949;36:798. (Abstr.).

[104] Tiku AR, Razdan MK, Raina SN. Production of triploid plants from endosperm cultures of *Phlox drummondii*. Biol Plant 2014;58(1):153–8.

[105] Sun DQ, Lu XH, Liang GL, Guo QG, Mo YW, Xie JH. Production of triploid plants of papaya by endosperm culture. Plant Cell Tissue Organ Cult 2011;104(1):23–9.

[106] Popielarska-Konieczna M, Kozieradzka-Kiszkurno M, Tuleja M, Ślesak H, Kapusta P, Marcińska I, et al. Genotype-dependent efficiency of endosperm development in culture of selected cereals: histological and ultrastructural studies. Protoplasma 2013;250(1):361–9.

[107] White PR. Potentially unlimited growth of excised tomato root tips in a liquid medium. Plant Physiol 1934;9:585–600.

[108] Stanley WM. Aucuba mosaic virus protein isolated from diseased, excised tomato roots grown *in vitro*. J Biol Chem 1938;126:125–31.

[109] Raggio M, Raggio N. A new method for the cultivation of isolated roots. Physiol Plant 1956;9(3):466–9.

[110] White PR. Vitamin B1 in the nutrition of excised tomato roots. Plant Physiol 2000;12:803–811.

[111] Lazzeri PA, Dunwell JM. Establishment of isolated root cultures of Brassica species and regeneration from cultured-root segments of *Brassica oleracea* var. italica. Ann Bot 1984;54(3):351–61.

[112] Raggio M, Raggio N, Torrey JG. The nodulation of isolated leguminous roots. Am J Bot 1957;44(4):325–34.

[113] Akashi R, Harris S, Hoffmann-Tsay SS, Hoffmann F. Plants from protoplasts isolated from a long-term root culture (super root) of *Lotus corniculatus*. J Plant Physiol 2000;157(2):215–21.

[114] Iwase A, Mitsuda N, Koyama T, Hiratsu K, Kojima M, Arai T, et al. The AP2/ERF transcription factor WIND1 controls cell dedifferentiation in *Arabidopsis*. Curr Biol 2011;21:508–14.

[115] Gautheret R. Sur la possibilité de réaliser la culture indéfinie des tissues de tubercules de carotte. C R Soc Biol Paris 1939;208:118–20.

[116] Nobécourt P. Sur la pérennité et l'augmentation de volume des cultures de tissues végétaux. C R Soc Biol Lyon 1939;130:1270–1.

[117] White PR. Potentially unlimited growth of excised plant callus in an artificial nutrient. Am J Bot 1939;26:59–64.

[118] Ball E. Differentiation in a callus culture of *Sequoia sempervirens*. Growth 1950;14(4):295–325.

[119] Tulecke W. A tissue derived from the pollen of *Ginkgo biloba*. Science (NY) 1953;117:599–600.

[120] Jablonski JR, Skoog F. Cell enlargement and cell division in excised tobacco pith tissue. Physiol Plant 1954;7: 16–24.

[121] Miller CO, Skoog F, Von Saltza MH, Strong F. Kinetin, a cell division factor from deoxyribonucleic acid. J Am Chem Soc 1955;77:1392.

[122] Miller CO, Skoog F, Okumura FS, von Saltza MH, Strong FM. Structure and synthesis of kinetin. J Am Chem Soc 1955;78:2662–3.

[123] Skoog F, Miller CO. Chemical regulation of growth and organ formation in plant tissue cultured *in vitro*. Symp Soc Exp Biol 1957;XI:118–31.

[124] Reinert J. Uber die kontrolle der morphogenese und die induktion von adventivembryonen an gewebekulturen aus karotten. Planta 1959;53:318–33.

[125] Steward FC. Growth and development of cultivated cells. III. Interpretations of the growth from free cell to carrot plant. Am J Bot 1958;45:709–13.

[126] Kato H, Takeuchi M. Morphogenesis *in vitro* starting from single cell soft carrot root. Plant Cell Physiol 1963;4:243–5.

[127] Gibbs JL, Dougall DK. The growth of single cells from *Nicotiana tabacum* callus tissue in nutrient medium containing agar. Exp Cell Res 1965;40(1):85–95.

[128] Murakishi HH. Survival of dissociated tomato callus cells inoculated with tobacco mosaic virus. Virology 1965;27(2):236–9.

[129] Furuya T, Kojima H, Syono K. Nicotine and anatabine in tobacco callus tissue. Chem Pharm Bull 1966;14(10): 1189–90.

[130] Hansen AJ, Hildebrandt AC. The distribution of tobacco mosaic virus in plant callus cultures. Virology 1966;28(1):15–21.

[131] Vasil V, Hildebrandt AC. Further studies on the growth and differentiation of single, isolated cells of tobacco *in vitro*. Planta 1967;75(2):139–51.

[132] Chandra N, Hildebrandt AC. Differentiation of plants from tobacco mosaic virus inclusion-bearing and inclusion-free single tobacco cells. Virology 1967;31(3):414–21.

[133] Wilmar C, Hellendoorn M. Growth and morphogenesis of asparagus cells culture *in vitro*. Nature 1968;217: 369–70.

[134] Heble MR, Narayanaswami S, Chadha MS. Diosgenin and beta-sitosterol: isolation from *Solanum xanthocarpum* tissue cultures. Science 1968;161(3846):1145.

[135] Kaul B, Stohs SJ, Staba EJ. Dioscorea tissue cultures. 3. Influence of various factors on diosgenin production by Dioscorea deltoidea callus and suspension cultures. Lloydia 1969;32(3):347–59.

[136] O'Hara JF, Street HE. Wheat callus culture: the initiation, growth and organogenesis of callus derived from various explant sources. Ann Bot 1978;42(5):1029–978.

[137] Chen WH, Davey MR, Power JB, Cocking EC. Control and maintenance of plant regeneration in sugarcane callus cultures. J Exp Bot 1988;39:251–61.

[138] Goren R, Altman A, Giladi I. Role of ethylene in abscisic acid-induced callus formation in citrus bud cultures. Plant Physiol 1979;63:280–2.

[139] Akiyoshi DE, Klee H, Amasino RM, Nester EW, Gordon MP. T-DNA of Agrobacterium tumefaciens encodes an enzyme of cytokinin biosynthesis. Proc Natl Acad Sci USA 1984;81:5994–8.

[140] Akiyoshi DE, Morris RO, Hinz R, Mischke BS, Kosuge T, Garfinkel DJ, et al. Cytokinin/auxin balance in crown gall tumors is regulated by specific loci in the T-DNA. Proc Natl Acad Sci USA 1983;80:407–11.

[141] Bourgaud F, Gravot A, Milesi S, Gontier E. Production of plant secondary metabolites: a historical perspective. Plant Sci 2001;161:839–51.

[142] Hu Y, Bao F, Li J. Promotive effect of brassinosteroids on cell division involves a distinct CycD3-induction pathway in Arabidopsis. Plant J 2000;24:693–701.

[143] Stobbe H, Schmitt U, Eckstein D, Dujesiefken D. Developmental stages and fine structure of surface callus formed after debarking of living lime trees (Tilia sp.). Ann Bot (Lond) 2002;89:773–82.

[144] Iwai H, Masaoka N, Ishii T, Satoh S. A pectin glucuronyltransferase gene is essential for intercellular attachment in the plant meristem. Proc Natl Acad Sci USA 2002;99:16319–24.

[145] Dewitte W, Riou-Khamlichi C, Scofield S, Healy JM, Jacqmard A, Kilby NJ, et al. Altered cell cycle distribution, hyperplasia, and inhibited differentiation in Arabidopsis caused by the D-type cyclin CYCD3. Plant Cell 2003;15:79–92.

[146] Udagawa M, Aoki S, Syono K. Expression analysis of the NgORF13 promoter during the development of tobacco genetic tumors. Plant Cell Physiol 2004;45:1023–31.

[147] Ohtani M, Sugiyama M. Involvement of SRD2-mediated activation of snRNA transcription in the control of cell proliferation competence in Arabidopsis. Plant J 2005;43:479–90.

[148] Eckardt N. A genomic analysis of tumor development and source-sink relationships in Agrobacterium-induced crown gall disease in Arabidopsis. Plant Cell 2006;18:3350–2.

[149] Umehara M, Ikeda M, Kamada H. Endogenous factors that regulate plant embryogenesis: recent advances. Jpn J Plant Sci 2007;1:1–6.

[150] Tooker JF, Rohr JR, Abrahamson WG, De Moraes CM. Gall insects can avoid and alter indirect plant defenses. New Phytol 2008;178:657–71.

[151] Atta R, Laurens L, Boucheron-Dubuisson E, Guivarc'h A, Carnero E, Giraudat-Pautot V, et al. Pluripotency of Arabidopsis xylem pericycle underlies shoot regeneration from root and hypocotyl explants grown in vitro. Plant J 2009;57:626–44.

[152] Chiappetta A, Michelotti V, Fambrini M, Bruno L, Salvini M, Petrarulo M, et al. Zeatin accumulation and misexpression of a class I knox gene are intimately linked in the epiphyllous response of the interspecific hybrid EMB-2 (Helianthus annuus x H. tuberosus). Planta 2006;223:917–31.

[153] Chiappetta A, Fambrini M, Petrarulo M, Rapparini F, Michelotti V, Bruno L, et al. Ectopic expression of LEAFY COTYLEDON1-LIKE gene and localized auxin accumulation mark embryogenic competence in epiphyllous plants of Helianthus annuus x H. tuberosus. Ann Bot (Lond) 2009;103:735–47.

[154] Sugimoto K, Jiao Y, Meyerowitz EM. Arabidopsis regeneration from multiple tissues occurs via a root development pathway. Dev Cell 2010;18:463–71.

[155] Hwang I, Sheen J, Müller B. Cytokinin signaling networks. Annu Rev Plant Biol 2012;63:353–80.

[156] Stroud H, Ding B, Simon SA, Feng S, Bellizzi M, Pellegrini M, et al. Plants regenerated from tissue culture contain stable epigenome changes in rice. eLife 2013;19(2):e00354.

[157] Xu L, Huang H. Genetic and epigenetic controls of plant regeneration. Curr Top Dev Biol 2014;108:1–33.

[158] Haberlandt G. Culturversuche mit isolierten Pflanzenzellen. Sitz-Ber Mat Nat Kl Kais Akad Wiss Wien 1902;111:69–92.

[159] Muir WH, Hildebrandt AC, Riker AJ. The preparation, isolation, and growth in culture of single cells from higher plants. Am J Bot 1958;45:589–97.

[160] Lindsey K, Yeoman MM. The relationship between growth rate, differentiation and alkaloid accumulation in cell cultures. J Exp Bot 1983;34:1055–65.

[161] Panda AK, Mishra S, Bisaria VS, Bhojwani SS. Plant cell reactors – a perspective. Enzyme Microb Technol 1989;11:386–97.

[162] Fowler MW. The large scale cultivation of plant cells. Prog Ind Microbiol 1982;17:207–29.

[163] Torrey JG, Reinert J. Suspension cultures of higher plant cells in synthetic media. Plant Physiol 1961;36(4):483–91.

[164] Earle ED, Torrey JG. Colony formation by isolated Convolvulus cells plated on defined media. Plant Physiol 1965;40(3):520–8.

[165] Torres KC. Tissue culture techniques for horticultural crops. New York: Avi-Van Nostrand Reinhold; 1989. 1–285.

[166] Bergmann L. Growth and division of single cells of higher plants in vitro. J Gen Physiol 1960;43(4):841–51.

[167] De Ropp RS. The growth and behavior in vitro of isolated plant cells. Proc R Soc Lond B 1955;144:86–93.

[168] Jones LE, Hildebrandt AC, Ritker AJ, Wu JH. Growth of somatic tobacco cells in microculture. Am J Bot 1960;47:468–75.

[169] Mustafa NR, Winter WD, Iren FV, Verpoorte R. Initiation, growth and cryopreservation of plant cell suspension cultures. Nature Protocols 2011;6:715–42.

[170] Vasil IK, Vasil V. Isolation and culture of protoplasts. Int Rev Cytol Suppl 1980;11B:1–19.

[171] Hanstein J.V. Das Protoplasma als Trager der pflanzlichen und thierischen Lebensverrichtungen. Für Laien und Sachgenossen dargestellt. From Sammlung von Vortragen fur das deutsche Volk. In: Frommel W, Pfaff F, Heidelberg (Winter); 1880, p. 125.

[172] Klercker JA. Eine methods zur isoliering lebender Protoplasten. Vetenskaps Adad Stockholm 1892;9:463–71.

[173] Klercker J. Eine Methode zur Isolierung lebender Protoplasten. Ofvers Vetensk Akad Forh Stock 1892;49: 463–75.

[174] Küster E. Über die gewinnung nackter. Protoplasten 1927;3(1):223–33.

[175] Chambers R, Hofler K. Microsurgical studies of the tonoplast of *Allium cepa*. Protoplasma 1931;12:338–51.

[176] Cocking EC. A method for the isolation of plant protoplast and vacuoles. Nature 1960;187:962–3.

[177] Nagata T, Takebe I. Plating of isolated tobacco mesophyll protoplasts on agar medium. Planta 1971;99:12–20.

[178] Carlson PS, Smith HH, Dearing RD. Parasexual interspecific plant hybridization. Proc Natl Acad Sci USA 1972;69:2292–4.

[179] Carlson PS. The use of protoplasts for genetic research. Proc Natl Acad Sci USA 1973;70(2):598–602.

[180] Potrykus I, Durand J. Callus formation from single protoplasts of petunia. Nat New Biol 1972;237(78):286–7.

[181] Frearson EM, Power JB, Cocking EC. The isolation, culture and regeneration of Petunia leaf protoplasts. Dev Biol 1973;33(1):130–7.

[182] Vasil V, Vasil IK. Regeneration of tobacco and petunia plants from protoplasts and culture of corn protoplasts. *In Vitro* 1974;10:83–96.

[183] Shepard JF, Totten RE. Isolation and regeneration of tobacco mesophyll cell protoplasts under low osmotic conditions. Plant Physiol 1975;55:689–94.

[184] Potrykus I, Harms CT, Lörz H, Thomas E. Callus formation from stem protoplasts of corn (*Zea mays* L.). Mol Gen Genet 1977;156(3):347–50.

[185] Potrykus I, Harms CT, Lörz H. Callus formation from cell culture protoplasts of corn (*Zea mays* L.). Theoret Appl Genet 1979;54(5):209–14.

[186] Hearn VM, Wilson EV, Mackenzie DWR. The preparation of protoplasts from *Aspergillus fumigatus* mycelium. Sabouraudia 1980;18(1):75–7.

[187] Glimelius K. High growth rate and regeneration capacity of hypocotyl protoplasts in some Brassicaceae. Physiol Plant 1984;61:38–44.

[188] Firoozabady E, Deboer DL. Isolation, culture, and cell division in cotyledon protoplasts of cotton (Gossypium hirsutum and G. barbadense). Plant Cell Rep 1986;5(2):127–31.

[189] Yamada Y, Yang ZQ, Tang DT. Plant regeneration from protoplast-derived callus of rice (*Oryza sativa* L.). Plant Cell Rep 1986;5(2):85–8.

[190] Wei ZM, Xu ZH. Plant regeneration from protoplasts of soybean (*Glycine max* L.). Plant Cell Rep 1988;7(5): 348–51.

[191] Lührs R, Lörz H. Initiation of morphogenic cell-suspension and protoplast cultures of barley (*Hordeum vulgare* L.). Planta 1988;175(1):71–81.

[192] Harris R, Wright M, Byrne M, Varnum J, Brightwell B, Schubert K. Callus formation and plantlet regeneration from protoplasts derived from suspension cultures of wheat (*Triticum aestivum* L.). Plant Cell Rep 1988;7(5): 337–40.

[193] Li Z, Murai N. Efficient plant regeneration from rice protoplasts in general medium. Plant Cell Rep 1990;9(4): 216–20.

[194] Hayashimoto A, Li Z, Murai N. A polyethylene glycol-mediated protoplast transformation system for production of fertile transgenic rice plants. Plant Physiol 1990;93(3):857–63.

[195] Arya S, Liu JR, Eriksson T. Plant regeneration from protoplasts of *Panax ginseng* (Meyer CA) through somatic embryogenesis. Plant Cell Rep 1991;10(6–7):277–81.

[196] Hayakawa T, Zhu Y, Itoh K, Kimura Y, Izawa T, Shimamoto K, et al. Genetically engineered rice resistant to rice stripe virus, an insect-transmitted virus. Proc Natl Acad Sci USA 1992;89(20):9865–9.

[197] Jain RK, Khehra GS, Lee SH, Blackball NW, Marchant R, Davey MR, et al. An improved procedure for plant regeneration from indica and japonica rice protoplasts. Plant Cell Rep 1995;14(8):515–9.

[198] Rosenbluh J, Singh SK, Gafni Y, Graessmann A, Loyter A. Non-endocytic penetration of core histones into petunia protoplasts and cultured cells: a novel mechanism for the introduction of macromolecules into plant cells. Biochim Biophys Acta 2004;1664(2):230–40.

[199] Yoo SD, Cho YH, Sheen J. Arabidopsis mesophyll protoplasts: a versatile cell system for transient gene expression analysis. Nat Protocols 2007;2:1565–72.

[200] Yang X, Tu L, Zhu L, Fu L, Min L, Zhang X. Expression profile analysis of genes involved in cell wall regeneration during protoplast culture in cotton by suppression subtractive hybridization and macroarray. J Exp Bot 2008;59(13):3661–74.

[201] Power JB, Cocking EC. A simple method for the isolation of very large numbers of leaf protoplasts by using mixtures of cellulase and pectinase. Biochem J 1969;111(5):33 p.

[202] Melchers G, Labib G. Somatic hybridization of plants by fusion of protoplasts. Mol Gen Genet 1974;135(4):277–94.

[203] Tempé J, Petit A, Holsters M, Montagu MV, Schell J. Thermosensitive step associated with transfer of the Ti plasmid during conjugation: possible relation to transformation in crown gall. Proc Natl Acad Sci USA 1977;74(7):2848–9.

[204] George EF, Hall MA, De Klerk G-J. The components of plant tissue culture media I: macro- and micro-nutrients. In: Plant Propagation by Tissue Culture, 3rd edition, vol. 1. The Netherlands, Springer. 2008;65–113.

[205] Murashige T, Skoog F. A revised medium for rapid growth and bio-assays with tobacco tissue cultures. Physiol Plant 1962;15:473–97.

[206] Hoagland, D., 1938. The water-culture method for growing plants without soil (Circular (California Agricultural Experiment Station), 347 ed.). Berkeley, CA: University of California, College of Agriculture, Agricultural Experiment Station. 2014.

[207] Hoagland and Arnon (Revised 1950). The water-culture method for growing plants without soil. Berkeley, CA: University of California, College of Agriculture, Agricultural Experiment Station.

[208] Knudson L. A new nutrient solution for germination orchid seed. Am Orchid Soc Bull 1946;15:215–7.

[209] Vacin EF, Went FW. Some pH changes in nutrient solutions. Bot Gaz 1949;110:604–13.

[210] Burkholder PR, Nickell LG. Atypical growth of plants. I. Cultivation of virus tumors of Rumex on nutrient agar. Bot Gaz 1949;110:426–37.

[211] Heller R. Researches on the mineral nutrition of plant tissues. Ann Sci Nat Bot Biol Vg, 11th Ser 1953;14:1–223.

[212] Reinert J, White PR. The cultivation in vitro of tumor tissues and normal tissues of Picea glauca. Physiol Plant 1956;9:177–89.

[213] White PR. The cultivation of animal and plant cells. 2nd ed. New York: Ronald Press; 1963.

[214] Linsmaier EM, Skoog F. Organic growth factor requirements of tobacco tissue cultures. Physiol Plant 1965;18:100–27.

[215] Eriksson T. Studies on the growth requirements and growth measurements of cell cultures of Happlopapus gracilis. Physiol Plant 1965;18:976–93.

[216] Gamborg OL, Miller RA, Ojima K. Nutrient requirements of suspension cultures of soybean root cells. Exp Cell Res 1968;50:151–8.

[217] Gamborg OL, Miller RA, Ojima K. Nutrient requirements of suspension cultures of soybean root cells. Exp Cell Res 1968;50:151–8.

[218] Nitsch JP. Experimental androgenesis in Nicotiana. Phytomorphology 1969;19:389–404.

[219] Schenk RU, Hildebrandt AC. Medium and techniques for induction and growth of monocotyledonous and dicotyledonous plant cell cultures. Can J Bot 1972;50:199–204.

[220] Gresshoff P, Doy C. Derivation of a haploid cell line from Vitis vinifera and the importance of the stage of meiotic development of anthers for haploid culture of this and other genera. Z Pftlanzenphysiol 1974;73:132–41.

[221] Chih-Ching C, Ching-Chu W, Ching-San S, Chen H, Kwang-Chu Y, Chih-Yin C, et al. Establishment of an efficient medium for anther culture of rice, through comparative experiments on the nitrogen sources. Sci Sin 1975;18:659–68.

[222] Kao KN, Michayluk MR. Nutritional requirements for growth of Vicia hajastana cells and protoplasts at a very low population density in liquid media. Planta 1975;126:105–10.

[223] Mitra GC, Prasad RN, Roychowdhury A. Inorganic salts and differentiation of protocorms in seed-callus of an orchid and correlated changes in its free amino acid content. Indian J Exp Biol 1976;14:350–1.

[224] Lloyd G, McCown B. Commercially-feasible micropropagation of mountain laurel, Kalmia latifolia, by use of shoot tip culture. Int Plant Propagat Soc Proc 1981;30:421–7.

[225] Lichter R. Anther culture of Brassica napus in a liquid culture medium. Z Pflanzenphysiol 1981;103:229–37.

[226] Driver JA, Kuniyuki AH. *In vitro* propagation of Paradox walnut rootstock. HortScience 1984;19:507–9.

[227] McGranahan GH, et al. In: Bonga JB, Durzan DJ, editors. Cell and tissue culture in forestry. Dordrecht: Martinus Nijhoff; 1987. p. 261–71.

[228] Hickok LG, Warne TR, Fribourg RS. The biology of the fern ceratopteris and its use as a model system. Int J Plant Sci 1995;156(3):332–45.

[229] Quoirin M, Lepoivre P. Improved media for *in vitro* culture of *Prunus* sp. Acta Horticult 1977;78:437–42.

[230] Quoirin M, Lepoivre P, Boxus P. Un premier bilan de 10 années de recherches sur les cultures de méristèmes et la multiplication *in vitro* de fruitiers ligneux. CR Rech (1976–1977), Stat Cultures Fruitières Maraîchères, Gembloux. 1977: p. 93–117.

[231] Coke JE. Basal nutrient medium for *in vitro* cultures of loblolly pines. US Patent: 1996; 5,534,434.

[232] Vuylstke DR. Shoot-tip culture for the propagation, conservation, and distribution of Musa germplasm. Ibadan, Nigeria: IITA; 1998. 82.

[233] Maliro MFA, Lameck G. Potential of cassava flour as a gelling agent in media for plant tissue cultures. Afr J Biotechnol 2004;3(4):244–7.

[234] Che P, Lall S, Nettleton D, Howell SH. Gene expression programs during shoot, root, and callus development in Arabidopsis tissue culture. Plant Physiol 2006;141(2):620–37.

[235] Gautheret RJ. Factors affecting differentiation of plant tissue grown *in vitro*. In: Beerman W, Nieuwkoop PD, Wolff E, editors. Cell differentiation and morphogenesis. Amsterdam: North-Holland Publishing; 1966. p. 55–95.

[236] Hicks GS. Patterns of organ development in plant tissue culture and the problem of organ determination. Bot Rev 1980;46:1–23.

[237] Stehsela ML, Caplina SM. Sugars: autoclaving sterile filtration on the growth of carrot root tissue in culture. Life Sci 1969;8(24):1255–9.

[238] Jacquiot C. Action of meso-inositol and of adenine on bud formation in the cambium tissue of *Ulmus campestris* cultivated *in vitro*. C R Acad Sci Paris 1951;233:815–7.

[239] Pollard JK, Shantz EM, Steward FC. Hexitols in coconut milk: their role in the nurture of dividing cells. Plant Physiol 1961;36:492–501.

[240] Watanabe K, Tanaka K, Asada K, Kasal Z. The growth promoting effect of phytic acid on callus tissues of rice seed. Plant Cell Physiol 1971;12:161–4.

[241] Loewus F.A., Loewus M.W. Myo-inositol: biosynthesis and metabolism. In: Stumpf, Conn, editors. The Biochemistry of Plants 3. New York: Academic Press; 1980. p. 43–76.

[242] Wood HN, Braun AC. Studies on the regulation of certain essential biosynthetic systems in normal and crown-gall tumor cells. Proc Natl Acad Sci USA 1961;47:1907–13.

[243] Murashige T, Serpa M, Jones JB. Clonal multiplication of *Gerbera* through tissue culture. HortScience 1974;9: 175–80.

[244] Barwale UB, Kerns HR, Widholm JM. Plant regeneration from callus cultures of several soybean genotypes via embryogenesis and organogenesis. Planta 1986;167:473–81.

[245] Inoue M, Maeda E. Control of organ formation in rice callus using two-step culture method. In: Fujiwara A, editor. 1982. p. 183–184 (q.v.).

[246] Joy IV RW, Patel KR, Thorpe TA. Ascorbic acid enhancement of organogenesis in tobacco. Plant Cell Tissue Organ Cult 1988;13:219–28.

[247] Drew RA, Smith NG. Growth of apical and lateral buds of pawpaw (*Carica papaya* L.) as affected by nutritional and hormonal factors. J Horticult Sci 1986;61:535–43.

[248] Overbeek JV, Conklin ME, Blakeslee AF. Cultivation *in vitro* of small *Datura* embryos. Am J Bot 1942;29: 472–7.

[249] Robbins WJ, Bartley MA. Vitamin B, and the growth of excised tomato roots. Science 1937;85:246–7.

[250] Bonner J, Addicott F. Cultivation *in vitro* of excised pea roots. Bot Gaz 1937;99:144–70.

[251] Skinner JC, Street HE. Studies on the growth of excised roots. II. Observations on the growth of excised groundsel roots. New Phytol 1954;53:44–67.

[252] Abraham F, Bhatt A, Keng Lai C, Indrayanto G, Shaida F. Effect of yeast extract and chitosan on shoot proliferation, morphology and antioxidant activity of *Curcuma mangga in vitro* plantlets. Afr J Biotechnol 2011;10(40):7787–95.

[253] Rangan TS, Murashige T, Bitters WP. *In vitro* initiation of nucellar embryos in monoembryonic *Citrus*. HortScience 1968;3:226–7.

[254] Rangan T.S. Clonal propagation: cell culture and somatic cell genetics of plants. In: Vasil IK, editor, vol. 1. New York: Academic Press; 1984. p. 68–73.

[255] Das T, Mitra GC, Chatterjee A. Micropropagation of *Citrus sinensis* var. mosambi: an important scion. Phytomorphology 1995;45:57–64.

[256] Dix L, Van Staden J. Auxin and gibberellin-like substances in coconut milk and malt extract. Plant Cell Tissue Organ Cult 1982;1:239–45.

[257] Carimi F, De Pasquale F, Puglia AM. *In vitro* rescue of zygotic embryos of sour orange, *Citrus aurantium* L., and their detection based on RFLP analysis. Plant Breed 1998;117:261–6.

[258] Chuang CC, Ouyang TW, Chia H, Chou SM, Ching CK. A set of potato media for wheat anther culture. Proceedings of the Peking Symposium Pitman, Boston, London, Melbourne. Plant Tissue Culture 1978:51–56.

[259] Van Staden J, Drewes SE. Identification of zeatin and zeatin riboside in coconut milk. Physiol Plant 1975;34:106–9.

[260] George EF, de Klerk GJ. The components of plant tissue culture media. I: Macro- and micro-nutrients. In: George EF, Hall MA, de Klerk GJ, editors. Plant propagation of tissue culture, 3rd ed. The background, 1. The Netherlands: Springer; 2008. p. 65–113.

[261] Jameson PE. Plant hormones in algae. In: Round FE, Chapman DJ, editors. Progress in phycological research, 9. Bristol: Biopress Ltd; 1993. p. 239–79.

[262] Ördög V, Stirk WA, Van Staden J, Novák O, Strnad M. Endogenous cytokinins in three genera of microalgae from the Chlorophyta. J Phycol 2004;40:88–95.

[263] Shantz EM, Steward FC. The general nature of some nitrogen free growth-promoting substances from *Aesculus* and *Cocos*. Plant Physiol 1956;30:XXXV.

[264] Went F. Auxin: the plant growth hormone. Bot Rev 1935;1:162–82.

[265] Hecht SM. Probing the cytokinin receptor site(s). In: Skoog F, editor. Plant Growth Substances 1979. Proceedings of the 10th International Conference on Plant Growth Substances. Berlin: Springer; 1980. p. 144–60.

[266] Entsch B, Letham DS, Parker CW, Summons RE, Gollnow BI. Metabolites of cytokinins. In: Skoog F, editor. Plant Growth Substances 1979. Proceedings of the 10th International Conference on Plant Growth Substances. Berlin: Springer; 1980. p. 109–18.

[267] De Fossard RA, Nitsch C, Cresswell R, Lee E. Tissue and organ culture of Eucalyptus. NZ J Forest Sci 1974;4:267–78.

[268] Rinkis G. Optimization of plant mineral nutrition. Riga: Zinatne; 1972. 355 p. (in Russian).

[269] Rinkis G, Nollendorfs V. Macro and micronutrients in balanced nutrition of plants. Riga: Zinatne; 1982. 202 p. (in Russian).

[270] Osvalde A. Optimization of plant mineral nutrition revisited: the roles of plant requirements, nutrient interactions, and soil properties in fertilization management. Environ Exp Biol 2011;9:1–8.

[271] Rinkis G. Interactions among nutrients during their uptake processes in plants in relation to soil properties. Dissertation thesis. Kaunas 1973; 40 (in Russian).

[272] Riņķis G, Paegle G, Kuņicka T, Osvalde A. Optimization system of plant mineral nutrition. The Quarterly Norleg International Newsletter Breakthrough, UK 1995:14.

[273] Riņķis G, Ramane H. Plant nutrition. Rīga: Avots; 1989. 151 p. (in Latvian).

[274] Riņķis G, Ramane H, Paegle G, Kuņicka T. Optimization system and diagnostic methods of plant mineral nutrition. Riga: Zinatne; 1989. 196p.

[275] Hildebrandt AC, Riker AJ, Duggar BM. The influence of the composition of the medium on the growth *in vitro* of excised tobacco and sunflower tissue cultures. Am J Bot 1946;33:591–7.

[276] George EF, Hall MA, De Klerk GJ. Plant propagation by tissue culture. Dordrecht, Netherlands: Springer Verlag; 2008.

[277] Gago J, Landín M, Gallego PP. A neurofuzzy logic approach for modeling plant processes: a practical case of *in vitro* direct rooting and acclimatization of Vitis vinifera L. Plant Sci 2010;179:241–9.

[278] Gallego PP, Gago J, Landin M. Artificial neural networks technology to model and predict plant biology process. In: Suzuki K, editor. Artificial neural networks – methodological advances and biomedical applications. Croatia: Intech Open Access Publisher; 2011. p. 197–216.

[279] Zielinska A, Kepczynska E. Neural modeling of plant tissue cultures: a review. Biotechnologia 2013;94:253–68.

[280] Gago J, Pérez-Tornero O, Landín M, Burgos L, Gallego PP. Improving knowledge on plant tissue culture and media formulation by neurofuzzy logic: a practical case of data mining using apricot databases. J Plant Physiol 2011;168:1858–65.

[281] George EF. The components of plant tissue culture media. II: Organic additions, osmotic and pH effects and support systems. Plant Propagat Tissue Cult 2008;115–73. 3rd ed.

3

Laboratory Organization

Saurabh Bhatia, Randhir Dahiya

3.1 INTRODUCTION

Plant tissue culture broadly refers to the *in vitro* cultivation of all plant parts under aseptic conditions.

The laboratory in which tissue culture techniques are performed must have following facilities:

- A general washing area and media preparation, sterilization, and storage area.
- An aseptic transfer area.
- Environmentally controlled incubators or culture rooms.
- An observation/data collection area.

These facilities can be designed in several ways.

Modern Applications of Plant Biotechnology in Pharmaceutical Sciences. http://dx.doi.org/10.1016/B978-0-12-802221-4.00003-0

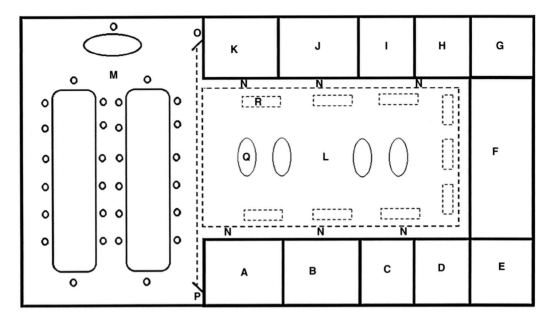

FIGURE 3.1 **Layout for organization of a tissue culture laboratory.** Media preparation room (A); with connected heat sterilization (B); autoclave room (C); washing area having washing stations and drying oven (D); dark room for highly sophisticated and light- and dust-sensitive equipment (e.g., electron microscope) (E); transfer room with UV cabinet, HEPA filter, air curtain, laminar air flow hood (F); store room for glasswares and chemicals (G); light room for daily use equipment such as centrifuge, pH meter, hot plate, stirrer, and balance (H); millipore and double distillation unit room having facility for keeping large vessels (canes) for storing water (I); store room for small equipment (weighing balance, compound microscope, etc.), glass wares and specialized facility room for germplasm conservation (it is essential to have lower temperature, and installation of cryopreservation units is a must) (J) change room for containing head and mouth masks, hand gloves, shoes, and sanitizers (K); transparent glass shielded culture room (L); with temperature regulating sensors and racks (R); with light adjustable fluorescent tubes and installed shaking machine (Q); main laboratory with laboratory bench and teacher's desk; gallery having two doors, exit (O) and entry(P), both having a double door system (air curtain) (M).

Figures 3.1, 3.2, 3.3, and 3.4 demonstrate the suitable way to organize all these facilities.

The following points need to be considered for the site selection of plant tissue culture laboratory establishment.

- The selected area should be relatively free from dust, smoke, molds, spores, and chemicals.
- The laboratory should be far away from a plant pathology laboratory and access to the laboratory should be through an outer room hall.
- Location should have well-maintained lawn and disease-free shrubs.

3.2 WASHING AREA

The washing area should contain large sinks with ample drying space including draining boards, racks, dryers, automated dishwashers, storage cabinets, and access to demineralized water, distilled water, and double-distilled water.

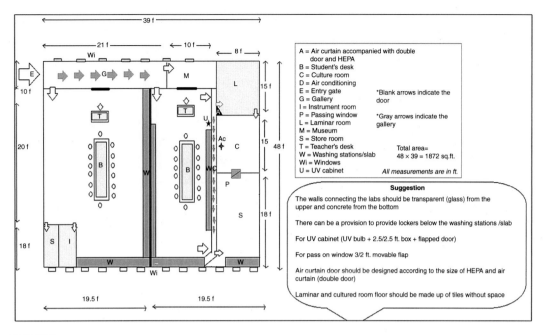

FIGURE 3.2   A simplified and conventional form of laboratory design in plant tissue culture.

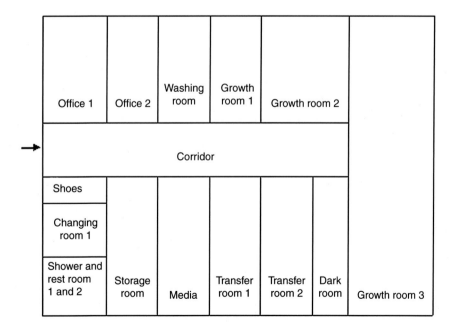

FIGURE 3.3   Incubation shelf.

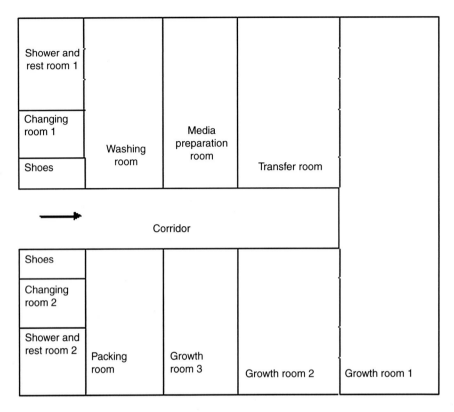

FIGURE 3.4   Alternative I: tissue culture lab with office. Layout of tissue culture facility.

The following are general guidelines for a washing area:

- Reusable glassware for tissue culture should be emptied immediately and should be soaked in water. Media or agar should not be allowed to dry on glassware.
- All glassware containing corrosive chemicals or fixatives should be separated from the rest of the tissue culture glassware and glassware contaminated with microorganisms should be autoclaved before washing.
- The contents of containers should be discarded immediately after completion of an experiment.
- Flasks or beakers used for agar-based media should be rinsed immediately after dispensing the media into culture vessels so as to prevent drying of the residual agar in the beaker prior to washing.

3.3 MEDIA PREPARATION AREA

The media preparation area should have ample storage space for the chemicals, culture vessels, closures, and glassware required for media preparation and dispensing. The minimum area required for media preparation, transfer, and primary growth shelves is approximately 130 sq. ft.

3.3.1 Mandatory Requirements for Media Preparation Room

- Refrigerator/freezer and high quality water
- Balances, hot plate/stirrer, pH meter, aspirator or vacuum pump
- Double-distillation assembly and autoclave
- Optional equipment such as dissecting microscopes, microwave, water baths, laboratory washers, ovens, automatic media (dispensers are helpful when pipetting large volumes of media)
- Bunsen burners with a gas source

The water used for preparation of media must be of highest purity and quality. Water used for plant tissue culture should be of type II reagent grade water, i.e., free from pyrogens, gases, and organic matter, and electrical conductivity should be less than 1.0 μmho/cm. The most common and preferred method of purifying water to type II standards is deionization treatment followed by one or two glass distillations. The deionization treatment removes most ionic impurities, and the distillation process removes large organic molecules, microorganisms, and pyrogens. Other methods to produce type II purity water are: absorption filtration, in which activated carbon removes organic contaminants and free chlorine; membrane filtration, in which particulate matter and most bacterial contamination are removed by filtration; and reverse osmosis, which removes approximately 9% of the bacterial, organic, and particulate matter as well as about 90% of the ionized impurities [1–3].

3.3.2 Chemicals for Culture Media

1. Inorganic elements:
   a. Macronutrient: The macronutrients are required in higher amounts in tissue culture media (Table 3.1) [4].
   b. Micronutrients: Micronutrients are essential for plant cell tissue growth (Table 3.2) [4].

TABLE 3.1 Description of the Macroelements Along with Their Form and Respective Function

Sr. no.	Name of the macronutrient	Available form	Function
1.	Nitrogen (N)	KNO_3, NH_4NO_3	Both a structural and functional role in protein synthesis
2.	Phosphorus (P)	KH_2PO_4	Activation in nucleotide synthesis
3.	Potassium (K)	KNO_3	Essential for activation of many enzymes, maintenance of ionic balance of the cell
4.	Calcium (Ca)	$CaCl_2 \cdot 2H_2O$	Acts as a cofactor and is largely bound to the cell wall and cell membrane, essential for cation–anion balance by counteracting organic–inorganic anions
5.	Magnesium (Mg)	$MgSO_4 \cdot 7H_2O$	Essential for photosynthesis and many other enzymatic reactions
6.	Sulfur (S)	$MgSO_4 \cdot 7H_2O$, K_2SO_4	Functional role in protein synthesis

TABLE 3.2   Description of the Microelements Along with Their Form and Respective Function

Sr. no.	Name	Available form	Function
1.	Zinc (Zn)	$ZnSO_4 \cdot 7H_2O$	Acts as a component of a number of enzymes, plays active role in protein synthesis, specifically in synthesis of tryptophan
2.	Manganese (Mn)	$MnSO_4 \cdot 4H_2O$	Helps in photosynthesis
3.	Copper (Cu)	$CuSO_4 \cdot 5H_2O$	Plays an important role in electron transport chain at the time of photosynthesis
4.	Molybdenum (Mo)		Participates in the conversion of nitrate to ammonium
5.	Boron (B)	H_3BO_3	Required for the synthesis of cell wall and cell membrane
6.	Iron (Fe)	$FeSO_4 \cdot 5H_2O$	Formation of protein, important for biosynthesis of chlorophyll
7.	Cobalt (Co)	$CoCl_2 \cdot 6H_2O$	Helpful for nitrogen fixation
8.	Chlorine (Cl)	$CaCl_2 \cdot 2H_2O$	Controls the osmoregulation of cell development

TABLE 3.3   Vitamins and Their Function in Plant Tissue Culture

Sr. no.	Name of the vitamin	Function
1.	Thiamine (vitamin B1)	
2.	Nicotinic acid B20	
3.	Pyridoxin-HCl (B6)	
4.	Folic acid	Promotion of cell growth and development
5.	Biotin	
6.	Riboflavin	
7.	Retinol (vitamin A)	

2. Organic components (Table 3.3):
   a. Vitamins: Normally plants synthesize vitamins endogenously. When plant cells and tissues are grown on *in vitro* some essential vitamins are required.
   b. Myoinositol: This has several functions like sugar transport, carbohydrate metabolism, and formation of membrane and cell wall.
   c. Sugar: This can be supplied in the form of sucrose, glucose, and fructose. It is a source of carbon.
   d. Amino acid: Cultured tissues are normally capable of synthesis of amino acid. Moreover, addition of amino acids to media is important for stimulating cell growth. Unlike inorganic nitrogen, amino acids are taken up more rapidly by plant cells. Glycine is the most common amino acid used in different tissue culture media. Some of the other amino acids like glutamine, asparagines, cysteine, etc. are also required for cell culture [3].

e. Plant growth regulators: Plant growth regulators are the organic molecules that have different regulatory effects on growth and development in plant tissues and plants. They are the most vital component of any culture media and without regulators, *in vitro* culture is often impossible. The following are plant growth regulators often used in plant tissue culture:

- Auxin: The major functions of auxin include cell division, cell elongation, and organogenesis. It is frequently used as a rooting hormone. The most frequently employed auxins are IAA (indole-3-acetic acid), IBA (indole-3-butyric acid), NAA (naphthalene acetic acid), and 2,4-D (2,4-dichlorophenoxyacetic acid). IAA is a naturally occurring auxin and is added in concentrations of 0.01–10 mg/L. The most effective auxin of callus proliferation for most cultures is 2,4-D, but unfortunately it strongly suppresses organogenesis and should not be used in experiments involving root and shoot initiation [6].
- Cytokinin: Cytokinins are derivatives of adenine, which promote cell division, and regulate growth and development in plant tissues. It is known as a shooting hormone essential for induction of axillary branching and adventitious shoot formation. The most widely used cytokinins are kinetin, zeatin, BAP (benzyladenine), and 2iP (2- isopentenyladenine) [6].
- Other regulators: Other types of hormones that may be used in plant tissue culture include gibberellins (GA3), which promote shoot elongation and internodal elongation, ethylene, and abscisic acid.

3.4 STERILIZATION ROOM

The sterilization room should be used in continuation with the media preparation room. The layout must be planned in such a way that it ensures the smooth movement of the containers from washing to the media preparation and sterilization room.

The sterilization room must have walls and floors that can withstand moisture, heat, and steam. An exhaust fan should be fitted to remove the warm and moist air. The exhaust fan should have an outer cover to prevent entry of outside air. The fan cover should open only when the fan is in operation. In small tissue culture facilities, costly autoclaves can be replaced by simple pressure cookers. However, for large volume media making, horizontal or vertical autoclaves should be installed. Double door autoclaves, which open directly into the media storage room, may be costly but reduce contamination. A cheaper alternative is to transfer the sterilized media to the adjoining room through a hatch window [1,2].

3.5 ASEPTIC TRANSFER AREA/INOCULATION ROOM

The most important work area is the culture transfer room where the core activity takes place. The transfer area needs to be as clean as possible and be a separate room with minimal air disturbance. Walls and floors of the transfer room must be smooth to facilitate frequent cleaning. The doors and windows should be minimal to prevent contamination, but within local safety codes. There is no special light requirement in the transfer room. The illumination of the laminar air flow chamber is sufficient for work. Sterilization of the instruments can be done with glass-bead sterilizers or flaming after dipping in alcohol, usually ethanol. The culture containers should be stacked on mobile carts (trolleys) to facilitate easy movement from the medium storage room to the transfer room, and finally to the growth room. Fire extinguishers and first aid kits should be provided in the transfer room as a safety measure. Special laboratory shoes and coats should be used in the working area. Ultraviolet (UV) lights are sometimes installed in transfer areas to disinfect the room; these lights should be used only when people and plant material are not in the room. Safety switches can be installed to turn off the UV lights when regular room lights are turned on. All the activities of sterile transfers are performed in this room. There must be a laminar air flow cabinet where precautions should be taken to prevent entry of any contaminant into the culture vial during the process of inoculation or subculture. Laminar air flow hoods are usually sterilized by switching on the hood and wiping the working surface with 70% ethyl alcohol for 13 min before initiating any operation under the hood.

3.6 CULTURE ROOM

This is the room where light, temperature, and humidity are maintained. All these environmental considerations vary according to the size of the growth room. The growth room is an equally important area where plant cultures are maintained under controlled environmental conditions to achieve optimal growth. It is advisable to have more than one growth room to provide varied culture conditions since different plant species may have different requirements of light and temperature during *in vitro* culture. All types of tissue cultures should be incubated under conditions of well-controlled temperature (temperature should be constant throughout the entire culture room, i.e., no hot or cold spots; 13 and 30°C, with a temperature fluctuation of less than ±0.3°C always with a temperature alert alarm system to monitor temperature fluctuations), humidity (range of 20–98% controllable to ±3%, air circulation), light quality (fluorescent lighting to reach 10,000 lux; the lighting should be adjustable in terms of quantity and photoperiod duration), and uniform forced-air ventilation. Both light and temperature should be programmable for a 24-h period. Protoplast cultures, low-density cell suspension cultures, and anther cultures are particularly sensitive to environmental cultural condition. Also, in the event of the failure of cooling or lighting in one room, the plant cultures can be moved to another room to prevent loss of cultures. In the growth room, the number of doors should be minimal to prevent contamination. There is no need for windows in the growth room, except when natural light is used. When artificial lighting is used, the external light can interfere with the photoperiod and temperature of the growth room [5].

Depending on the amount of available space and cost, the culture containers can be placed on either fixed or mobile shelves. Mobile shelves have the advantage of providing access to cultures from both sides of the shelves. The height of the shelves should not exceed 2 m (Fig. 3.5). High shelving requires step-up stools to place and remove cultures, which can be dangerous and time consuming. The primary source of illumination in the growth room is normally from the lights mounted on the shelves. Overhead light sources can be minimized, as they would be in use only while working during the dark cycle. Plant cultures might not receive uniform light from the conventional downward illumination. Lights directly fitted

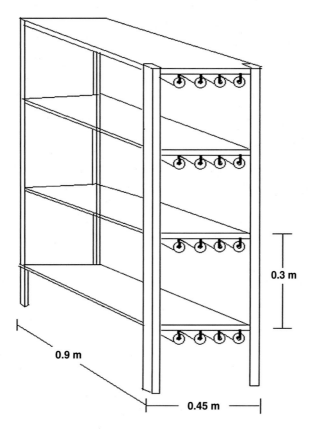

FIGURE 3.5 Alternative II: tissue culture without office. In this case an independent office should be available within the premise of the laboratory.

to the racks create uneven heat distribution. This leads to high humidity within the culture containers, which in turn can cause hyperhydricity. Sideways illumination is an alternative, which requires fewer lights, and provides more uniform lighting. Some of the essential requirements of a culture room are highlighted below.

3.6.1 Sterile Transfer Room

Tissue culture techniques can be successfully performed under sterile conditions on an open laboratory bench. However, it is advisable that a laminar flow hood or sterile transfer room accompanied by a source of electricity, gas, compressed air, and vacuum be utilized for making transfers. The laminar flow hood should be equipped with an ultraviolet light, fluorescent and visible light, and a positive-pressure ventilation unit. The ventilation unit should be equipped with a high-efficiency particulate air (HEPA) filter. A 0.3-μm HEPA filter of 99.97–99.99% efficiency works well. HEPA filters or regular furnace filters can be installed over air intakes to the laboratory or on furnaces. In a sterile transfer room, large numbers of cultures are being utilized and screened for their further processing.

3.6.2 Vertical Flow Unit or Horizontal Flow Unit

Another type of transfer area is a laminar flow hood. Air is forced into the unit through a dust filter then passed through a HEPA filter. The air is then either directed downward (vertical flow unit) or outward (horizontal flow unit) over the working surface. The constant flow of bacteria-free filtered air prevents nonfiltered air and particulate matter from settling on the working surface.

3.6.3 Glove Box

The simplest type of transfer area suitable for tissue culture work is an enclosed plastic box commonly called a glove box. This type of culture hood is sterilized by an ultraviolet light and wiped down periodically with 93% ethyl alcohol when in use. This type of unit is used when relatively few transfers are required.

3.6.4 Primary Growth Room and the Aseptic Transfer Area

This should be designed in such a way that there is no direct entry from outside a building and the media preparation area, glassware washing area, or storage area should be located outside these rooms.

3.7 DATA COLLECTION AREA

Culture room is prepared by glass wall. Qualitative data can be collected from outside the glass wall, whereas quantitative data can be collected from inside the culture room by following aseptic rules and regulations. In the data collection area, information based on regular observations of growth and development of tissue cultured *in vitro* under aseptic conditions may be collected using a laminar.

3.8 ACCLIMATIZATION AREA

Plants regenerated from *in vitro* tissue cultures are transplanted to vermiculite pots. The potted plants are ultimately transferred to greenhouses or growth cabinets and maintained for further observations under controlled conditions of light, temperature, and humidity [1,2].

The following are general rules to be followed in a tissue culture laboratory:

1. A laboratory should have an inventory and updated records of all equipment along with their operating manuals and chemicals including the name of manufacturer and grade.
2. All chemicals should be assigned to specific areas preferably in alphabetical order and strong acid and bases should be stored separately. Chloroform, alcohol, phenol, which are volatile or toxic in nature, must be stored in a fume hood whereas chemicals that are hygroscopic in nature must be stored in desiccators in order to avoid caking.
3. Chemicals kept in refrigerators or freezers should be arranged either alphabetically or in small baskets.

3.9 SAFETY RULES

1. Eating, smoking, and drinking are strictly prohibited in the tissue culture laboratory.
2. Toxic chemicals must be handled with appropriate precautions and should be discarded into separate labeled containers, e.g., organic compounds, halogens, etc.
3. Broken glass and scalpel blades must be disposed of in individual marked containers.
4. Pipettes, tips, Pasteur pipettes, and other items used in the laboratory should be first collected in autoclavable bags and then finally autoclaved and disposed of in a safe place.
5. Laboratories should be equipped with first aid kits and fire extinguishers.

3.10 DESIGN AND LAYOUT OF TISSUE CULTURE LABORATORY

Correct design of a laboratory not only reduces contamination, but also achieves a high efficiency in work performance [7]. A tissue culture laboratory should be planned to reduce both operational and energy costs. It should accommodate the equipment used in the various stages of micropropagation in the most efficient manner. The availability of good quality access roads, and reliable telephone, electricity and water supplies are taken as the most important consideration while choosing a location. Not only a convenient location but also sufficient working rooms with partitioned walls and sealed ceilings are taken into account in setting up a commercial micropropagation unit. Walls and ceilings should be insulated and covered inside with water-resistant material. Windows should be placed wherever convenient in the media preparation and glassware washing rooms. The heating system should be capable of maintaining a room temperature at 20°C during the coldest winter season. Water supply pipes should be connected to a septic system and sanitary sewer. Air conditioning requirements should be carefully estimated. Electrical service capacity for equipment, lights, and future expansion are calculated. For safety reasons, the electrical installation should be carried out professionally. The media preparation room, inoculation room, and growth chambers should be isolated as "clean zones." The office, storage area, staff center, and packaging rooms should be maintained under ordinary conditions. The working areas should be demarcated according to the activities involved in the facility. To minimize contamination, cleanliness is the major consideration of a plant tissue culture laboratory. A positive pressure module should be installed to circumvent air intake from outside. An enclosed entrance and sticky mats should be used to collect dirt from shoes.

3.11 AUTOMATION IN PLANT TISSUE CULTURE

Nowadays plant tissue culture is known to be a best technology for the production of large numbers of identical plants. There are two biological methods, organogenesis and embryogenesis, which have been exploited in plant tissue culture for several years. Choice of the either method depends on the cost, species, success rate of method for producing plants at a realistic cost, and local laboratory conditions. The requirements of intensive labor and special environment make plant tissue culture more expensive than other forms of propagation. Automation of all or some of the stages of either organogenesis or embryogenesis is envisaged as a way of reducing the handling of the tissue, thereby reducing labor input and hence cost of the plantlet/somatic seedling. In recent years, there has been extensive research interest in automation of tissue culture to achieve bulk handling of the tissue (e.g., bioreactors, encapsulators) and automatic assessment (image analysis), cutting, transport, and planting through the use of robots or other devices. However, some processes are already automated, e.g., nutrient media preparation, environmental control of incubators/greenhouses that contain cultures and plantlets, and computer management of laboratory and greenhouse. Unaccountably, currently employed automatic systems are still ineffective such as:

- Systems are not cost effective when compared with manual methods
- Failure to adequately address the biological and engineering constraints
- Unacceptable tissue or plantlet quality
- Requirement of skilled professionals, e.g., tissue culture researcher and engineers

On this basis there are two types of automation:

1. Total automation: This is a totally automated process where little or no human intervention is required. The involvement of a tissue culture vessel in this process may be automatic presentation of small vessels by conveyors or by providing tissue in bulk form as a reactor. The Toshiba plant tissue culture robot is one example of total automation.
2. Semiautomation: This type of automation involves human operators contributing to any stage of the process. This is the most commonly researched type of automation. Automated advancements suffer from various contamination, vitrification, and abnormal plant development in liquid media, repeatability and synchronization, cost effectiveness, and selection of method [8].

References

[1] Bhojwani SS, Razdan MK. Plant tissue culture: theory and practice – a revised edition, 5. Amsterdam: Elsevier Publications; 1996. p. 19–38.
[2] Mageau OC. Laboratory design. In: Debergh PC, Zimmerman RH, editors. Micropropagation: technology and application. London: Kluwer Academic Publishers; 1991. p. 15–9.
[3] Trigiano RN, Gray DJ, editors. Plant tissue culture concepts and laboratory exercises. 2nd ed. Florida, USA: CRC Press; 1999.
[4] Ramage CM, Williams RR. Mineral nutrition and plant morphogenesis. *In Vitro* Cell Devel Biol-plant 2002;38:116–24.
[5] Murashige T. Plant propagation through tissue cultures. Annu Rev Plant Physiol 1974;25:135–66.
[6] George EF, Hall MA, De Klerk F Greet-Jan, editors. Plant propagation by tissue culture. 3rd ed. New York: Springer Publications; 2008. p. 175–204.
[7] Bridgen MP, Bartok JW. Designing a Plant Micropropagation Laboratory. Comb Proc Int Plant Prop Soc 1987;37:462–7.
[8] Chawla HS. Introduction to plant biotechnology. 2nd ed. USA: Science Publishers; 2002.

4

Concepts and Techniques of Plant Tissue Culture Science

Saurabh Bhatia, Randhir Dahiya

Modern Applications of Plant Biotechnology in Pharmaceutical Sciences. http://dx.doi.org/10.1016/B978-0-12-802221-4.00004-2

4.1 INTRODUCTION

Plant tissue culture science forms the basis of various areas such as agriculture, horticulture, and plant biotechnology. It is an area of applied science that provides a broad platform for the aseptic culture of cells, tissues, organs, and their components under defined chemical and physical *in vitro* conditions. This science follows a basic concept in which the plant body or organ or any tissue can be dissected into smaller parts called "explants" and any explants can be further developed into a whole plant. This concept led to the development of an effective technique called *in vitro* propagation. Plant regeneration forms the basis of *in vitro* propagation. Totipotency and genetic and cellular machinery information of the plant cell are essentially required to generate the whole plant. Therefore, this *in vitro* science includes several concepts and techniques that can be utilized to produce a higher number of plants that are genetically similar to a parent plant as well as to one another. To understand the regeneration potential of plant cell culture an in-depth knowledge of concepts like plasticity and totipotency is required. Additionally, plants themselves hold certain key features that favor their growth and development. Features like longer life span and sessile nature of plant cells enhance plant tolerance power and adaptability to extreme conditions. Thus, processes that are involved in the growth and development of the plant cell always run parallel to the environmental conditions. When plant cells or tissues are exposed to *in vitro* conditions most of the cells generally exhibit a very high degree of plasticity, which allows one type of organ or tissue to be initiated from another type. Following this principle, the whole plant can be regenerated. Thus, totipotency is the regeneration process acquired by the plant to preserve its genetic potential. Furthermore, artificial nutrient medium plays a vital role in regeneration by supplementing organic and inorganic nutrients. Success of the culture is much dependent on the appropriate composition of the medium. Manipulation of the culture media is a usual practice to check the growth pattern of implanted explants. The mixture of salts, organic supplements, and sucrose (source of fixed carbon) concentration varies from media to media. Each medium has its different composition, which can be later manipulated according to the designed study. Supplementation of appropriate concentration of hormones (auxin and cytokinin) always decides the growth pattern of the implanted explants. Selection of organ or tissue segment called the explant, which can potentially induce *in vitro* propagation of the explants on a supporting solidified nutrient medium under sterile conditions, is also an important step to begin the desired full *in vitro* propagation in tissue culture studies. Culturing of such explants in an appropriate medium gives rise to an unorganized, growing, and dividing mass of cells called callus. During callus formation a degree of dedifferentiation happens both in morphology and metabolism. One of the major consequences of dedifferentiation is that most plant cultures lose their ability to perform photosynthesis. Addition of other components such as carbon and vitamins to the culture media, apart from the unusual mineral nutrients, enhances the cell photosynthetic and regeneration power. All these processes include various basic concepts and techniques that lead to the successive development of callus and finally establishment of the desired full cell line of the plant, which could be experimented on again for various research purposes. Selection of an appropriate protocol that involves basic procedures designed by applying the most advanced concept with the latest technology provides germination to cell lines that have a long life and are equipped with the needed full features. This selection leads to the transformation of any part of the plant organ or tissues into a dedifferentiated mass called callus.

There are various concepts and techniques that are frequently practiced in plant tissue culture science. In modern biotechnology, most of the concepts and techniques deal with the genetic study of plants. In modern plant biotechnology the gene of interest is extracted from the genome with the help of a restriction enzyme. This gene of interest is then inserted into cloning vector such as a cosmid or plasmid with the help of a *ligase* enzyme. Cloned vectors are then introduced into the host cell and selected and cultured in fermenters. The desired products are extracted using a downstream process (this refers to the recovery and purification of biosynthetic products, particularly pharmaceuticals, from natural sources such as animal or plant tissue or fermentation broth, including the recycling of salvagable components and the proper treatment and disposal of waste). The basic concepts and techniques involved during these processes are stated in Fig. 4.1. Developments in conventional concepts led to

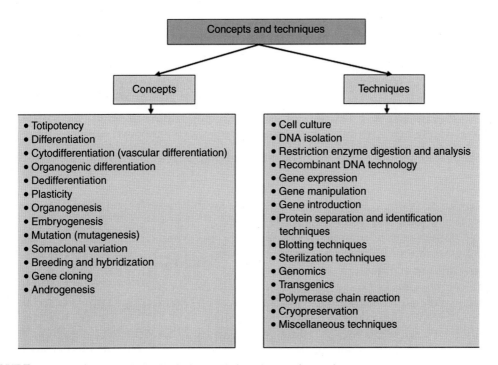

FIGURE 4.1 **Various concepts and techniques of plant tissue culture science.**

the origin of contemporary technologies. In general terms, concepts can be captured from any natural mechanism though techniques are applied on those concepts for their improvement or to evaluate the application of that concept. In a similar manner, we have successfully differentiated the concepts and techniques separately (Fig. 4.1). Techniques that are frequently utilized in plant tissue culture are shown in Table 4.1.

4.2 CULTURING TECHNIQUES

Plant cell, tissue, and organ culture is a set of techniques designed for the growth and multiplication of the cells and tissue using nutrient solution in aseptic and controlled environmental conditions. This technology explores conditions that promote cell division and genetic reprogramming to develop a potent and stable plant cell line with distinguishing features. Various scientific studies, for example physiology, biochemistry, and molecular biology, of primary and secondary metabolism, developmental regulation, and cellular responses to pathogens and stress can be performed by using different culturing techniques under *in vitro* conditions. These *in vitro* studies provide an excellent opportunity to investigate the properties and potentialities of plant cells, which may help in understanding the function of plant cells in particular tissues or organs. Culturing technique allows the exploration of molecular pathways involved in cellular metabolism and other essential processes of plant cells. In addition, such techniques also assist in studying the processes that are involved in the synthesis of secondary metabolites. Various applications such as mutant selection and crop improvement have also been explored. Furthermore, culturing techniques explore growing individual cell systems within a population of cultured cells, and invariably show cytogenetically and metabolic variations. This variation is called spatial heterogeneity (which explores the differences in the karyotype and ability to accumulate secondary metabolites during morphogenesis among various clones regenerated from a single cell). Therefore, they provide a tool to study and operate the plant cell under suitable conditions. All culturing techniques are described in Chapter 2. The cell culturing technique includes several steps that are always followed during *in vitro* propagation of different plants as mentioned subsequently:

- Isolation of the plant cell from (mechanical method/enzymatic method) the cultured tissue
- Growth and subculture of suspension cultures (batch and continuous cultures)
- Selection and optimization of culture medium for cell suspension culture
- Synchronization of suspension cultures
- Physical (selection by volume and temperature shock) and chemical methods (starvation, inhibition, mitotic arrest)
- Measurement of growth in suspension cultures
- Cell counting, packed cell volume, cell fresh, and dry weight
- Viability of cultured cells (phase contrast microscopy, reduction of tetrazolium salts, fluorescein diacetate method, Evans blue staining)
- Culture of isolated single cells [plating technique (to culture isolated single cell), filter paper raft nurse technique, microchamber technique (to culture low-density cell cultures), and scale-up technique (bioreactors are used for large-scale cultures)]

TABLE 4.1 Several Techniques that are Frequently Utilized in Plant Tissue Culture Science

Name of technique	Types of technique	
Culturing techniques	• Suspension culture • Callus culture • Hairy root culture • Seed culture (embryo, endosperm)	• Protoplast culture • Ovary culture • Root, shoot, and leaf culture • Flower culture (ovary, anther, pollen)
Protein separation and identification techniques	• Agarose gel electrophoresis • Pulsed field electrophoresis • Field inversion gel electrophoresis • Vertical pulse field gradient electrophoresis	• Counter clamped homogeneous electric field gel electrophoresis • Polyacrylamide gel electrophoresis • Isoelectric focusing • 2-D gel electrophoresis • Microarray
Blotting techniques	• Nucleic acid blotting • Southern blot analysis • Northern blot analysis	• Protein blotting • Dot blot technique • Autoradiography
Sterilization techniques	• Steam sterilization • Dry sterilization • Filter sterilization • Ultraviolet sterilization	• Alcohol sterilization • Flame sterilization • Chemical sterilization
Genomics	• Patterns of gene expression • Mapping and sequencing techniques used for eukaryotes and prokaryotes • DNA chip technology • SAGE	• Gene overexpression regulation • Gene inactivation • Metabolomics • Metabolic fingerprinting • Metabolic profiling • Proteomics
Transgenics	Insect resistance	• Resistance gene from microorganisms • (Bt toxin gene) • Resistance gene from higher plants • (Proteinase inhibitors and lectins)
	Virus resistance	• Nonstructural protein-mediated cross-protection • Defective interfering RNAs • Antisense and sense-mediated resistance • Satellite RNA protection • Coat protein-mediated cross-protection • Pathogen-targeted resistance

(Continued)

TABLE 4.1 Several Techniques that are Frequently Utilized in Plant Tissue Culture Science *(cont.)*

Name of technique	Types of technique		
	Disease resistance	• Pathogenesis-related proteins • Antimicrobial proteins • Manipulation of disease resistance gene • Phytoalexins	
Gene transfer techniques	Vector-mediated transfer method	Bacteria mediated	• *Agrobacterim*-mediated gene transfer
		Virus mediated	• Virus-mediated gene transfer
	Vectorless or direct transfer method	Physical methods	• Biolistics/particle bombardment/microprojectile • Microinjection • Macroinjection • Electroporation • Liposome-mediated method • Silicon carbide fiber-mediated transformation • Ultrasound-mediated gene transformation
		Chemical methods	• Calcium phosphate coprecipitation • Polycation DMSO technique • DEAE dextran procedure • PEG-mediated transformation
Gene expression	Marker genes	Reporter genes	Opine synthase Chloramphenicol acetyl transferase Beta glucuronidase Bacterial luciferase Firefly luciferase Green fluorescent protein Anthocyanins
		Selectable markers	Antibiotic resistance markers Antimetabolite resistance markers Herbicide resistance markers

TABLE 4.1 Several Techniques that are Frequently Utilized in Plant Tissue Culture Science *(cont.)*

Name of technique	Types of technique	
	Regulation of transfer gene expression	• Gene silencing • Detection of intrusive DNA • Causes of gene silencing • DNA methylation • Homology-dependent gene silencing suppression by antisense gene • Silencing by RNA interference
	Methods for the removal of marker genes	• Cotransformation • Removal of marker genes by transposases
PCR	• Inverse PCR • Reverse transcriptase-mediated PCR	
	• Non-PCR-based techniques	RFLP

	PCR-based techniques	• Random amplified polymorphic DNA
		• DNA amplification fingerprinting
		• Arbitrarily fragmented length polymorphism
		• Simple sequence repeats or microsatellites
		  ◦ Microsatellite-directed PCR: unanchored primers
		  ◦ Microsatellite-directed PCR: anchored primers
		  ◦ Random amplified microsatellite polymorphism
		  ◦ Selective amplification of microsatellite polymorphic loci
		• Retrotransposon-based markers
		  ◦ Sequence specified amplified polymorphism
		  ◦ Inter-retro transposon amplified polymorphism
		  ◦ Retrotransposon microsatellite amplified polymorphism
		  ◦ Retrotransposn-based insertional polymorphism

(Continued)

TABLE 4.1   Several Techniques that are Frequently Utilized in Plant Tissue Culture Science *(cont.)*

Name of technique	Types of technique	
	• Single nucleotide polymorphism	
	• Targeted PCR and sequencing	• Sequence-targeted microsatellites • Sequence-characterized amplified regions • Cleaved amplified polymorphic sequences • Sequence-related amplification polymorphism
Cryopreservation	• Determination of viability or survival	• TTC method of staining • Evans blue staining
Miscellaneous techniques	Protoplast fusion techniques, transposon tagging in heterologous species, techniques used for single cell cultures (Bergmann cell plating technique), immobilization technique, artificial seed technology, chromosome elimination technique, recombinant DNA technology, spectrophotometry (quantitation, enzyme kinetics), nucleic acid purification and molecular weight determinations, cell separation methods, protein separation and quantitation, liquid scintillation (double label) counting, autoradiography (cellular and gross), restriction enzyme mapping, gene expression, and oligonucleotide synthesis	

4.2.1 Suspension Culture Technique

As described in Chapter 2, suspension cultures are those cultures in which cells are suspended in a liquid medium and mixed at a certain speed to expose the cells to uniform nutrient media from all directions, which could prevent the aggregation of cells and eventually increase the absorption of nutrients by promoting the growth of the cells. These cultures are maintained by the subculturing of the cells in the early stationary phase to a fresh medium. In the incubation period cell division and cell enlargement increase, which provides rapid growth to the cells. Due to exhaustion of some factors or the accumulation of toxic substances in the medium the viability of cells in the suspension after the stationary phase is decreased, which further decreases the growth rate of whole culture. This step is followed by addition of aliquot of the cell suspension to the freshly prepared medium of the original composition. Examination of the incubation period from culture initiation to the stationary phase is primarily determined by cell density, duration of lag phase, and growth rate of the cell line. As discussed in Chapter 2, there are two types of suspension culture: batch culture and continuous culture. Cultures that are continuously maintained by propagating a small aliquot of the inoculums in the moving liquid medium and transferring it to a fresh medium at regular intervals are called batch cultures. On the contrary, continuous cultures are those cultures that are propagated at a larger level under controlled conditions for longer periods by adding fresh medium and draining out the used medium in a number of specially designed culture vessels; these are known as continuous or mass cultures. There are two types of continuous culture: open and closed types. In the closed type, the equilibrium of the medium is maintained by addition of fresh medium to balance the outflow of the old medium. Whereas in the open type the inflow of the medium is accomplished by a balancing return of an equal quantity of the culture medium and cells. *Chemostat* and *turbidostat* are the two major types of open cultures. Constant inflow of fresh medium is maintained steadily in chemostat whereas in turbidostat the input of the medium is intermittent as it is mainly required to control the rise in turbidity due to cell growth. Basic techniques that are involved during the process are:

- Techniques for conditioning and agitation of the medium: slow rotating culture, spinning culture, shaking culture, stirred culture, and continuous culture.
- Synchronization of cell – physical method: selection by volume and temperature shock; chemical method: starvation, inhibition, and mitotic arrest.
- Techniques to measure the growth in suspension culture: cell counting, packed cell volume, cell fresh weight, cell dry weight.
- Techniques to measure viability of the cultured cells: phase contrast microscopy, reduction of tetrazolium salts, fluorescein diacetate method, Evans blue staining.
- Techniques to immobilize the plant cell: various techniques for cell immobilization are described in Chapter 7.
- Techniques to grow single cell cultures from either plant organs or cell suspension: platting technique, medium manipulation, filter paper raft nurse culture and microchamber technique, bioreactors for large-scale cultures (described in Chapter 7).
- Techniques to increase the secondary metabolite production (described in Chapter 7).

Success in the establishment of a cell suspension culture depends to a great extent on the availability of "friable" callus tissue. Such a system is much more amenable for biochemical studies and process development than calli, since they generally grow at a faster rate and allow cells to be in direct contact with the medium nutrients. Suspensions or liquid cultures of plant cells are usually grown as microbial cells. However, plant cell dimensions are much larger than those of bacteria or fungi, ranging from 20 to 40 μm in diameter and from 100 to 200 μm in length (central vacuole occupies a large portion of the mature cell volume). Hence, the plant growth pattern is comparatively slower than others. Plant cell cultures tend to contain clumps, formed by a variable number of cells. These clumps arise as a result of the failure of new cells to separate after division or from the adherence of free cells among themselves. In some cases, such clumps (also known as aggregates) may contain up to 200 cells, and reach up to 2 mm in diameter. Although cell stickiness can be overcome by modifying the culture medium, as a rule cells in culture become "sticky" in the late lag phase of growth. Methods to obtain suspensions composed largely of free cells include the use of cell wall degrading enzymes and sieving. Unfortunately, once established, a fine cell suspension has a tendency with time to revert to a clumped condition.

4.3 STERILIZATION TECHNIQUES

Microorganisms promote their growth by absorbing the entire essential nutrients from the medium. A medium that is usually made for plant cell culture, when attacked by microorganisms, can excrete substances in the medium that may often be toxic or inhibitory to the plant cell. Association of such microorganisms with plant cells causes contamination.

Some microorganisms are beneficial for plant growth and hence do not interfere with the *in vitro* growth of plant cell and form a symbiotic relationship. But due to the large difference in growth rate pattern of plant (slow) and microorganisms (rapid), plant cell culture growth is suppressed and does not show any type of growth in the medium. Moreover, microorganisms often utilize plant tissue as a substratum to proliferate their further development. Explants and environment are the two major sources of microbial contaminant. Microbial contaminants may influence the behavior of the tissues *in vitro* by releasing metabolites and proteins that affect the plant tissues and alter the composition and/or pH of the culture medium. Microbial contamination of plant tissue cultures is foremost due to the high nutrient availability in the almost universally used MS (Murashige and Skoog) medium. Therefore, biological contamination is one of the frequently encountered reasons that hinder the *in vitro* propagation of plant tissue culture. Apart from biological contamination there are other types of contamination (physical, chemical, radiation, cross-culture, etc.) that must be avoided to allow the proper growth of implanted explants (Figs 4.2 and 4.3). The management of contamination in tissue culture involves three stages: indexing explants (detection of contaminants by using various media or screening methods) and cultures for contaminants, identifying the source of contaminants or disease, identifying or characterizing the contaminants and eliminating the contaminating organisms with improved cultures (Figs 4.2 and 4.3) [1].

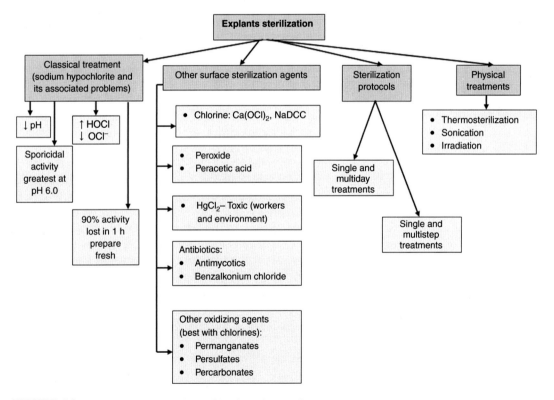

FIGURE 4.2 Sterilization protocols used in plant tissue culture.

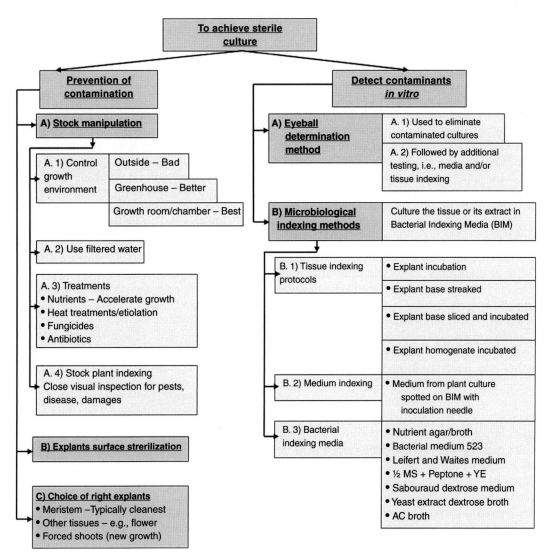

FIGURE 4.3 Prevention and detection of contaminants to furnish sterile culture.

For *in vitro* propagation studies, plant tissue when brought in from the outside environment should be sterilized first to avoid contamination. Sterilization provides a germ-free environment that allows the proper growth of the tissue under aseptic environmental conditions. The maintenance of aseptic or sterile conditions is essential for successful tissue culture procedures. Modern plant tissue culture is performed under aseptic conditions under filtered air. Several techniques are employed for the sterilization of glassware, instruments, liquids, and plant material (Figs 4.2 and 4.3). Methods such as dry heat, wet heat, and ultrafiltration are widely used during tissue culture studies. Environmentally contaminated living tissue should be sterilized on their surfaces to eliminate microorganisms present at the periphery. Sodium or calcium hypochlorite and mercuric chloride are the most common surface sterilizing agents (Figs 4.2 and 4.3). Mercuric chloride is rarely used as a plant sterilant these days as it is dangerous to use and difficult to dispose of. It is only utilized when the other sterilizing agents are found to be ineffective (Figs 4.2 and 4.3). Chemically sterilized explants are then usually placed on the surface of a solid culture medium, but are sometimes placed directly into a liquid medium, particularly when cell suspension cultures are desired. Sterilization procedures have some additional positive effects, e.g., autoclaving seems to hydrolyze sucrose into more efficiently utilizable sugars such as fructose. Sucrose was reported to act as a morphogenetic trigger in the formation of auxiliary buds and branching of adventitious root. In contrast, sterilization can sometimes also have ill effects on tissue culture media, e.g., sterilization of coconut milk and any other natural sources leads to decline in potential of whole media. Some media are highly unstable at high temperature and must be sterilized at room temperature. Several chemicals employed in plant tissue culture media degrade on exposure to steam sterilization, e.g., gibberellins are rapidly degraded at elevated temperature, whereas auxins, NAA, IAA, and 2,4-D are thermostable. Furthermore, vitamins have a varying degree of thermostability. In general, the addition of vitamins prior to autoclaving is not advisable (filter sterilization at room temperature is preferable). Surface sterilization sometime causes lot of damage to the tissue, e.g., calcium hypochlorite was found to be one of the effective and least injurious agents whereas sodium ions (sodium hypochlorite) may induce abnormal development in the seedlings (Figs 4.2 and 4.3).

Solid and liquid media are generally composed of inorganic salts plus a few organic nutrients, vitamins, and plant hormones, which can, if not sterilized at particular conditions, become damaged. Solid media are prepared from liquid media with the addition of a gelling agent, usually purified agar (Figs 4.2 and 4.3). Although sterilization of culture media is best carried out in a steam autoclave at temperatures between 121°C and 134°C, it has to be recognized that damage is caused to the media by the heating process. The composition of the medium, particularly the plant hormones and the nitrogen source (nitrate versus ammonium salts or amino acids) has profound effects on the morphology of the tissues. Heat treatment of complex culture media, which contain peptides, sugars, minerals, and metals, results in nutrient destruction, either by direct thermal degradation or by reaction between the media components. A general instruction for sterilizing culture media in volumes up to 1 L at 121°C for 20 min is given on each label. Overheating is a common cause of pH drift, darkening, precipitation, and poor gel strength. Overheating effects will occur if agar media are allowed to gel in bottles and are later steamed to melt the agar. They will also occur if molten media are held at 50°C for more than 3 h before use. Agar media with pH values at or below 5.0 are very sensitive to overheating in any form because the agar is hydrolyzed and the gel strength fails. It is recommended to sterilize the agar of media with a pH lower than 5.0 separately. Reports also suggested that media that contain reducing sugars (glucose) should be sterilized with care as there is a possibility of Maillard reaction (during sterilization at 121°C) due to amino acid in the nitrogen source [2]. This auto-oxidation of sugar in phosphate buffer produces reactive oxygen species in the medium [3]. Therefore, while preparing semidefined media (i.e., minimal salt media), organic nitrogen sources (yeast extract/malt extract) should be autoclaved separately.

Aseptic techniques are widely utilized in a different manner for each process. Their utilization depends on nature of the explant. Some of the basic aseptic techniques that are commonly used in plant tissue culture are highlighted in Table 4.2. Health hazards associated

TABLE 4.2   Sterilization Techniques Used in Plant Tissue Culture

Technique	Chief characteristics	Materials sterilized
Steam sterilization/ Autoclaving (121°C at 15 psi for 20–40 min)	• Simple, fast, causes destruction of viruses • Disadvantages are change in pH by 0.3–0.5 units, • Components can separate out and chemical reactions can occur resulting in a loss of activity of media	Nutrient media, culture vessels, glassware, and plastic ware • Test tubes/flasks: 20–50 mL; media: 20 min, –120°C; 15 psi • Flasks 50–500 mL; nutrient media: 25 min, –120°C; 15 psi • Flasks 500–5000 mL; nutrient media: 35 min, –120°C; 15 psi • Propylene, polymethylpentene, Tefzel, ETPE, and Teflon FEP 20–50 mL; nutrient media: 20 min, –120°C; 15 psi
Dry heat (160–180°C for 3 h)	An exposure of 160°C dry heat for 2 h is regarded as equivalent to moist heat sterilization at 121°C for 15 h	Instruments (scalpel, forceps, needles, etc.), glassware, pipettes, tips, and other plastic ware
Flame sterilization	Instruments are soaked in 70–80% alcohol followed by flaming on a burner in the laminar air flow hood	Instruments (scalpel, forceps, needles, etc.), mouth of culture vessel
Filter sterilization	Asbestos and asbestos paper discs, sinter glass filters, microfilters, depth filters, cellulose membrane filters (membrane filter made of cellulose nitrate or cellulose acetate of 0.45–0.22 μm pore size)	Thermolabile substances like growth factors, amino acids, vitamins, and enzymes
Alcohol sterilization	For hand wash 70% alcohol is quite effective	Workers' hands, laminar flow cabinet
Surface/ chemical sterilization	Different sterilants with their exposure time in minutes and their degree of effectiveness: • 1–1.4% sodium hypochlorite (5–30 m), 9–10% calcium hypochlorite (5–30 m), and 1–2% bromine water are very effective • 10–12% hydrogen peroxide (5–15 m), 1% silver nitrate (5–30 m), and 4–50 mg/L antibiotics (30–60 m) are effective • 0.01–1% mercuric chloride (2–10 m) gives satisfactory response	Plant material can be surface sterilized by using various sterilants. The optimal condition for plant tissue against the sterilants should be determined to prevent its toxic or lethal effect. After treatment with sterilants each explant must be rinsed several times with distilled water to remove the noxious chemicals
Radiation sterilization	*UV sterilization*: This is hardly used for sterilization of tissue culture media as it is more expensive than the autoclave method *Microwave sterilization*	Disposable plastic ware is generally sterilized. UV irradiation may generate PCR inhibitors and ruin plastic ware and pipettes For small quantity of media
Antibiotic- mediated sterilization	Amino glycosides (streptomycin), actams (penicillin), quinolones (nalidixic acid), polymyxin (rifampicin)	For sterilizing various plant tissue cultures

with hypochlorite solutions (should not be used under UV and never use a mouth pipette for such solutions), fire (ethanol is highly inflammable), UV irradiation (serious health risks), lysol 3.5% (causes burning and irritation on the skin), mercury chloride (highly volatile at room temperature, can cause mercury poisoning), and gas sterilization (ethylene dioxide should not be used without supervision) should always be considered before designing any sterilization protocol [4].

4.4 GENETIC ENGINEERING TECHNIQUES

4.4.1 DNA Isolation Technique

For any molecular studies the isolation of pure, intact, and high-quality DNA is very crucial. However, secondary metabolites by excessive contamination interfere with DNA isolation. Unlike animals and microbes, plants contain a variety of secondary metabolites. These metabolites vary from plant to plant species and even in each plant tissue. Therefore, DNA isolation methods need to be adjusted according to the nature of metabolites. Several protocols have been developed for obtaining the best quality and highest yield of DNA from plants containing high levels of secondary metabolites. Some plants (e.g., mangrove and salt marsh) are specially adapted to harsh environments and exposed to higher stress conditions, and hence synthesize high amounts of polysaccharides, polyphenols, and other secondary metabolites such as alkaloids and flavonoids, which could always impede DNA extraction. Many factors can cause shearing of DNA, such as (i) degradation during extraction of DNA due to endonucleases, (ii) inhibition of Taq polymerase and restriction enzyme activity under the influence of large amounts of polysaccharides, and (iii) browning of DNA due to covalently binding with oxidized forms of polyphenols and presence of polysaccharides in the DNA sample. Currently, several commercial kits are also accessible to extract genomic DNA from plants with sufficient quality. Extraction of genomic DNA (nuclear material) without degradation involves initial mechanical grinding of the sample, which is carried out in the presence of liquid nitrogen. Various toxic, hazardous, and expensive chemicals (e.g., phenol) are used to separate cellular molecules and debris from the DNA. For high throughput DNA extraction several researchers have attempted to eliminate the use of hazardous chemicals, expensive kits, equipment, and labor-intensive steps. Most of the developed methods have demerits such as limited shelf-life, low purity, low recovery, and poor amplification. Therefore, DNA extraction protocols recommend fresh biological samples for genomic DNA isolation; however, due to various reasons it is very difficult always to obtain fresh samples. There is a tremendous demand on processes or technology for isolating DNA from dried leaf samples. Recently, a CTAB (cetyltrimethylammonium bromide) protocol has been developed, which enables the isolation of high-quality genomic DNA amenable to RAPD (random amplified polymorphic DNA), restriction digestion, and amplification of plant barcode genes (matK and rbcl) with reduced cost and health concerns [5,6]. Various other techniques are also involved in the isolation of DNA of interest. For genomic cloning, isolation of high molecular weight chromosomal DNA should be done from a tissue which is free of organelle DNA and RNA. For the isolation of chromosomal DNA, nucleus DNA is separated from the organellar

DNA and other cellular components. For the separation of DNA from RNA *ribonuclease* are added, which causes the digestion of RNA, while the solution is made free of *deoxyribonuclease* by heat treatment. This makes DNA available in a purified and stable form. The size of chromosomal DNA can be measured by agar gel electrophoresis [5]. DNA isolation totally depends on the experimental organisms, but somehow these techniques have the following characteristics:

- Treatment for opening the cells and releasing their DNA
- Methods of inactivating and removing the enzymes that degrade the DNA
- Methods of separating the DNA from proteins and other molecules that contaminate the DNA

Alcohol precipitation is a common method of isolation whereas DNA isolation kits are also available on the market.

4.4.2 DNA Transformation Techniques

Exposing plant cells to any stress ruptures its physical strength and avails the various fragmented DNA with different molecular sizes. Vectors, *Agrobacterium*, microinjection, polyethyleneglycol (PEG)-mediated gene transfer, silicon carbide whiskers, particle gun (biolistics), electroporation, liposome-mediated gene transfer, ultrasonication, incubation, chemical transfection, and *in planta* transformation are the transformation methods that are reported in genetic engineering. These transformation methods allow the genetic improvement of plants for regulating its differentiation and development [7,8].

4.4.3 Restriction Enzyme Digestion and Analysis Technique

An enzyme that cuts DNA at specific recognition nucleotide sequences (with Type II restriction enzymes cutting double-stranded DNA) is called a restriction enzyme. Such types of enzymes are usually found in bacteria and archaea and provide a better defense mechanism against invading viruses. A restriction enzyme works inside the bacterial host in such a manner that it selectively cuts up foreign DNA in a process called restriction. To provide protection from their own restriction enzyme's activity, host DNA is methylated by a modification enzyme called *methylase*. Restriction enzymes recognize particular sequences of bases in a double stranded DNA and cut the DNA molecule either in blunt (cutting at opposite sites in the two strands of DNA) or staggered form (cutting at asymmetrical positions). Hence, these two processes form the basis of a restriction modification system. The exact mechanism is described in Fig. 4.4.

4.4.4 Genetic Manipulation

Genetic manipulation is a process to identify a gene that controls a trait of interest or modifies an existing gene. Isolation of genes of interest is now a routine process. Based on desired phenotype, genes of interest or target genes must be carefully chosen. Gene manipulation has the following functions.

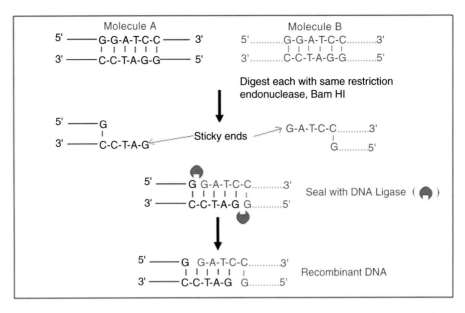

FIGURE 4.4   **Restriction of DNA by restriction enzyme.**

4.4.4.1 Glyphosate (Roundup®) Resistance

In 1970s, glyphosate was discovered to be an herbicide by world's largest seed corporation, Monsanto [9]. It was brought to the market under the trade name "Roundup" with the composition of glyphosate as active ingredient, along with water, surfactant, and polyoxyethylene alkyl amine [9]. Surfactant allows better adhesion of herbicide and penetration to the leaves. Roundup was the first glyphosate-based herbicide sold on the international market. Owing to the increase in the planting of Roundup Ready GM Crops it has become the number one selling herbicide worldwide. Recently, various human health-related ill effects have been found using glyphosate-based herbicides [10]. Several reports suggested that glyphosate may be a direct causative factor in the inhibition of cytochrome P450 (CYP) enzymes and development of celiac disease (impairment with gut ecology), but still Monsanto continues to sell glyphosate products under the brand name Roundup [11]. In crops glyphosate binds with the active site of the EPSP synthase enzyme (synthesizes 3-enolpyruvylshikimic acid-5-phosphate and acts as a essential precursor to aromatic amino acids). This binding is responsible for the development of a group of aromatic amino acids, subsequently inhibits the synthesis of amino acids, and ultimately the plants die because protein synthesis is severely disrupted [12]. Genetic interference with EPSP synthase prevents glyphosate binding, which makes the plant survive when sprayed with the herbicide. Therefore, genetically engineered EPSP synthase protects Roundup Ready crops and allows them to produce enough aromatic amino acids to survive [12]. Established examples of genetically engineered crops are corn, soy, canola, cotton, sugar beets, and most recently alfalfa. These crops have altered DNA, which allows them to survive against a glyphosate called Roundup Ready feature or Roundup Ready technology. Crops that are developed by such technology are called

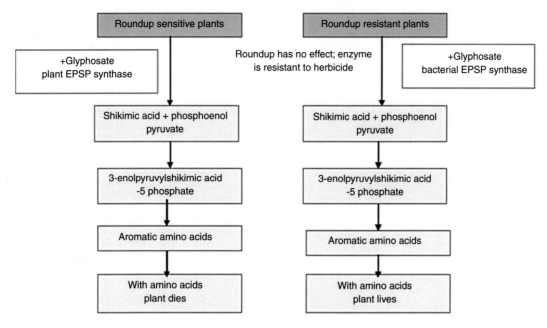

FIGURE 4.5 Protocol for genetic introduction of resistant EPSP synthase gene in crops.

"glyphosate tolerant crops" [13]. The exact protocol for the introduction of the resistant EPSP *synthase* gene in crops is described in Fig. 4.5.

4.4.4.2 Increased Vitamin A Content

The problem with vitamin A deficiency is the second major plant biotechnology issue that was raised to address its ill effects such as blindness and affects the severity of many diseases and conditions including diarrhea and measles throughout the world. More than 100 million children are affected by this problem worldwide [14]. Distribution of vitamins among deficient children and desirable regions is a simple solution. Improvement of vitamin A content in widely consumed and readily available product can again prove to be a better solution. To increase the level of the precursor to vitamin A, genetic transformation in rice was proved to be a promising solution for the development of transgenic rice plants. Because of the variation in color (yellow rather than white) and other properties of this crop is called "Golden Rice" or GMO crop [14].

Color variation from white to yellow is due to β-carotene, a precursor to vitamin A abundantly present in the seed. In contrast to the single-step Roundup Ready pathway, synthesis of the β-carotene pathway involves several enzymes. Due to the absence of four key enzymes, the vitamin A precursor cannot be synthesized in rice. Due to this β-carotene deficiency, the precursor is not made, and the plant contains white kernels. Therefore, with the help of genetic engineering a complete, functioning, β-carotene biosynthetic pathway was designed and inserted into the rice plant. This was done by introducing a functional gene called daffodil gene. Such insertion produces functioning versions of the first and last enzymes of the

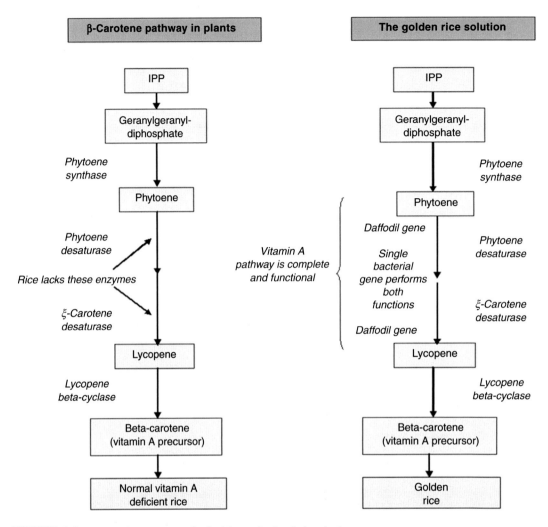

FIGURE 4.6   Genetic improvement in the biosynthesis of vitamin A.

pathway [15]. In addition, a single bacterial gene that provides the same function as the second and third enzymes of the pathway was introduced. Once the pathway is activated or functioned, the production of the vitamin A precursor β-carotene is increased, which gives a product called "Golden Rice" having a characteristic yellow color [15]. Introduction of the daffodil gene improves the biosynthesis of the vitamin by resembling the function of enzymes involved in the formation of vitamins as mentioned in Fig. 4.6.

4.4.5 Gene Introduction

In this process the gene is introduced by a technique called transformation, which forms transgenic organisms. This genetic element contains a recombination site and a gene creates a transformation cassette. Crops that are developed through genetic modification are referred to as genetically modified crops, transgenic crops, or genetically engineered crops and the process is known as transgenesis. Plant tissue culture science covers the development of transgenic crops in greater depth. Stable organization of a suitable gene cassette or mobile genetic element (which contains a gene of interest and a recombination site) is essential for the successful introduction of the cassette into the plant. Transformation cassettes are composed of three main regions: gene of interest (coding region and its controlling elements), selectable marker (distinguishes transformed/untransformed plants), and insertion sequences (aids *Agrobacterium* insertion).

4.4.5.1 *Gene of Interest*

This is the specified or actual gene introduced to provide a new function to the plant. After the development of a suitable transformation cassette, numerous plant tissues are treated with these cassettes. Only some tissues will successfully receive the cassette and transform into the desired plants. Successful transformation is checked by a selectable marker, which distinguishes transformed (those that contain the gene) from nontransformed (those that do not) plants. *Agrobacterium*-mediated gene transfer is the most common method of introducing the transformation cassette. For efficient transformations it is essential that the constructed transformation cassette contain insertion sequences that are used by the bacteria [16].

The transformation cassette is composed of several components such as coding region, which encodes the protein product (e.g., EPSP, β-carotene genes), and the gene of interest, which contains two important controlling regions (promoter region and transit peptide) [8,16]. The promoter region is located just before the coding region, designed in such a way that it decides and controls the expression of the gene of interest. This region also helps to determine when, where, and to what degree the gene of interest will be expressed. There are two types of promoter region: constitutive promoter and specific expression promoter [17]. A constitutive promoter directs expression in virtually all tissues and their expression is normally not conditioned by endogenous factors, which lead to a relatively high level of gene expression [17,18].

The expression of the 35S RNA of the cauliflower mosaic virus is the most often used constitutive promoter and is abbreviated to CaMV35S promoter [18]. The first constitutive promoters used for the expression of transgenes in plants were isolated from plant pathogens. Constitutive promoters have several advantages in expression vectors that are used in plant biotechnology:

- High level of production of proteins (used to select transgenic cells or plants) and transcription factor (which is part of a regulatory transcription system)
- High level of expression of reporter proteins (allowing easy detection and quantification)
- Production of compounds that requires ubiquitous activity in the plant and compounds that are required during all stages of plant development

The most widely used constitutive promoters are shown subsequently:

- Plant pathogen promoters: CaMV 35S promoter and opine promoters
- Monocot promoters: Plant ubiquitin promoter (Ubi), rice actin 1 promoter (Act-1) and maize *alcohol dehydrogenase* 1 promoter (Adh-1)

The specific expression promoter (glutelin-1 promoter) directs a very specific expression pattern, e.g., during the specific time of seed development the glutelin-1 promoter directs the expression of the glutelin storage protein in the rice endosperm. In this case if the gene of interest is led by the CaMV35S promoter, it will be expressed in all tissues at all times [18,19]. On the other hand, if the gene of interest is controlled by the glutelin-1 promoter then the expression of the target gene could be limited to the endosperm [20]. There are only some genes that encode proteins that are functional in the plant organelles such as chloroplasts and mitochondria. Such protein control participates in processes like photosynthesis and carbon and lipid metabolism. A short amino acid sequence (found before the coding region) called transit peptide is required to ensure delivery of these proteins to the appropriate organelle [21]. This peptide sequence is recognized by proteins that are present in the outer membranes and this recognition process leads to the import of the protein into the organelle. Therefore to allow the entry of the whole transformation cassette into the organelle, an appropriate transit peptide must be required. In general, transit peptides are responsible for the transport of a protein encoded by a nuclear gene to a particular organelle. One of the best examples of transit peptide is to target RbCS (RUBISCO small subunit) to the correct organelle (chloroplast target) [21].

4.4.5.2 Selectable Marker

A gene that encodes a protein product is called a selectable marker. Such marker genes are introduced into the plant genome to express a protein generally with an enzymatic activity, which allows transformed cells to be distinguished from nontransformed cells. In plant cells, genes that are presenting resistance to selective agents such as antibiotics or herbicides are widely employed to select transformants [22]. These markers are particularly effective for selection and providing a means of rapidly identifying transformed cells that express the selectable gene product. For their expression they require a constitutive promoter region (CaMV35S RNA promoter). A selectable marker controls a gene that encodes a protein, which allows transformed plants to survive in toxic environments, while nontransformed cells and tissues die [22]. Kanamycin and hygromycin (bacterial antibiotics), and herbicide glufosinate are the most often used selective agents. The protein encoded by the selectable marker genes usually renders these selective agents harmless to the transgenic plant. The most popular examples of a gene that breaks down a toxic compound are: *aphIV* [hygromycin (bacterial antibiotic) resistance], *bar* [glufosinate (herbicide) resistance], and *nptII* [kanamycin (bacterial antibiotic) resistance] [22]. Various examples of selectable markers with their respective traits are highlighted in Table 4.3.

TABLE 4.3   Prominent Traits/Genes and Their Examples

Trait	Gene
Roundup ready	Bacterial EPSP
Golden rice	Complete pathway
Plant virus resistance	Viral coat protein
Male sterility	Barnase
Plant bacterial resistance	*p35*
Salt tolerance	*AtNHX1*

4.4.5.3 *Insertion Sequences*

Insertion sequences are part of transposons (sequences of DNA that can move around to different positions within the genome of a single cell in a process called transposition), which use insertion sequences to insert into another or another part of the genome. Transposons will carry other genes with them, e.g., genes for antibiotic resistance. Transposon exchange mutagenesis is known to be a potent tool for studying pathogen/plant interaction. The main advantage of transposon mutagenesis over chemical or irradiational mutagenesis is its ability to mark the location of genetic change caused (which is difficult to determine in chemical or irradiational mutagenesis). The insertion sequences include the selectable marker and the gene-of-interest coding region. During transformation these insertion sequences are used by *Agrobacteria* to create a DNA molecule (of desirable trait), which is inserted into the nucleus of a cell in the recipient plant tissue. Inactivation of transgene expression has often been observed in plants and seems to be especially problematic in cereal crops. A recent report suggested the transposition of insertion sequences (IS136) of *Agrobacterium tumefaciens* can cause the inactivation of the transgene [23]. Therefore, successful transformation is required for the stable expression of the transgene, which may further cause a proper cell developmental pathway to form a new plant, having stable existence as well as expression of sequences in each cell of the transformed tissue.

4.5 SCREENING METHOD OF GENOMIC LIBRARY

Genetic screening is one of the most powerful methods available for gaining insights into complex biological processes [24]. The principal use of cloning technology is to isolate specific a gene from the entire genome. For a 99% probability of getting one fragment each per clone, 1500 cloned fragments are needed with *Escherichia coli*, 4600 with yeast, and 800,000 with mammals. Techniques like chromosomal walking and colony hybridization [24] are employed for selecting a particular genome as follows.

4.5.1 Colony Hybridization

This is a type of DNA hybridization in which a radioactive probe is used to detect DNA sequence on a nitrocellulose filter. Sometimes this is also called a "colony filter" because in this process a filter is placed on the surface of agar plate and bacterial colonies are transferred to grow on the filter. In this method there is no need to purify the DNA from bacterial cells as bacterial colonies are directly grown and lyse on the nitrocellulose filters [24]. During lysing (alkali hydrolysis) DNA is denatured and binds directly to the filter. Radioactive probes are added to the filter discs. Hybridization takes place followed by washing of the filter to remove unbound probes [24]. The colonies that contain sequences complementary to the probe will bind the radioactive DNA. Hybridized probes can be visualized when the resulting filters are exposed to X-ray film. Finally, the desired colonies will be lit up on the autoradiograph.

4.5.2 Chromosome Walking

Primer walking is a method to determine the sequence of DNA up to the 1.3–7.0 kb range whereas chromosome walking is used to produce the clones of already known sequences

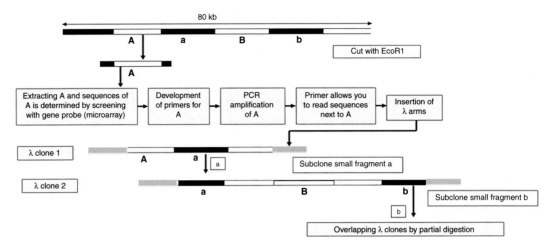

FIGURE 4.7   Chromosomal walking of DNA.

of the gene. Chromosome walking is a technique used to clone a gene (e.g., disease gene) from its known closest markers (e.g., known gene) and hence is used in moderate modifications in cloning and sequencing projects in plants, fungi, and animals. In another words, it is used to identify, isolate, and clone a particular sequence present in close vicinity of the gene to be mapped. Libraries of large fragments, mainly bacterial artificial chromosome libraries, are mostly used in genomic projects. To identify the desired colony and to select a particular clone the library is screened first with a desired probe. After screening, the clone is overlapped with the probe and overlapping fragments are mapped. These fragments are then used as a new probe (short DNA fragments obtained from the 3′ or 5′ ends of clones) to identify other clones. A library approximately consists of 96 clones and each clone contains a different insert. Probe one identifies λ1 and λ2 as it overlaps them (Fig. 4.5). Probe two derived from λ2 clones is used to identify λ3, and so on. Orientation of the clones is determined by restriction mapping of the clones. Thus, new chromosomal regions present in the vicinity of a gene could be identified. Protocol for chromosomal walking of DNA is described in Fig. 4.7. Since chromosomal walking is very tedious, chromosome landing is preferred for gene identification. This approach requires the identification of the marker that is tightly linked to mutant locus [25].

4.5.3 Blotting Techniques

In molecular biology and genetics, a blot is a method of transferring proteins, DNA or RNA, on a carrier (nitrocellulose polyvinylidene fluoride or nylon membrane). Blotting involves four major steps: (i) immobilization of samples (nucleic acid, proteins) on a solid support (nylon or nitrocellulose membranes; (ii) electrophoretic separation of nucleic acids in a gel, (iii) transfer of the separated components to a membrane; and (iv) detection of specific sequences by probing the membrane. Transfer and immobilization on the membrane make the nucleic acids available to probes used for detection, which do not readily enter the gel.

Southern and northern blotting are the two most common nucleic acid blotting techniques. Southern blotting is used to detect a sequence in a DNA mixture, and northern blotting detects a sequence in an RNA mixture. In contrast, western blotting is used for the separation of proteins.

4.5.3.1 Southern Blot Analysis

British biologist Edwin Southern (1975) gave the method for detecting DNA fragments in an agarose gel by blotting on a nylon or nitrocellulose membrane followed by detection with a probe of complementary DNA or RNA sequence [26]. In this method, DNA molecules are fragmented by restriction endonucleases and its fragments are separated on the basis of their size by agarose-gel electrophoresis. The fragments are denatured by alkali treatment and transferred to a nitrocellulose filter after their immobilization by heat treatment. Filter paper containing DNA fragments is incubated with radiolabeled probes in a buffer solution. Hybridized DNA can be visualized by autoradiography. The blotting technique has not changed since its first description, except for the availability of increasingly sophisticated blotting membranes, kits for labeling, and apparatus for electrophoresis transfer. Membranes originally used for DNA transfer were made of nitrocellulose. Due to the high nucleic acid binding capacity and physical strength, nylon-based membranes are preferred.

4.5.3.2 Northern Blot Analysis

This method was developed by George Stark et al. [27] at Stanford University. Protocols involved in southern and northern blotting analysis are quite similar except that RNA rather than DNA is blotted on the membrane. Northern blot involves the blotting of RNA separated by gel electrophoresis on nylon or nitrocellulose membranes followed by hybridization with nucleic acid (RNA or DNA) sequences. Blotting is carried out in such a way that the maximum amount of RNA sequences are bound covalently on chemically reactive paper. The RNA was blotted/immobilized on diazotized cellulose. As like southern blotting northern hybridization does not require denaturation of DNA before blotting, which makes the process less time consuming.

4.5.3.3 Immunoblotting or Proteins Blotting or Western Blotting

This technique was developed by Harry Towbin at the Friedrich Miescher Institute. Later on the name western blot was given to the technique by W. Neal Burnette [28,29]. Blotting of electrophoresed protein bands from a sodium dodecyl sulfate (SDS)-polyacrylamide gel on to nylon or nitrocellulose membrane and their detection with antibody probes is called western blotting. Western blotting is a method by which proteins that have been physically separated and subsequently immobilized on the surface of a membrane are probed for reactivity with different types of affinity reagents, such as antibodies and receptors, and are tested for the presence of interacting proteins in pure preparations or complex mixtures. Western blot analysis can analyze any protein sample whether from cells or tissues including recombinant proteins synthesized *in vitro*. Western blot is dependent on the quality of affinity reagents used to probe the protein of interest, and how specific they are for this protein. According to the protein of interest such reagents are commercially available. Availability of antibody or affinity reagent is obligatory for new proteins. For this process, a small amount of protein (either purified from cell extracts or made as a recombinant) and its respective antibody or affinity reagent are required. These vital antibodies specifically bind to the protein of interest instead of the thousands of proteins on the western blot. During the first step (electrophoresis), proteins are separated according to their differences in size, which results in the development of series of bands. Due to the large size of antibodies, a gel matrix does not allow them to enter, hence the sample proteins are transferred to a solid support. Superimposition of gel with nitrocellulose or nylon sheet under the application of an electric field leads to the migration of proteins from the gel to the sheet where they become bound. This step furnishes membranes of nitrocellulose having a similar pattern of proteins as in the gel. This technique has vast applications in the immune detection of proteins.

4.5.4 Dot Blot Technique

This technique is generally used to detect, analyze, and identify proteins. It is a simplified form of blotting technique in which biomolecules to be detected are not first separated by electrophoresis. This process assures the presence or absence of biomolecules that can be detected by the DNA probes or the antibody. However, it offers no information on the size of the target biomolecules. This process involves application of dot and subsequently hybridization and detection of proteins. DNA does not bind well to the filters, thus it is essential to denature the proteins. This technique is both easier to use and significantly less time consuming than other techniques. One of the recently reported applications of this technique was found in the detection of potato viruses and viroids, which is one of the major constraints for the improvement of potato (*Solanum tuberosum* L.) production worldwide [30]. By using the dot blot technique, spindle tuber viroids were recently detected in potato leaf tissue.

4.5.5 Techniques for Detection of Specific Proteins

4.5.5.1 Hybrid-Arrested Translation (HART)

The process of identification of recombinant DNA clones by their ability to hybridize and prevent the translation of a specific messenger RNA in a cell-free system is called HART [31]. In this technique, the mRNA molecule is incubated with recombinant plasmid DNA, which contains a sequence complementary to mRNA. As a result DNA/RNA hybrids are produced. A fraction of the mRNA acts as a probe, which will pick up the clones. After positive selection, a negative selection can be done by using mRNA from the same organisms but from a cell that does not represent the desired sequence. Any positively selected colonies that hybridize with negative probes are discarded. Even hybrids formed by positive selection could not be translated. The plasmids thus identified by the probe are missing from the translation product.

4.5.5.2 Hybrid-Released Translation (HRT)

Many situations arise in recombinant DNA research in which it is necessary to identify the mRNA encoded by a particular cloned DNA sequence. Cloned DNA fragments can be characterized by hybridization to mRNA, which is being further identified by translation *in vitro*. There are two different approaches for this procedure: (i) hybrid-arrest translation and (ii) hybrid-release translation. In the former, hybridization of cloned DNA to an mRNA population in solution can be used to identify the complementary mRNA, since the mRNA/DNA hybrid will not be translated *in vitro*. In the latter, cloned DNA bound to a solid support is used to isolate the complementary mRNA, which can then be eluted and translated *in vitro*. This technique is more sensitive than hybrid-arrested translation. The plasmid is fixed on a filter and incubated with mRNA, which is used as a probe. Washing is done to remove unbound probes. The bound mRNA is eluted and translated. This technique exploits the presence of a specific protein encoded by it [31].

4.5.6 *In vivo* RNA Interference

Nowadays, various improvement strategies and tools for genetic manipulation have become available. This results in the existence of powerful "toolboxes" for each model organism. RNA interference (RNAi) provides a powerful reverse genetics approach to analyze gene functions both in tissue culture and *in vivo* [32]. After the discovery of double-stranded RNAs (dsRNAs), RNAi-based methods were added to the toolboxes of various organisms. These methods have several advantages such as relative ease, and provide a powerful reverse genetic approach especially for organisms in which genetics is difficult. In plants such as *Caenorhabditis elegans* RNAi is both systemic and heritable [32]. The focus of *in vivo* RNAi applications in plants is directed toward the improvement of plant productivity and/or nutritional value. Among the exciting applications in which RNAi could have a major impact in agriculture is the improvement of essential food crops such as corn and rice.

4.6 ELECTROPHORESIS TECHNIQUES

4.6.1 Agarose Gel Electrophoresis

Agarose gel electrophoresis is one of several physical methods for determining the size of DNA. In this method, DNA is forced to migrate through a highly cross-linked agarose matrix in response to an electric current. In solution, the phosphates of the DNA are negatively charged, and the molecule will therefore migrate to the positive (red) pole. There are three factors that affect migration rate through a gel: size of the DNA, conformation of the DNA, and ionic strength of the running buffer. Construction of agarose electrophoresis is mentioned in Fig. 4.8.

4.6.2 Pulsed Field Electrophoresis

Recently, there has been great demand for those techniques that can easily analyze the entire genomes. Apart from *Arabidopsis* and rice genome analysis, progress in determining the complete genome in plants is slow. Among the successful techniques, pulsed field gel electrophoresis (PFGE) is currently used. Schwartz and Cantor introduced PFGE for the purpose of separation of several megabase-sized DNA molecules [33]. Foundation of this technology is based on standard agarose gel electrophoresis, used for separation of nucleic acids. This conventional agarose-mediated separation cannot resolve fragments greater than 20 kb. Because of the incapability of large DNA to migrate through agarose gel matrix like smaller ones, simple agar electrophoresis fails to separate the large or long DNA molecules. A steady

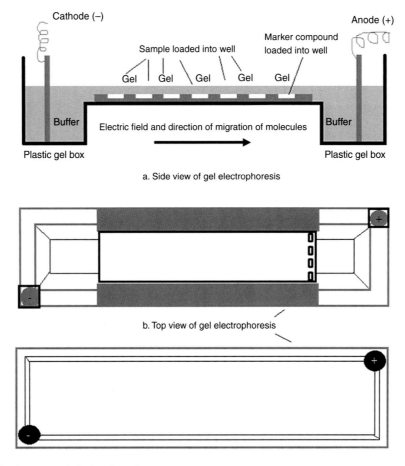

FIGURE 4.8   **Agarose gel electrophoresis.**

electric field is one more factor that stretches them out so that they travel in a snake-like fashion. This mode of migration is called as repatation. Agarose gel with low concentrations of agarose (0.1–0.2%) is capable of resolving extremely large DNA. However, such gels are quite fragile and must be run very slowly; and even then they are incapable of resolving linear DNA molecules larger than 750 kb in length. In the PFGE method by pulsed alternating orthogonal electric fields, DNA molecules are forced to reorient before continuing to move snake-like through the gel. This type of electric field, when applied to gel, forces the molecule to reorient before continuing in a snake-like fashion through the gel. During this reorientation period larger DNA molecules take longer to move slowly through the gel. Large DNA molecules become trapped in their reptation tubes and the electric field is altered every time. The larger the DNA molecule, the longer the time required for this alignment. However, in conventional electrophoresis a single electric field is required, which limits the separation range to kilobases. Separation in PFGE is achieved by applying twin-perpendicularly oriented electric fields in an alternating mode to separate chromosome up to 2000 kb.

4.6.3 Field Inversion Gel Electrophoresis

This technique was introduced by Carle et al. [34] using apparatus in which there was a provision of periodic inversion of a single electric field. The applied field is uniform in both directions. The forward pulse is slightly longer than the reverse pulse resulting in the movement of the DNA along a perfectly straight track. This technique resolves DNA fragments up to 2000 kb in length.

4.6.4 Vertical Pulse Field Gradient Electrophoresis

This was designed and developed by Gardiner et al., using two oppositely positioned electrodes in such a manner that when electric field is switched DNA moves toward another set of electrodes, which results in a zigzag movement of DNA from the traveling point to the bottom of the gel. There is no horizontal distortion of the DNA because the entire DNA is exposed to an equivalent electric field [35].

4.6.5 Counter Clamped Homogeneous Electric Field Gel Electrophoresis

In this technique the electric field is generated from various electrodes that are arranged in a square or hexagonal contour around the horizontal gel and are clamped to predetermined potential [36]. This leads to the development of a homogeneous electric field, which makes it possible to resolve DNA molecules up to 5000 kb in length.

4.6.6 Polyacrylamide Gel Electrophoresis

Chemically inert polyacrylamide gel (porous gel) is formed by polymerization of acrylamide at a particular concentration in the presence of cross-linking agent (methylene bisacrylamide), which can further control the pore size of the gel. In this process proteins are applied to porous polyacrylamide gel and separated in an electric field. When proteins are placed in an electric field they are separated on the basis of their size and net electric charge. Since the whole process is carried out in a gel, this type of separation serves as a molecular sieve, i.e., small molecules move faster through the pores as compared to large molecules.

4.6.7 Isoelectric Focusing

The isoelectric point is the point at which the overall charge of the protein is zero (a neutral charge). Separation of proteins at the isoelectric point is called isoelectric focusing. In isoelectric focusing a gradient of pH and an electric potential are applied across the gel, making one end more positive than the other. Separation occurs on the basis of the positive or negative groups present on the molecule. If they are positively charged, they will be pulled toward the more negative end of the gel and if they are negatively charged they will be pulled to the more positive end of the gel. The proteins applied in the first dimension will migrate through the gel and will accumulate at their isoelectric point. At this stage the protein net charge is zero and therefore does not move in an electric field.

4.6.8 2-D Gel Electrophoresis

In 2-D gel electrophoresis a sample is first subjected to isoelectric focusing and then sodium dodecyl sulfate polyacrylamide gel electrophoresis (SDS-PAGE) to obtain very high resolution separations. Sample proteins are first placed on the strip of gel containing polyampholytes where proteins are separated on the basis of isoelectric focusing. This process begins with 1-D electrophoresis when sample proteins/molecules lie along a lane followed by the 2-D electrophoresis when the sample is spread out across a 2-D gel and separation of the molecules occurs in a direction 90° from the first. Generally, electrophoresis separation is based on the properties of the protein molecules that are meant for separation, e.g., mass and charge. During the separation a single band/spot is produced if either the mass (SDS-PAGE) or charge (isoelectric focusing) of two different proteins is similar. Therefore, combination of these techniques provides 2-D separation of the proteins, which is more effective than 1-D electrophoresis.

4.7 POLYMERASE CHAIN REACTION

Polymerase chain reaction (PCR) is an amplification technique for cloning the specific or targeted parts of a DNA sequence to generate thousands to millions of copies of DNA of interest. It is based on cell-free *in vitro* fast cloning and replication of both strands of DNA in the test tube rather than the living cell like *E. coli*. This technique was conceived by Kary Mullis of Cetus Corporation in 1983 and was awarded the Nobel Prize in 1993 [37]. The key feature of the PCR technique is the exponential nature of amplification. This rapid amplification and production of pure DNA of interest is achieved by a repetitive series of thermal cycling, which involves three major steps: denaturation of DNA duplex at 94°C, annealing of oligonucleotide primers to the target sequences of separated DNA strands, and DNA synthesis from the 3-OH end of each primer by DNA polymerase at 72°C. In order to perform PCR we must know the portion of DNA sequence that we wish to replicate. Afterwards short DNA fragments or primers (short oligonucleotides) are synthesized from the nucleotides' base pair. These primers are complementary to the sequence of the DNA that is to amplified. Four kinds of deoxyribonucleotides and primers, which contain a complementary sequence of the target sequence, are added to the solution. This process is conducted in an Eppendorf tube and later placed in an automated piece of equipment called a thermocycler in which thermal cycling, consisting of cycles of repeated heating and cooling reaction for DNA melting and enzymatic replication of the DNA, occurs. Primers enable selective and repeated amplification of the targeted sequence. As PCR progresses, the DNA generated is itself used as a template for replication, setting in motion a chain reaction in which the DNA template is exponentially amplified. PCR can be extensively modified to perform a wide array of genetic manipulations. This technique has become an advantageous tool to amplify a selected DNA sequence in a multifold genome without involving the bacterial cells. It is completely performed *in vitro*. PCR is a much faster method than gene cloning. This process can only be initiated when the complementary sequence of the targeted sequence is known. A heat stable enzyme DNA polymerase, which is functional at 50–70°C, catalyzes these reactions. DNA polymerase is extracted from species of a bacteria living in hot springs at a temperature of 90°C. It is added to the solution

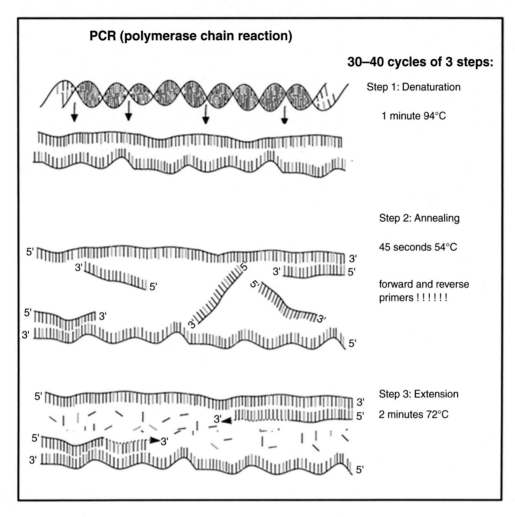

PCR (polymerase chain reaction)

30–40 cycles of 3 steps:

Step 1: Denaturation

1 minute 94°C

Step 2: Annealing

45 seconds 54°C

forward and reverse
primers ! ! ! ! ! !

Step 3: Extension

2 minutes 72°C

FIGURE 4.9   Polymerase chain reaction.

of Tris-HCl buffer containing the double-stranded DNA with targeted nucleotide sequence.
The whole technique is described in Fig. 4.9.

The polymerase reaction proceeds in the following steps:

- The DNA is heated for 30 s to separate its strands at 94°C.
- The separated strands of DNA are allowed to cool for 1.5 min at 52°C, which facilitates
  binding of primers by hydrogen bond at the ends of the target sequences.
- DNA polymerase or Taq DNA polymerase catalyzes the addition of nucleotides to the
  primers by taking the longer DNA sequence as templates. This process completes in 1
  min at 72°C. This reaction cycles for more than 20 min. The products of the first cycle of
  replication are denatured, annealed to oligonucleotide primers, and replicated with DNA

polymerase. This reaction is recycled until sufficient amplification of targeted sequence is achieved.

- This whole process is repeated, which results in four copies. The process is repeated at least 20 times or more depending upon the desired quantity of targeted sequence of DNA, resulting in eight after three cycles, 16 after four cycles, 1024 after 10 cycles, and so on.

Objectives of gene cloning and PCR are quite similar. PCR is very fast and takes less time (1 day) in isolating the gene than gene cloning (which usually takes 2–3 months). But still, PCR acquires some disadvantages such as: for designing primers the nucleotide sequences of the targeted part of the DNA should be known, slight contamination of the DNA sample can furnish inaccurate results, and it is difficult to amplify long stretches through PCR.

4.8 MICROARRAY

DNA microarray, DNA chips, gene chips, or biochip is a collection of high-density microscopic single-stranded DNA attached to a solid surface by biochemical analysis. The microarray was introduced by Chang [38]. It is derived from either cDNA (cDNA microarray) or synthesized short oligonucleotides (oligonucleotide microarray). In this technique cDNA or RNA (molecules of known sequences or probe, reporters, oligos, or antisense RNA) covalently attached on the solid surface. Each DNA spot contains picomoles (10^{-12} moles) of a specific DNA sequence. The experimental DNA or RNA (unknown sequences or test, target, or sample DNA or RNA) are tagged with fluorescent dye and poured over the probe area for hybridization. Probe-target hybridization is usually detected and quantified by techniques like autoradiography, laser scanning, fluorescence, and enzyme detection devices. Such techniques can be used to read the chip surface and hybridization pattern. The outline of a microarray is highlighted in Fig. 4.10. Scientists use DNA microarrays to measure the expression levels of large numbers of genes or their multiple regions simultaneously. Several approaches (photolithography, mechanical microspotting, and ink jetting) are used to manufacture microarrays for exploring their diverse applications in gene expression analysis, DNA sequencing, characterization of mutants, diagnostics and genetic mapping, proteomics, and agricultural biotechnology.

4.9 CRYOPRESERVATION

Generally, cryopreservation is a method of storing sperm cells in order to preserve them for artificial insemination during animal breeding programs [39]. Regular extinction of rare and economic plant species demands a modern technique for preserving genetic resources of the plant kingdom especially agricultural/medicinal plants. Old methods used for the storage of genetic resources are restricted since they fail to prevent losses caused by climatic and natural disorders, pathogens and pest attack, and economic and political grounds. In addition the viability of short-lived seeds of economic plants could not be saved by the conventional methods, e.g., coffee species, rubber (*Hevea brasiliensis*), oil palm (*Elaeis guineensis*),

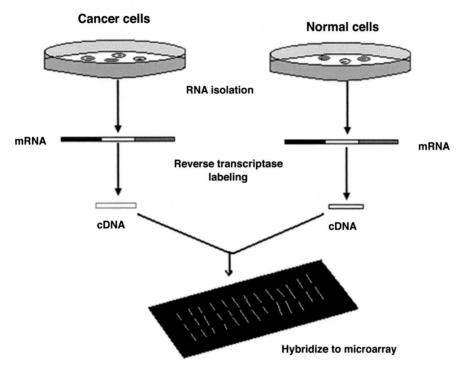

FIGURE 4.10 Microarray.

and various citrus species. The introduction of various methods such as the slow growth method, cryopreservation (Greek *krayos*, meaning frost), and various other freezing methods allows the long-term preservation of germplasms without affecting their viability. In cryopreservation, cells are preserved in the frozen state by bringing the plant cells and tissue cultures to a zero metabolism or nondividing state. This is achieved by reducing the temperature in the presence of cryoprotectants. Meristematic, thin-walled, highly cytoplasmic, and small nonvacuolated cells with small aggregates and high cell density are always selected for cryopreservation. In plant tissue culture cryopreservation is generally used for the storage of germplasm at very low temperature. This low temperature could be achieved by using solid carbon dioxide (at $-79°C$), low temperature deep freezers (at $-80°C$), nitrogen vapor (at $-150°C$), and liquid nitrogen (at $-196°C$). Among these the most commonly used method of cryopreservation is by employing liquid nitrogen. The cells stay in a completely inactive state at the temperature of liquid nitrogen (at $-196°C$) and thus can be conserved for a prolonged period. Various types of tissue can be used for cryopreservation, e.g., ovules, seeds, cultured plant cells, protoplasts, calli, meristems, embryos, and endosperms. Compounds like DMSO (dimethyl sulfoxide), mannose, glucose, praline, acetamide, glycerol, ethylene, propylene, sucrose, etc., are added during cryopreservation. Such compounds that prevent cryodestruction (by freezing or thawing) by reducing the freezing point and supercooling point of water are called cryoprotectants. Cryoprotectants are always used in combination at low concentrations as a single cryoprotectant at high concentration could be toxic. During the course of treatment, the cultures should be maintained in ice to avoid deleterious effects. This freeze preservation technique is based on the transfer of water present in the cells from a liquid to solid state. Due to the presence of salts and organic molecules in the cells, the cell water requires a much lower temperature ($-68°C$) to remain in the liquid state. Storage at such a low temperature slows down or halts the metabolic process and biological deteriorations in the cells/tissues. For freezing the specimen a degree of intracellular freeze tolerance and ice crystal formation within the cell should always be considered. Regulated rate of cooling or prefreezing is done to avoid this problem. Nowadays, programmed freezers that allow the uniform decrease in temperature at a desired rate (not less than $1°C$ per minute) are also available. During the storage stage, cells are stored at sufficiently low temperature to stop all metabolic activity and avoid additional injury to the cultures. Storage of frozen materials for longer periods is achieved when the temperature is lower than $-130°C$. This can be simply achieved with the help of liquid nitrogen, which keeps the temperature at $-196°C$. Afterwards thawing is required for releasing the vials containing cultures from the frozen state to elevate the temperature between 35 and $40°C$. Thawing is done rapidly to avoid overheating. The vials are transferred into a water bath at $0°C$ when the last ice crystal disappears. After thawing the plant materials are washed to remove the toxic effects of the cryoprotectants. This process includes dilution, resuspension, centrifugation, and removal of cells. Determination of cell viability in growth medium at this stage is essential as some cells die due to storage stress and only the most stable ones survive. Regeneration of plantlets is achieved by culturing viable cells on nonspecific growth media. Bajaj has demonstrated the list of works on cryopreservation of cells, tissue, and organ culture of various plants, e.g., potato, cassava, sugarcane, soybean, groundnut, carrot, cotton, citrus, coconut, etc. [40].

Cryopreservation has been successfully applied to germplasm conservation of vegetatively propagated crops, recalcitrant producing plants, rare plant species, medicinal, horticultural and forest plants, and VAM fungi in liquid nitrogen on a long-term basis. This can be achieved by the establishment of a plant cell bank (i.e., germplasm bank and cell cryobank). Collaboration of some germplasm-producing institutes at national and international levels is also required. This collaboration could be responsibility for the storage, maintenance, distribution, and exchange of these disease-free germplasms of the important plants. These types of institutes are called germplasm banks, where the facilities of on demand cryopreservation of genetic resources of a variety of plants are available. Large sized cylinders (30–50-liter capacity) of liquid nitrogen are present in these banks to preserve genetic stocks of plants. In addition to germplasm banks, pollen grain storage in liquid nitrogen and pollen bank establishment have also been suggested to retain their viability for various lengths of time. This type of conservation facilitates maintenance of germplasm and enhancement of longevity and hybridization between plants with flowering at different times and growth at different places, reducing the dissemination of diseases by pollination vectors [40]. An outline of cryopreservation and its applications is highlighted in Figs 4.11 and 4.12.

Various problems do occur, such as the high specific feature of plant cells (large size, strong vacuolization, and abundance of water); chances of cell damage/dehydration during freezing and subsequent thawing; gradual large crystals formation (greater than 0.1 mm may rupture many cell organelles and membranes); increase in concentration of intracellular solute; and leakage of vital solutes during the freezing process. Reduced temperature and presence

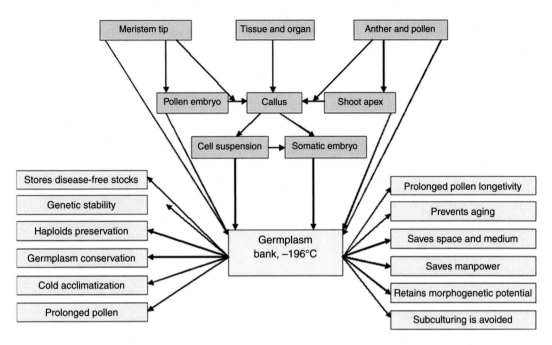

FIGURE 4.11 Potential and prospects of cryopreservation of plant cell, tissue, and organ, and establishment of the germplasm bank.

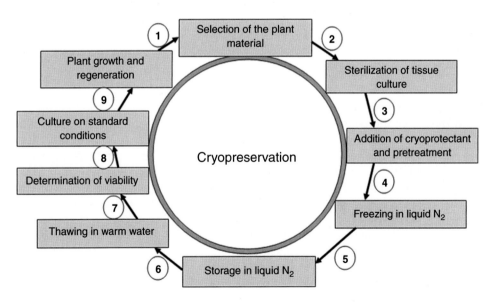

FIGURE 4.12 Steps (1–9) involved in cryopreservation.

TABLE 4.4   Applications of Cryopreservation in Plant Tissue Culture

Sr. no.	Type of cryopreservation	Cryopreserved material/specimen
	Cryopreservation of cell lines	Cell suspensions (soybean, tobacco, *Datura*, carrot) and somatic hybrid protoplasts (rice × pea, wheat × pea)
	Cryopreservation of pollen and pollen embryos	Fruit crops, trees, mustard, carrot, peanut, etc.
	Cryopreservation of excised meristems	Potato, sugarcane, chickpea, peanut, etc.
	Cryopreservation of germplasm of vegetatively propagated crops	Potato, sugarcane, etc.
	Cryopreservation of recalcitrant seeds and embryos	Large sized seeds that are short lived and abortive, such as oil palm, coconut, walnut, mango, and cocoa

of cryoprotectants favor the marked dehydration (free water has enough time to leave the cells) and protoplast shrinkage of plant cells.

4.9.1 Applications

Bajaj reported a variety of plant materials, namely root/shoot tip propagules (tubers), pollen grains, cell suspension clones, calli, tissues, somatic embryos, etc. which can be successfully cryopreserved in liquid nitrogen for prolonged periods and tested for their survival and regeneration potential [40] (Table 4.4).

4.10 AUTORADIOGRAPHY

In general terms visualization of the pattern of distribution of radiation is called radiography. In the conventional X-ray technique the sample to be examined was placed between the source of radiation and the film. Thereafter, absorption and scattering of radiation by the sample produces its image on the film. However, in autoradiography X-ray, gamma (γ) or beta (β) rays form the radiation and the recording medium is a photographic film. The sample itself is the source of the radiation, which originates from radioactive material incorporated into it. The medium used for the recording, which makes visible the resultant image, is usually, though not always, photographic emulsion. Now, any biological compound can be labeled with radioactive isotopes opening up many possibilities in the study of living systems. Autoradiography has tremendous applications in plant science. In this respect the utilization of this technique for discovering the path of carbon in photosynthesis was first made by Melvin Calvin, who received the Noble Prize in 1961 [41]. Calvin discovered the path of carbon in photosynthesis and reported that ribulosebisphosphate was the first acceptor of CO_2 and phosphoglyceric acid was the first stable compound produced. Using this technique of autoradiography, Calvin found that ^{14}C turned up in glucose molecules within 30 s after the start of photosynthesis. This was a major breakthrough in the field of plant science. Later on autoradiography was widely utilized in biology at the macroscopic level to study the uptake of radioactive tracers by both plant and animal organs.

4.11 OTHER TECHNIQUES

The following is a list of other plant tissue culture techniques: recombinant DNA and monoclonal antibody procedure; column chromatography; immunocytochemistry; ELISA; spectrophotometry (quantitation; enzyme kinetics); nucleic acid purification and molecular weight determinations; cell separation methods; protein separation and quantitation; liquid scintillation (double label) counting; autoradiography (cellular and gross); restriction enzyme mapping; gene expression; and oligonucleotide synthesis.

References

[1] Reed BM, Tanpraser P. Detection and control of bacterial contaminants of plant tissue cultures. A review of recent literature. Plant Tiss Cult Biotechnol 1995;3:137–42.

[2] Baumgartner JG. Heat sterilised reducing sugars and their effects on the thermal resistance of bacteria. J Bacteriol 1938;36:369–82.

[3] Mackey BM, Derrick CM. Peroxide sensitivity of cold-shocked Salmonella typhimurium and *Escherichia coli* and its relationship to minimal medium recovery. J Appl Bacteriol 1986;60:501–11.

[4] Dodds JH, Roberts LW. Experiments in plant tissue culture. 2nd ed. Cambridge, UK: Cambridge University; 1985. p. 29-31.

[5] Khanuja SPS, Shasany AK, Darokar MP, Kumar S. Rapid isolation of DNA from dry and fresh samples of plants producing large amounts of secondary metabolites and essential oils. Plant Mol Biol Rep 1999;17:1–7.

[6] Semagn K, Bjørnstad Å, Ndjiondjop MN. An overview of molecular marker methods for plants. Afr J Biotechnol 2006;5(25):2540–68.

[7] Jha TB, Ghosh B, editors. Plant tissue culture basic and applied. New Delhi, India: University Press; 2005. p. 163–4.

[8] Veluthambi K, Gupta KA, Sharma A. The current status of plant transformation technologies. Curr Sci 2003;84(3):368–80.

[9] US patent 3799758, Franz JE, 'N-phosphonomethyl-glycine phytotoxicant compositions', issued 1974-03-26, assigned to Monsanto Company.

[10] Richard S, Moslemi S, Sipahutar H, Benachour N, Seralini GE. Differential effects of glyphosate and Roundup on human placental cells and aromatase. Environ Health Perspect 2005;113(6):716–20.

[11] Samsel A, Seneff S. Glyphosate, pathways to modern diseases II: celiac sprue and gluten intolerance. Interdiscip Toxicol 2013;6(4):159–84.

[12] Schönbrunn E, Eschenburg S, Shuttleworth WA, Schloss JV, Amrhein N, Evans JN, Kabsch W. Interaction of the herbicide glyphosate with its target enzyme 5-enolpyruvylshikimate 3-phosphate synthase in atomic detail. Proc Natl Acad Sci USA 2001;98(4):1376–80.

[13] Funke T, Han H, Healy-Fried ML, Fischer M, Schönbrunn E. Molecular basis for the herbicide resistance of Roundup Ready crops. PNAS 2006;1039(35):13010–5.

[14] Avni A, Blazquez M. Can plant biotechnology help in solving our food and energy shortage in the future? Curr Opin Biotechnol 2011;22:1–2.

[15] Kirakosyan A, Cseke LJ, Kaufman PB. The Use of Plant Cell Biotechnology for the Production of Phytochemicals. In: Kirakosyan A, Kaufman PB, editors. Recent Advances in Plant Biotechnology. Springer; 2009. p. 15–33.

[16] Liu W, Yuan JS, Stewart JCN. Advanced genetic tools for plant biotechnology. Nat Rev Genet 2013;14:781–93.

[17] Singh KB. Transcriptional regulation in plants: the importance of combinatorial control. Plant Physiol 1998;118:1111–20.

[18] Mitsuhara I, Ugaki M, Hirochika H, Ohshima M, Murakami T, Gotoh Y, et al. Efficient promoter cassettes for enhanced expression of foreign genes in dicotyledonous and monocotyledonous plants. Plant Cell Physiol 1996;37(1):49–59.

[19] Anuar MR, Ismail I, Zainal Z. Expression analysis of the 35S CaMV promoter and its derivatives in transgenic hairy root cultures of cucumber (*Cucumis sativus*) generated by *Agrobacterium rhizogenes* infection. Afr J Biotechnol 2011;10(42):8236–44.

[20] Qu LQ, Xing YP, Liu WX, Xu XP, Song YR. Expression pattern and activity of six glutelin gene promoters in transgenic rice. J Exp Bot 2008;59(9):2417–24.

[21] Bruce BD. The paradox of plastid transit peptides: conservation of function despite divergence in primary structure. Biochim Biophys Acta (BBA) – Mol Cell Res 2001;1541(1–2):2–21.

[22] Sundar IK, Sakthivel N. Advances in selectable marker genes for plant transformation. J Plant Physiol 2008;165:1698–716.

[23] Rawat P, Kumar S, Pental D, Burma PK. Inactivation of a transgene due to transposition of insertion sequence (IS136) of *Agrobacterium tumefaciens*. J Biosci 2009;34(2):199–202.

[24] Campbell TN, Choy FYM. Approaches to library screening. J Mol Microbiol Biotechnol 2002;4(6):551–4.

[25] Arencibia A, editor. Plant genetic engineering: towards the third millennium. Amsterdam: Elsevier Science; 2000. p. 65.

[26] Southern EM. Detection of specific sequences among DNA fragments separated by gel electrophoresis. J Mol Biol 1975;98:503–17.

[27] Alwine JC, Kemp DJ, Stark GR. Method for detection of specific RNAs in agarose gels by transfer to diazobenzyloxymethyl-paper and hybridization with DNA probes. Proc Natl Acad Sci USA 1977;74(12):5350–4.

[28] Towbin H, Staehelin T, Gordon J. Electrophoretic transfer of proteins from polyacrylamide gels to nitrocellulose sheets: procedure and some applications. Proc Natl Acad Sci USA 1979;76(9):4350–4.

[29] Burnette WN. Western blotting: electrophoretic transfer of proteins from sodium dodecyl sulfate-polyacrylamide gels to unmodified nitrocellulose and radiographic detection with antibody and radioiodinated protein A. Analyt Biochem 1981;112(2):195–203.

[30] Bernardy MG, Jacoli GG, Ragetli HWJ. Rapid detection of potato spindle tuber viroid (PSTV) by dot blot hybridization. J Phytopathol 1987;118(2):171–80.

[31] Dudley K. Hybrid-arrested translation. Methods Mol Biol 1988;4:39–45.

[32] Perrimon N, Ni JQ, Perkins L. *In vivo* RNAi: today and tomorrow. Cold Spring Harb Perspect Biol 2010;2(8). a003640.

[33] Schwartz DC, Cantor CR. Separation of yeast chromosome sized DNA by pulse field gradient gel electrophoresis. Cell 1984;37:67–75.

[34] Carle GF, Frank M, Olson MV. Electrophoretic separation of large DNA molecules by periodic inversion of large DNA molecules by periodic inversion of electric field. Science 1986;232:65.

[35] Gardiner A, Lass RW, Patterson D. Function of large mammalian DNA restriction fragments using vertical pulse field gradient gel electrophoresis. Somat Cell Mol Gene 1986;12:185.

[36] Chu G, Vollrath D, Davis RW. Separation of large DNA molecule by contour clamped homogeneous electric fields. Science 1986;234:1582–5.

[37] Bartlett JMS, Stirling D. A short history of the polymerase chain reaction. PCR Protocols 2003;226:3–6.

[38] Chang TW. Binding of cells to matrixes of distinct antibodies coated on solid surface. J Immunol Meth 1983;65(1–2):217–23.

[39] Polge C. Low-temperature storage of mammalian spermatozoa. Royal Society of London 1957;147(929):498–508.

[40] Bajaj YPS. Cryopreservation of plant cell cultures and its prospects in agricultural and forest biotechnology. In: Natesh S, editor. Biotechnology in agriculture. New Delhi, India: Oxford & IBH Publishing Co. Pvt. Ltd; 1987. p. 109–31.

[41] Calvin M. The photosynthetic cycle. Bull Soc Chim Biol 1956;38(11):1233–44.

5

Application of Plant Biotechnology

Saurabh Bhatia

Modern Applications of Plant Biotechnology in Pharmaceutical Sciences. http://dx.doi.org/10.1016/B978-0-12-802221-4.00005-4

5.1 INTRODUCTION

Plant cells maintain totipotency and developmental plasticity in the differentiated state. They have the ability to dedifferentiate, proliferate, and subsequently regenerate into mature plants under appropriate culture conditions. The concept of *in vitro* growth of plant cells was introduced by Haberlandt [1]. This concept recently evolved into a powerful tool utilized throughout the plant sciences. In response to the optimum culture condition plants can initiate cell proliferation and development from diverse tissues. *In vitro* experimentation of plant cell and tissue culture provides enormous applications in basic and applied research (Fig. 5.1). These applications can be exploited in diverse areas. Plant tissue culture was earlier utilized for basic research to study cell division, plant growth, and biochemistry. Over the years the technology has grown and is being widely implemented on a more applied scale. The strategy of media manipulation is a frequent way to experiment its diverse applications. The advent of the latest technology diversifies tissue culture applications in several areas. Advancement in genetic engineering provides several genetic tools for deriving more applications from tissue culture science. These tools can be utilized to understand the molecular pathways or plant physiology or variation (somaclonal variation) in plant cell or tissue during its development under *in vitro* conditions. Such research forms the fundamental applications of *in vitro* technology so as to study tissue morphology and its biochemical and somatic cell genetics. Furthermore, concepts like transgenesis, somatic hybridization, mutant selection, metabolic engineering, somatic embryogenesis, organogenesis, molecular pharming, and phytoremediation enhance the further utilization of *in vitro* technology in plant science. Exploration and categorization of such broad applications allow the maximum though specified utilization of this technology. Plant tissue culture is a vast area and hence it covers vast applications (Fig. 5.1).

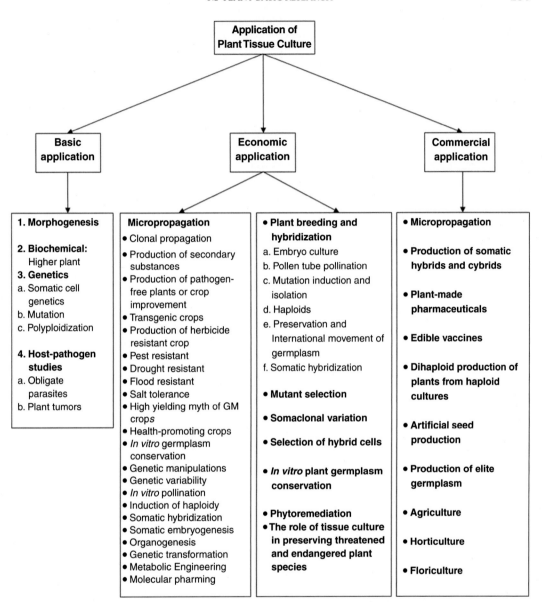

FIGURE 5.1 Illustration of several applications of plant tissue culture in the basic and applied research.

5.2 PLANT BASIC RESEARCH

5.2.1 Morphological Aspects

In vitro experimentation on plant cell or tissue is a good means of understanding the factors responsible for cell differentiation and organ formation. In contrast to animal cells, plant cells are highly mature and differentiated, retain the ability to change to a mersitematic state, and differentiate into a whole plant. Cultures of such cells offer valuable information on morphogenesis and plant development. During this process when explants (differentiated tissue) are implanted on an artificial nutrient medium, its nondividing, differentiated, quiescent cells first undergo changes to achieve the meristematic state. Cells of the meristematic state derived from mature cells further form a mass of cells called *callus* and the process is called *dedifferentiation*. As the cells of the explants are multicellular, the callus formed will be heterogeneous. The potential of the callus cell to differentiate into whole plant or an organ is called as *redifferentiation*. As illustrated in Fig. 5.2, morphological variation under *in vitro* conditions depends on the extent of transitions between these events. Development of plant cells *in vitro* begins with vascular differentiation, which is also called *cytodifferentiation* followed by organogenic and embryogenic differentiation (Figs 5.3 and 5.4). Vascular differentiation is governed by various factors. This process involves an array of steps that begins with cell elongation of parenchymatous cells followed by cell wall thickening and cell autolysis, and finally formation of tracheary elements. Since the process promotes xylem formation it is also known as *xylogenesis*. Depending upon the growth conditions organogenic differentiation leads to the formation of either shoot bud or embryo (Figs 5.3 and 5.4). Thus, whole studies on molecular, physiological, and biochemical aspects of cells in culture have contributed to an in-depth understanding of cytodifferentiation, organogenesis, and somatic embryogenesis. Several theories have been proposed (Skoog and Miller; hormonal control in organogenesis) [2]. These theories are also helpful in understanding the morphological application of plant biotechnology. Another important application of plant tissue culture is micropropagation. In a continuous process hundreds of cultures are raised from small amounts of tissue. Ball successfully raised transplantable

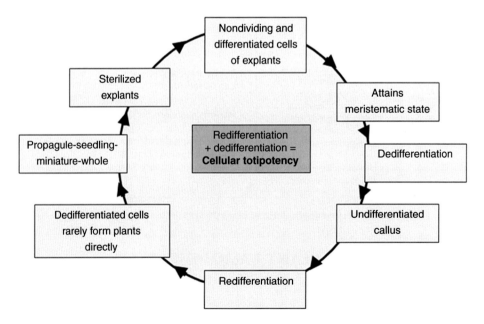

FIGURE 5.2   Development state of plant during its *in vitro* growth.

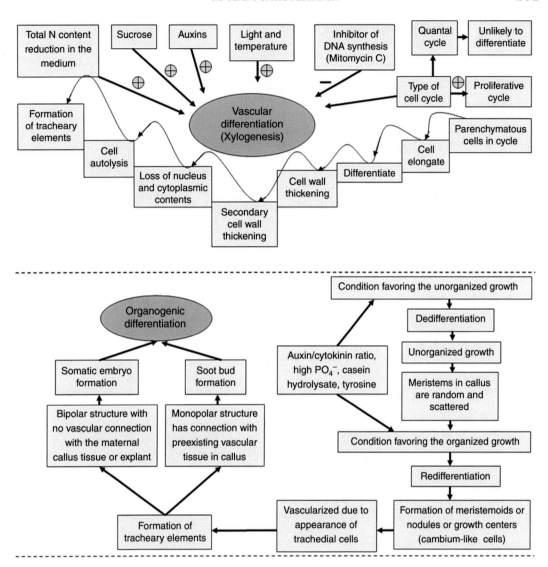

FIGURE 5.3 Illustration demonstrating the factors affecting the vascular differentiation and events involved in cytogenesis (vascular differentiation) and organogenesis.

whole plant of *Lupines* and *Tropaeolum* by culturing their shoot stem [3]. The potential of this for rapid propagation of orchids was soon realized by Morel [4]. The advantage of using this method was that about 4 million genetically identified plants could be obtained from a single bud. In the United States Murashige [5] has developed standard methods of propagation in *in vitro* species in which cytokinin supplementation led to the formation of lateral branches in shoot culture. This was exploited intensively by the horticulture and nursery

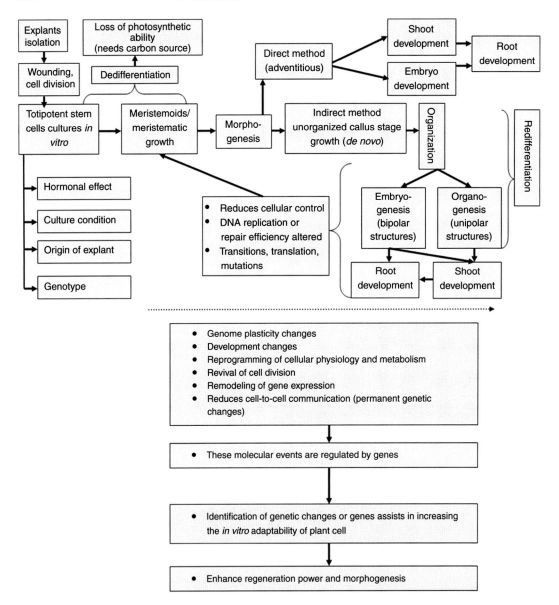

FIGURE 5.4   Molecular events followed by the plant during *in vitro* growth representing its genomic variation due to cellular reprogramming and many other processes.

industry for rapid clonal propagation of many dicotyledons, monocotyledons, and gymnosperms. Attempts are also directed at development of somatic embryogenesis systems for mass propagation of plants. Rapid multiplication is only possible in automated bioreactors with low inputs. These embryos can be singly encapsulated in suitable chemical composition for use as synthetic seeds.

5.2.2 Biochemical Studies

Biochemical attributes are indicators of morphogenetic potential, growth, and differentiation, representing differential gene action/expression or change in endogenous level of growth regulators in cell cultures and are used for analysis of gene function and metabolic regulation. Biochemical studies also facilitated in-depth understanding of organogenesis, cell cycle, and chromosomal changes in cultured cells and also reexamined neoplastic growth in cell culture [6–10]. Plant regeneration from *in vitro* cell and tissue culture is confined to a limited number of cells in some regions. Hence, selection of morphogenetically competent cell lines is important for plant regeneration. Changes in various biochemical parameters such as enzymes (peroxidase, IAA oxidase, β-amylase, α-amylase, glucose 6-phosphatase), hormones (auxins, cytokines, gibberellins, and others), and water soluble proteins affect the growth and development of plants, for example, marked reduction in number of attributes such as starch, protein, amylase, invertase, malate dehydrogenase, peroxidase, and phosphorylase with a subsequent increase in sugar level and amino acid content precedes in *in vitro* shoot propagation. Some of the key biochemicals that precedes the onset of embryogenesis/organogenesis can serve as markers of the differentiation process that brings about, morphological, developmental, and functional specialization. Thus, plant science sets a relationship between these biochemicals and their respective growth; therefore, identification of these key biomarkers is necessary for promoting specific growth in plants.

5.2.3 Somatic Cell Genetics

The study of mechanisms of inheritance in plants by using cells in culture is called *somatic cell genetics*. In such cells, chromosomes and genes can be reprogrammed by parasexual methods, rather than having to depend upon chromosome segregation and genetic recombination (which occur during the meiotic cell divisions preceding gamete formation and sexual reproduction). Genetic analysis is concerned with the role of genes and chromosomes in the development and function of individuals and the evolution of species. Genetic analysis of complex multicellular organisms classically required multiple-generation families, and fairly large numbers of progeny of defined matings, to be scored. As a result, analysis of plants with long generation times, small families, or lack of controlled matings was difficult and slow. Somatic cell genetics circumvents many of these limitations. It has enhanced the scope and speed of genetic analysis in higher plants, especially when combined with the powerful techniques of molecular biology to generate fertile plants from single cultured cells. With these methods, every gene in any species of interest can be identified and mapped to its position on a particular chromosome, its functions determined, and its evolutionary relationships to genes in other species revealed. Some of the important methods used in somatic cell genetics are mutant isolation, somatic hybridization, and transformation.

5.2.3.1 Mutant Isolation

The capability of applying biochemical selection to a large, nearly homogenous population of cells grown in a dish allows efficient recovery of rare events like genetic mutants. In this manner, mutants of immediate application, such as herbicide-resistant strains, have been isolated. In other instances, mutants altered in biochemical pathways have been found. These are useful in studying the normal cellular processes and can serve as genetic markers for somatic hybridization and transformation experiments.

5.2.3.2 Somatic Hybridization

Besides the nucleus, cytoplasm also contains genetic information that is located in subcellular bodies (organelles) such as chloroplast and mitochondria. Thus, somatic hybridization is the simplest way to combine the genetic information of two cells through fusion of their protoplasts. The resulting product is the sum of the two nuclear and cytoplasmic genomes.

5.2.3.3 Transformation

In this method, cells or protoplasts are treated or injected with DNA containing material to transfer the encoded genetic information to the recipient cell. The major advantage of transformation over protoplast fusion is that far smaller amounts of DNA are transferred, even single genes.

5.2.3.4 Somatic Cell Gene Manipulations

Somatic cell genetic manipulation can be successfully accomplished by considering the type of genetic variations that occur in somatic cells. While regenerating these variations cause the reprogramming of whole cells leading to establishment of new cell lines. However, due to lack of knowledge of fundamental processes of plant development, gene regulation, and poor development of many important crop plants *in vitro*, it is not easy to manipulate and induce the desirable changes into plant cells, for example, corn protoplasts usually cannot divide and soybean callus does not regenerate to plants [11]. Once the gene and its associated regulatory processes are identified, they can be manipulated and transferred through a suitable vector in the desired plant cell, although its safety is a concern and a critical issue in plant cells because at times it may cause side effects or cell death. Thus, manipulated gene expression and regulation should be properly studied before its transfer to a suitable host cell.

5.2.4 Polyploidy

Genetic changes associated with tissue culture are stochastic, nonreproducible, and unpredictable. These genetic changes originate from source/explants or during the culture process (*de novo*). Variation such as changes in chromosome number represents the major change during *in vitro* proliferation and differentiation. The number of sets in a given cell corresponds to the ploidy level of that cell. Polyploid cells and organisms are those containing more than two paired (homologous) sets of chromosomes [12]. Most eukaryotic species are diploid, meaning they have two sets of chromosomes – one set inherited from each parent. However, polyploidy is found in some organisms and is especially common in plants. Polyploidy refers to a numerical change in a whole set of chromosomes. An organism in which a chromosome is either missing or an extra chromosome is present is known as an *aneuploidic organism* and the process is called as *aneuploidy* [13]. Therefore, the aneuploidy refers to a numerical change in part of the chromosome set, whereas polyploidy refers to a numerical change in the whole set of chromosomes. The induction of polyploidy is a common technique to overcome the sterility of a hybrid species during plant breeding, for example, triticale is the hybrid of wheat (*Triticum turgidum*) and rye (*Secale cereale*) [14,15]. It combines sought-after characteristics of the parents, but the initial hybrids are sterile. After polyploidization, the hybrid becomes fertile and can thus be further propagated to become triticale. Polyploidy can be induced in cell culture by a chemical called *colchicine* (an antimitotic agent that blocks or suppresses cell division by inhibiting mitosis, the division of a cell's nucleus), which can result in chromosome doubling, though its use may have other less obvious consequences as well [16]. Colchicine is derived from the plant *Colchicum autumnale* (Liliaceae). Polyploid plants produced by this chemical are more robust than diploids. Usually plants that are stronger and tougher are more suitable for inducing polyploidy. Thus, many crops have unintentionally been bred to a higher level of ploidy. The major application of polyploidy in plant tissue culture is during plant breeding programs. In plant breeding programs, polyploid plants have been used to develop superior varieties and to restore the fertility of interspecific or intergeneric hybrids. Furthermore, the leaves, stems, roots, and flowers in polyploid plants are usually bigger than those of the diploid plants. Thus, the polyploid plants may have an increased biomass and yield. The technique of *in vitro* polyploid induction with colchicine has been employed in many crops, such as tomato and *Citrus sinensis* [17]. However, only a few cases of the generation of polyploid medicinal plants have been reported to date. Compared with diploids, tetraploid plants of *Datura stramonium* have up to twice the alkaloid content in leaves, stems, and roots [18]. The tissue culture-mediated induction of polyploid plants is advantageous, because when compared with traditional methods, tissue culture can obtain a large number of materials for induction, and is more effective and convenient.

5.2.5 Mutation

In vitro cell cultures represent many advantages for isolation of mutants in higher plants. Mutant plant cell cultures can be useful in the study of the physiology and genetics of plants, as well for the improvement of crops. The isolation of mutants is a necessary first step in any genetic program to provide strains that can be distinguished from one another. Mutant cell lines have been isolated for disease resistance, herbicide resistance, and sodium chloride resistance from cultured tissue. Efficient mutagenesis of plant cell cultures is possible when the cells are uniformly treated with physical or chemical mutagens. Several mutation techniques have been employed to improve yield, quality, disease, and pest resistance in crops. Ethyl methane sulfonate is the most commonly used chemical mutagen in plant tissue culture. Tissue culture makes it more efficient by allowing the handling of large populations and by increasing mutation induction efficiency, the possibility of mutant recovery, and speediness of cloning selected variants. Some vegetatively propagated species are recalcitrant to plant regeneration, which can be a limit for the application of gene transfer biotechnology, but not for mutation induction breeding [19]. Mutagenesis offers the possibility of altering only one or a few characters of an already first-rate cultivar, while preserving the overall characteristics. Traits induced by mutagenesis include plant size, blooming time and fruit ripening, fruit color, self-compatibility, self-thinning, and resistance to pathogens. *In vitro* culture combination with induced mutations is relatively inexpensive, simple, efficient, and can speed up breeding programs, from the generation of variability, through selection, to multiplication of the desired genotypes. In some vegetatively propagated species, mutations in combination with the *in vitro* culture technique may be the only method of improving an existing cultivar [19]. The availability of suitable selection methods could improve its effectiveness and potential applications. The molecular marker technology available today already provides tools to assist in mutation induction protocols by investigating both genetic variation within populations and early detection of mutants with desired traits. Once identified and isolated, the genes that encode agronomically important features can be either introduced directly into crop plants or used as probes to search for similar genes in crop species. However, cost still represents a major limitation to their application [19].

5.2.6 Host Pathogen Studies

Libbert et al. have shown that the majority of indole-3-acetic acid (IAA) extracted from plants is not a product of plants but of the epiphytic bacteria [20]. Further, the ability of plants or crude enzymes prepared therefrom to convert the tryptophan to IAA is mainly the action of epiphytic bacteria. Such investigations led to the promotion of a separate branch called phytopathology where plant hosts with one or more pathogens are tested *in vitro* [21]. Recently it has been found that plant inoculation with endophytic bacteria, which normally live inside the plant without harming the host, is a highly promising approach for biological disease control, for example, resistance induction by an endophytic *Methylobacterium* sp. in potato toward *Pectobacterium atrosepticum* [22]. Soil-borne bacteria, fungi, and oomycetes infect roots and enter the water-conducting xylem vessels where they proliferate and obstruct the transportation of water and minerals, and cause the most destructive plant diseases in annual crops and woody perennials known as *vascular wilts* [23]. Hence, genetic resistance is the most effective control strategy to regulate this group of plant pathogens [23]. Similarly, several crops are subject to attack by pathogenic viruses, fungi, and bacteria. Plant tissue cultures are now well recognized as valuable experimental systems for use in the study of host/pathogen interactions. Study of plant/pathogen interaction by *in vitro* tissue culture can help in producing disease-free and disease-resistant plants. These techniques have obvious major advantages for the examination of obligatory biotrophic fungi and also those with a necrotrophic lifestyle, and it is in these areas that much research effort has been concentrated. In this research, a pathogenic explant is cocultured with a healthy plant explant to examine its biochemical, morphological, and genetic changes. A tissue culture system grown under controlled conditions of nutritional, hormonal, and environmental factors provides the use of simplified methods permitting the assessment of disease resistance or susceptibility. The elucidation of the disease resistance and host/pathogen specificity is complex and varies according to the culture system used as hosts, whether organ, callus, cell suspension, or protoplast culture and their ploidy status (Fig. 5.5). *Agrobacterium*-mediated plant transformation [24], production of phytoalexins (well-characterized defense mechanisms against attack by microorganisms at the site of infection) [25], and molecular biology of viroid/host interactions are the most reported topics in phytopathology of plant tissue cultures [26].

5.3 APPLIED RESEARCH

5.3.1 Micropropagation

Micropropagation is the practice of rapidly multiplying stock plant material to produce a large number of progeny plants, using modern plant tissue culture methods. Micopropagation can also be defined as the plant propagation of selected genotypes using *in vitro*

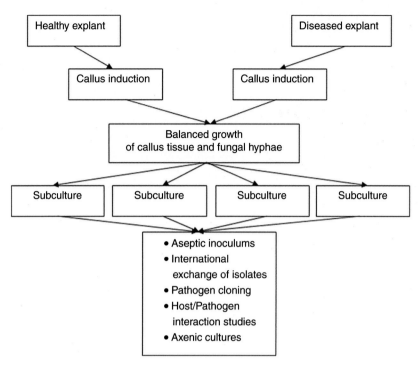

FIGURE 5.5 Schematic representation of the establishment of dual culture of obligatory biotrophic plant pathogens, either from the healthy explants that are subsequently inoculated or from diseased explants.

culture techniques. Micropropagation is a regeneration of whole plant through tissue culture where a callus mass has been initiated from a single explant, and within a very short time, a large number of plantlets can be produced from a callus tissue. By means of subculturing it is also possible to produce a large number of calli from single explants. And hundreds of plantlets can be produced from each callus obtained after subculturing. It is also used to provide a sufficient number of plantlets for planting from a stock plant that does not produce seeds, or does not respond well to vegetative reproduction. The most obvious advantage of micropropagation is the production of large numbers of seedlings in a short period of time. Various advantages and disadvantages of micropropagation are mentioned in Table 5.1. Different types of methods used in micropropagation are illustrated in Fig. 5.6.

These methods could be employed for either virus elimination from infected plants or for rapid multiplication. Exposing plants or cultures to high temperature (32–40°C) is the only method of ridding infected cultivars of their viruses. Currently the most frequently used micropropagation method for commercial production utilized enhanced axillary shoot proliferation from cultured meristems. Multiplication rates also tend to be slow initially but later, if cultural conditions are satisfactory, a rapid multiplication can be achieved.

TABLE 5.1   Merits and Demerits of Micropropagation

Merits	Demerits
• Rapid multiplication of true plants throughout the year.	• Culture methods are not viable (male sterility) or not available easily (e.g., banana) and in plants where propagation by conventional methods are expensive (e.g., orchid).
• Facilitates long distance transport of propagation material.	• The cost involved in setting up and maintenance of laboratory is very high and normally may not justify their use in all the horticultural plants.
• Long-term storage of clonal materials.	• Tissue culture techniques require skill and manpower.
• Large number of plants can be produced in culture tubes in small space with uniform growth and productivity.	• Slight infection may damage the entire crop of plants.
• A new plant can be regenerated from a miniature plant part.	• Some genetic modification (mutation) of the plant may develop with some varieties and culture systems that may alter the quality of the produce.
• Plants raised are free from diseases.	• The seedling grown under artificial conditions may not survive when placed under environmental conditions directly if proper conditions (optimum light, temperature, humidity, nutrition etc.) are not given.

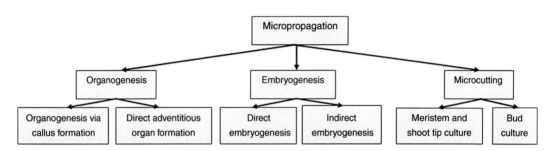

FIGURE 5.6   Illustration of types of micropropagation in plant tissue culture.

5.3.1.1 Production of Secondary Metabolite

Plant secondary metabolites are the most valuable phytochemicals of plant secondary metabolism and possess sufficient chemical or structural complexity so that artificial synthesis is difficult or not currently possible. Various culturing techniques used for the production of secondary metabolites are mentioned in Table 5.2. Occurrence, availability, and structural diversity of these active principals vary according to environmental conditions. Yield of these therapeutic compounds from different plant sources has been a major concern over last few decades. In addition factors that regulate or affect their metabolism require a basic *in vitro* model where plant sample can be experimented on to increase the yield of these active principals. Plant cell culture holds much promise as a method for producing complex secondary

TABLE 5.2 Strategies for Improving the Yield of Secondary Metabolites

Sr. No.	Strategies for improving the yield of secondary metabolites
1.	Culture conditions and their optimization
2.	Media optimization
3.	Optimization of sterilization protocol
4.	Hormonal supplementation and its optimization
5.	Elicitation
6.	Precursor feeding
7.	Immobilization and permeabilization
8.	Metabolic engineering: alteration of metabolic pathways (metabolomics)
9.	Dependent on type of explants (elite variety) and type of culture (organ, cell, callus, embryo, etc.)
10.	Identification of genes and expression of encoding key enzymes for secondary metabolite synthesis
11.	Genetic manipulation
12.	Scale-up technique: bioreactors (engineering considerations and their optimization)
13.	Role of endophytes
14.	Role of differentiation (cytodifferentiation and cellular organization)
15.	Type of culturing technique
16.	Hairy root culture
17.	Nature of explants
18.	Biotransformation
19.	Use of mutagen

metabolites *in vitro*. A breakthrough in cell culture methodology occurred with the successful establishment of cell lines capable of producing high yields of secondary compounds in cell suspension cultures [27]. In plant cell biotechnology, metabolic engineering is an emerging branch that plays a vital role in triggering specific pathways for the production of secondary metabolites (metabolomics). For the production of specific secondary metabolite, activation of a specific path way is necessary. This may occur when transcription triggers the expression of a specific gene to participate in production of those proteins that are further taking part in biosynthetic pathways as activator molecules for triggering specific secondary metabolites. This whole process requires a combined knowledge of transcriptonomics, genomics, proteomics, and metabolomics. Metabolic engineering is a branch to engineer/optimize parameters involved in the high production of secondary metabolites by using various tools such as proteomics, genomics, transcriptonomics, and metabolomics. The primary purpose involved here is to produce high-quality secondary metabolites with improved yield. Metabolic engineering also creates a good understanding of biosynthetic pathways and their respective end products. Various reports on secondary metabolite production through *in vitro* techniques are mentioned in Table 5.3.

TABLE 5.3   Some Reported Secondary Metabolites Produced by Plant Tissue Culture

Secondary metabolite	Plant species	Culture condition	Culture type	Biological action	Reference
L-Ephedrine	*Ephedra* sp.	MS + kinetin + 2,4-D	S	Sympathomimetic	[28]
Amarogentin	*Swertia japonica*	MS + IAA	HR	Bitter tonic and hepatoprotective	[29]
Anthocyanin	*Vitis vinifera*	MS + BAP + NAA	S	Protects against myriad of human diseases	[30]
Anthraquinones	*Cassia acutifolia*	MS + 2,4-D + kinetin	S	Purgative	[31]
Artemisinin	*Artemisia* spp.	MS + IAA + kinetin	HR	Antimalarial	[32]
Asiaticoside	*Centella asiatica*	MS + 2,4-D	HR	Wound healing	[33]
Azadirachtin	*Azadirachta indica*	MS + 2,4-D	S	Insecticidal	[34]
Berberine	*Coscinium fenestratum*	MS + IAA + BAP	C	Antibacterial, anti-inflammatory	[35]
Betacyanin	*Phytolacca americana*	MS + 2,4-D	S	Antioxidant	[36]
Caffeine	*Coffea arabica*	MS + 2,4-D + kinetin	C	CNS stimulant	[37]
Camptothecin	*Ophiorrhiza rugosa*	MS + BA + kinetin	Sc	Anticancer	[38]
Capsaicin	*Capsicum annuum*	MS + 2,4-D + kinetin	S	Cures rheumatic pain	[39]
Cardenolides	*Digitalis purpurea*	MS + BA	S	Cardioactive property	[40]
Catechin	*Rheum ribes*	MS + IBA + BA	C	Antioxidant	[41]
Catharanthine	*Catharanthus roseus*	MS + 2,4-D + UV-B radiation	S	Nicotinic receptor inhibitor, anticancer property	[42]
Cathin	*Brucea javanica*	MS + IAA + GA3	S	Psychoactive drug	[43]
Codeine	*Papaver* spp.	LS + BA + NAA		Analgesic	[44]
Cryptosin	*Cryptolepis buchanani*	B5 + 2,4-D + kinetin	C	Cardioactive property	[45]
Diosgenin	*Dioscorea deltoidea*	MS + 2,4-D	S	Synthesis of medicinal steroids	[46]
Eleutherosides	*Eleutherococcus senticosus*	MS + 2,4-D	S	Antidiabetic effects	[47]
Forskolin	*Coleus forskohlii*	MS + IAA + kinetin	HR	Anticancer, glaucoma	[48]
Glycyrrhizin	*Glycyrrhiza glabra*	MS + 2,4-D + GA3	HR	Expectorant and treatment of peptic ulcer	[49]
Gymnemic acid	*Gymnema sylvestre*	MS + 2,4-D + IAA	C	Antidiabetic	[50]
Hyoscyamine	*Datura stramonium*	MS + IAA	HR	Anticholinergic, antispasmodic	[51]
Hypericins	*Hypericum perforatum*	MS + BA + IAA	ML	Antidepressant	[52]
Indole alkaloid	*C. roseus*	MS + 2,4-D + GA3 + vanadium	S	Anticancer	[53]

TABLE 5.3   Some Reported Secondary Metabolites Produced by Plant Tissue Culture *(cont.)*

Secondary metabolite	Plant species	Culture condition	Culture type	Biological action	Reference
Isoflavones	*Psoralea corylifolia*	MS + TDZ + BAP	ML	Antioxidant	[54]
Lignan	*Linum flavum*	MS + IAA + GA3	HR	Anti-inflammatory and antioxidant effects	[55]
Lupeol, Rutin	*Hemidesmus indicus*	MS + BAP + NAA	Sc	Antioxidant	[56]
Plumbagin	*Plumbago rosea*	MS + CaCl2	C	Antimicrobial, anti-inflammatory	[57]
Quercetin	*Pluchea lanceolata*	MS + NAA + BAP	C	Antioxidant	[58]
Quinine	*Cinchona ledgeriana*	MS + kinetin	S	Antimalarial	[59]
Reserpine	*Rauvolfia serpentina*	MS + IAA + Cu^{2+}	C	Hypotensive	[60]
Resveratrol	*Vitis vinifera*	MS + IAA + GA3 + UV	C	Cardiac and anticancer effects	[61]
Rutin	*Fagopyrum esculentum*	MS + NAA	HR	Antioxidant Treatment of capillary bleeding	[62]
Shikonin	*Lithospermum erythrorhizon*	MS + 2,4-D + kinetin	HR	Anti-HIV therapeutic agents	[63]
Silymarin	*Silybum marianum*	MS + IAA + GA3	HR	Hepatoprotective	[64]
Umbelliferone	*Ammi majus*	MS + BAP	SL	Sunscreen agent	[65]
Valepotriates	*Centranthus ruber*	MS + IAA + kinetin	HR	Putative anxiolytic effect	[66]
Vincristine	*Catharanthus roseus*	MS + 2,4-D + GA3	S	Anticarcinogenic	[67]
Withanolide A	*Withania somnifera*	MS + IAA + kinetin	HR	Sedative and antirheumatic	[68]

S: Suspension; HR: Hairy root; C: Callus; Sc: Shoot culture; SL: Shootlet; ML: Multiple shoots

5.3.1.2 *Production of Pathogen-Free Plants or Crop Improvement*

Plant tissue culture is constantly exploring its applications in agricultural science. One of the major impacts of plant tissue culture is in the area of crop improvement. There are several significances of plant tissue culture and genetic engineering in crop production such as: developing new hybrid crops based on genetic male sterility, exploiting transgenic apomixes to fix hybrid vigor in inbred crops, increasing resistance to insect pests, diseases, and abiotic stress factors, improving effectiveness of biocontrol agents, enhancing nutritional value (vitamin A and iron) of crops and postharvest quality, increasing efficiency of soil phosphorus uptake and nitrogen fixation, improving adaptation to soil salinity and aluminum toxicity, understanding the nature of gene action and metabolic pathways, increasing photosynthetic activity, sugar, and starch production, and production of pharmaceuticals and vaccines. Eradication of virus has been a tremendous contribution to tissue culture technology. White gives his opinion that meristem was deprived of virus and therefore it was possible to eliminate the pathogen provided the transfer part does not contain sufficient amounts of old tissue [69]. Morel and Martin recovered virus-free *Dahlia* and potato from cultures obtained by cultivating the shoot meristem of infected plants [70]. This showed that even in infected plants the cells of shoot tip cells are either free of virus or carry a negligible amount of pathogen. This technique is economical and used frequently. This is also coupled with chemotherapy or thermotherapy for virus eradication. The important applications in crop improvement are production of new mutants, genomic combinations, and selection of new combinants by anther culture for haploid production (to produce embryos with half the number of chromosomes). When such haploid embryos are treated with chromosome doubling agent, for example, colchicines, the normal number is restored and the resulting plants are pure lines.

5.3.1.3 *Production of Herbicide-Resistant Crop*

The use of herbicides has developed weed control in many crop production systems. Production of herbicide-resistant crops is largely dependent on cell culture and selection, type of mutagenesis and transgenesis, and stability and expression of transgene. However, scientists are still unable to set up a clear relation between herbicides and their targeted resistant gene [71]. This is because most of the gene target sites responsible for herbicide-resistant effects are still unexplored. Approaches to maintain the efficiency of chemical weed control include the discovery of new herbicide target sites in plants and the discovery/synthesis of new, more potent herbicidal molecules (Table 5.4). However, these approaches are expensive to execute, take a considerably long time to succeed, and may lead to increased chemical loads in the environment [71].

5.3.1.4 *Pest-Resistant ("Bt Concept" Pest-Resistant Transgenic) Plants*

Genetic transformation provides direct access to a vast pool of useful genes not previously accessible to plant breeders. The first transgenic plants with *Bacillus thuringiensis* (Bt) genes were produced in 1987, while most of the insect-resistant transgenic plants have been developed by using Bt endotoxin gene [72]. *B. thuringiensis*, or Bt, is a bacterium that has attracted much attention for its use in pest control. The soil bacterium produces a protein that is toxic to various herbivorous insects. The protein, known as Bt toxin, is produced in an inactive, crystalline form. When consumed by insects, the protein is converted to its active, toxic form (delta endotoxin), which in turn destroys the gut of the insect. Bt preparations are commonly used in organic agriculture to control insects, as Bt toxin occurs naturally and is completely safe for humans. More than 100 different variations of Bt toxin have been identified in diverse strains of *B. thuringiensis*. The different variations have different target insect specificity. For example, Cry-type toxins from Bt gene are effective against various worms [73]. Researchers have used genetic engineering to take the bacterial genes needed to produce Bt toxins and introduce them into plants. If plants produce Bt toxin on their own, they can defend themselves against specific types of insects. This means farmers no longer have to use chemical insecticides to control certain insect problems. Critics claim that in some cases the use of insect-resistant crops can harm beneficial insects and other nontarget organisms. Extensive ecological impact assessments have been addressing these issues. In the field, no significant adverse effects on nontarget wildlife or long-term effects of higher Bt concentrations in soil have yet been observed. Successful expression of Bt genes has been achieved in tomato, potato, brinjal, groundnut, and chickpea.

TABLE 5.4 Strategies for Production of Herbicide-resistant Crops and Their Applications [71]

Strategies	Herbicide binding/ inhibitory site	Herbicide-resistant genes and mutagenesis	Applications
Engineering resistance to photosystem II (PSII) inhibitors	PSII electron transport cascade Function	Gene (bxn) from bacterium, *Klebsiella ozaenae*	Dicot crops
Engineering tolerance to growth regulator herbicides	Unknown target site	tfdA from plasmid of 2,4-D degrading bacteria is *Ralstonia eutropha*	Wheat, corn, sorghum and pasture crops, cotton, wine grapes
Engineering tolerance to glyphosate	Inhibits the enzyme 5-enolpyruvyl-shikimate phosphate (EPSP) synthase	EPSP synthase gene (cp4) and glyphosate oxidoreductase (*gox*) gene from *Pseudomonas* sp. strain (LBr)	Soybeans, corn, canola, cotton
Engineering tolerance to plant pigment biosynthesis inhibitors	Inhibits protoporphyrinogen oxidase and phytoene desaturase	PPO gene, hemY from *B. subtilis*	Tobacco, rice, maize, corn
Engineering resistance to acetolactate synthase (ALS) inhibitors	Acetolactate synthase	Mutations and oligonucleotide-mediated gene manipulation	Cotton, soybeans, rice
Engineering tolerance to mitotic disruptor herbicides	Binds to the tubulin protein subunits, and inhibits tubulin polymerization into microtubules	Overexpression of mutant and β-tubulin proteins	Maize calli
Multiherbicide tolerance	Overexpression of a plant ATP-binding efflux protein and the apyrase protein in *Arabidopsis*	Mammalian cytochrome P_{450} monooxygenase genes	Potatoes and rice

5.3.1.5 Drought Resistance

Major physiological responses of plants against drought are leaf wilting, a reduction in leaf area, leaf abscission, and thereby reducing water loss through transpiration, and increasing the rate of photosynthesis in relation to drought. These drought-related stresses can be alleviated by various molecular and genetic approaches such as gene manipulation and transgenesis. Traditional breeding also plays an important role in fighting against drought stress. The biotechnology industry has been working on drought-tolerant and water-saving crops for more than a decade, and the results so far, while useful, are underwhelming compared to conventional techniques like breeding. Despite all the hyperbole about the promise of genetically modified (GM), drought-resistant crops, it took until December 2011 for the first GM drought-resistant crop to be approved for marketing anywhere in the world [74]. That crop is Monsanto GM drought-resistant maize (Monsanto is the largest hybrid seeds producer in the world) for cultivation in the United States [74]. By contrast, non-GM plant breeding has achieved success after success in producing a variety of drought-resistant crops, including a whole series of drought-resistant maize varieties, and these have been made available in many countries, including developing countries that are particularly vulnerable to drought [74].

5.3.1.6 Flood Resistance

Floods are a major hazard to crops worldwide. Flooding imposes a severe selection pressure on plants principally because excess water in their surroundings can deprive them of certain basic needs, notably oxygen, carbon dioxide, and light for photosynthesis. It is one of the major abiotic influences on species distribution and agricultural productivity worldwide. Flood-tolerant crops as expected are able to survive flooding. Through genetic modification they can be completely submerged under water for about 2 to 3 weeks. There is a mechanism through which reduced oxygen levels are sensed. The mechanism controls key regulatory proteins called transcription factors, which can turn other genes on and off. It is the unusual structure of these proteins that predestines them for destruction under normal oxygen levels, but when oxygen levels decline, they become stable. Their stability results in changes in gene expression and metabolism that enhance survival in the low oxygen conditions brought on by flooding. When the plants return to normal oxygen levels, the proteins are again degraded, providing a feedback control mechanism [75]. Some of the available flood-resistant crops are highlighted in Table 5.5.

TABLE 5.5 List of Reports on Flood-Resistant Crops

Year	Reports on flood-resistant crops
October, 2007	Indigenous rice better than GM for dealing with stress: A New Delhi-based NGO, together with farmers from nine Indian states, has developed a register documenting over 2000 indigenous rice varieties. They say GM rice strains are not only costly to cultivate but also are a poor match to the native strains in fighting pests, diseases, and environmental fluctuation.
February, 2009	Flood-resistant non-GM rice: At the Philippines-based International Rice Research Institute (IRRI), scientists have developed a rice variety with high tolerance to submersion under water for extended periods.
August, 2009	"Snorkel" rice can survive deep water flooding: This rice, which withstands flooding by shooting up in height, has been hyped in many press stories as a triumph of GM.
September, 2010	Indian farmers adopt flood-tolerant rice at unprecedented rates (http://irri.org/news/media-releases).
March, 2011	BBC News published a report on "Flood-resistant rice also has drought-proof trait" stating that the researchers found that the gene, *Sub1A*, allowed plants to survive by growing fresh shoots after a period of drought. (Mark Kinver, Science and Environment Reporter. Flood-resistant rice also has drought-proof trait. BBC News (http://www.bbc.co.uk/news/science-environment)).

5.3.1.7 Salt Tolerance

A major abiotic stress in the agriculture industry is salinity of soil, which creates various problems in plant cultivation and propagation. Development of salt-tolerant plants by transgenesis is known to be the best alternative for crop improvement [76]. However, selection of a suitable genetic model is again a difficult task. A recently discovered halophytic plant species, *Thellungiella halophila* (also known as *T. salsuginea*), has emerged as a new model plant for the molecular elucidation of abiotic stress tolerance [77]. Because of its morphological and genetic similarity with *Arabidopsis* it allows utilization of *Arabidopsis* genetic information to investigate *Thellungiella* responses against different stresses [77]. A salt tolerance gene isolated from mangrove (*Avicennia marina*) has been cloned, and can be transferred to other crop plants [78]. The *gutD* gene from *Escherichia coli* can also be used to provide salt tolerance [79]. These genes hold great potential for increasing crop production in marginal lands [80].

5.3.1.8 High Yielding GM Crops

High yielding GM crops are those crops that give better yield than the already existing variety. These types of crops have high commercial value and hence are commercialized according to the needs of the market. But it is a myth among cultivars and consumers that GM crops are known to be high yielding crops, because until now no GM crop has shown better yield results. Yet in the case of the most widely grown GM crop, GM soybeans, there has been evidence of consistently lower yields for over a decade. Controlled comparative field trials of GM/non-GM Soya suggest that 50% of the drop in yield may be due to the genetic disruption caused by the GM transformation process [81,82]. A US Department of Agriculture report confirms the questionable yield performance of GM crops, stating that "GE crops available for commercial use do not increase the yield potential of a variety. In fact, yield may even decrease…. Perhaps the biggest issue raised by these results is how to explain the rapid adoption of GE crops when farm financial impacts appear to be mixed or even negative."

On the contrary, Monsanto reports estimated that approximately 95% of the soybeans and 75% of corn in the United States are GM. More than 95% of soybeans in Argentina and half the soybeans grown in Brazil are GM. In 2009, Monsanto released a line of soybeans in the United States that has been shown in field trials to increase yields by 7–11% (http://www.monsanto.com/newsviews/Pages/do-gm-crops-increase-yield.aspx). Monsanto claims related to the increase yield of GM (RR2) soybeans were proven false in 2010, during which period West Virginia had launched a probe into Monsanto for consumer fraud for false advertising claims. Thus, there are two critical issues (speculation that supports and opposes GM crops and their related technologies), though no strong evidence has been found yet that favors either side.

5.3.1.9 Health-Promoting Crops

Plants that have health-promoting traits that are beneficial to producers and consumers are called GM plants of commercial importance. Golden rice is an outstanding example, which explores the health-promoting properties of GM crops. Furthermore, technologies like metabolic engineering and metabolomics (comprehensive analysis of plant biochemicals) also assist in screening various GM clones that have potent chemical components with health-promoting properties. Another most popular example is GM tomatoes with supposed anticancer properties. Current (2012) licenses for commercial (international) releases of GM crops such as canola (*Brassica napus* L.) and cotton (*Gossypium hirsutum* L.) with modified traits such as insect and herbicide resistance have been issued to Monsanto Australia Ltd, Bayer Crop Science Pty Ltd, and Dow Agro Sciences Australia Pty Ltd. (http://www.ogtr.gov.au/internet/ogtr/publishing.nsf). In addition, various other genetically engineered vegetables, crops, and plants have been used for commercial use such as alfalfa, corn, soya, tomato, potato, rice, cantaloupe, sugar beet, radicchio, flax, papaya, squash, oilseed rape, and wheat (http://www.psrast.org/gefonmarket.htm). To date these crops have not been commercialized successfully and due to some serious health effects some have been withdrawn from the market.

The revolution in genetic engineering has brought lots of strategies to design or select a gene of interest for its further transformation in plant cells. Selectable markers, analysis of biosynthetic pathways (metabolic engineering), and cDNA library trait analysis assist in selection and proper designing of desirable genes. Genetic transformation of desirable genes with desirable traits produces crops with improved characteristics (Table 5.6 and Fig. 5.7).

TABLE 5.6 Improved Characteristics of GM Plants by Genetic Transformation

New trait	Genetic transformation	Examples	Reference
Development of plants with improved sugar and starch metabolism	• Sucrose phosphate synthase (SPS) is a key enzyme in the regulation of sucrose metabolism • Modification of TCA (tricarboxylic acid) cycle and hexokinases • Introduction of *E. coli* inorganic pyrophosphatase and a class of cupin protein	Changing the chemical composition of food grains	[83–85]
Reduction in the production of cytokinin causes leaf senescence	Introduction of stay green trait (farnesyl transferase and isopentenyl transferase genes) delays senescence	Sorghum, alfalfa	[86]
C3 photosynthesis suffers from O_2 inhibition	To introduce the C4 type of photosynthesis into C3 plants by phosphoenolpyruvate carboxylase	Arabidopsis and potato	[87]
Production of edible vaccines	Introduction of human antigen in plants causes the production of antigenic proteins that retain the immunogenic properties upon purification	Anticancer antibodies expressed in rice and wheat	[88]
Genetic or cytoplasmic male sterility leads to the suppression of production of viable pollen	Due to dysfunction of mitochondria by chimeric protein. Biotechnological approaches can be used to transfer CMS from within a species or from one species into another	*Z. mays, S. bicolor, Pennisetum glaucum*, and *Helianthus annuus*	[89]
Apomixis produces a large number of nucellar offspring, which are genetically similar to the female parent	Apomictic gene can be introduced by genetic engineering to fix genetic variation. This may produce similar crops with high productivity and better food quality	Citrus, sorghum, maize, turf grass, and other crop plants	[90]

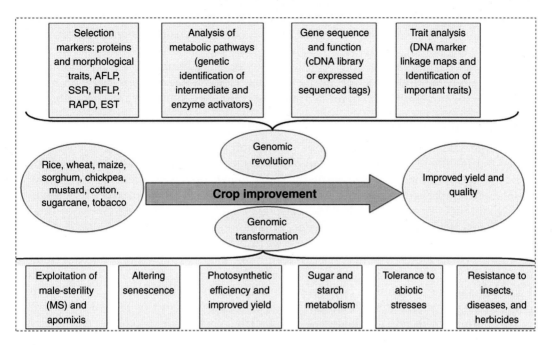

FIGURE 5.7 **Biotechnological applications in crop improvement.** Restriction fragment length polymorphism (RFLP); Inter-simple sequence repeats markers (ISSR); Random amplified polymorphic DNA (RAPD); Microsatellites or simple sequence repeat (SSR); Polymerase chain reaction–restriction fragment length polymorphism (PCR–RFLP); Amplified fragment length polymorphism (AFLP).

5.3.1.10 In vitro *Germplasm Conservation*

In the earlier times, plant germplasms were stored in the form of seeds, bulbs, tubers, roots, buds, corns, cuttings, etc. Greenhouses, fields, plots, and nurseries are other sources of maintaining gene banks or germplasms. This type of storage causes various problems for some important species that produce recalcitrant seeds (those seeds that are not stored for any length of time or that suffer from early embryo degradation). Further disadvantages such as maintenance of fields, nurseries, and greenhouses raise unnecessary expense in this process. Additionally, vulnerability of plants against various infections and climatic hazards causes serious damage to germplasms. According to reports about 2000 species are believed to be rare and threatened with extinction. Plant tissue culture is being used to develop an effective means of germplasm conservation since a low maintenance *in vitro* germplasm storage collection provides a cost-effective alternative to growing plants in fields, nurseries, or greenhouses.

5.3.1.11 *Genetic Manipulations*

Improvement of crops by use of genetics generates a separate section for genetic manipulation, which yields genetically engineered or transgenic plants, having distinguished characters such as herbicide, pathogen, drought, salt, and disease resistance. Due to simple genotypes (monocots) and strong redifferentiation power, plant systems act as the most suitable host to study the genetic interference for a specific gene. That is why genetic engineering of plants is much easier than that of animals. *Agrobacterium*-mediated transformation is rapidly used for the genetic engineering of plants. But there are some plant species that remain highly recalcitrant to this bacterium infection. Selection of suitable bacterium and genetic manipulation of such plants (identifying the specific gene with their expression) opens a new approach for improving the transformation of recalcitrant, but commercially important, crops [91].

5.3.1.12 *Genetic Variability*

In earlier times pollination and cross-fertilization were the only alternatives left to bring genetic variability to new generations of plants. But nowadays plant biotechnology is known to be the most promising area to create the stable genetic diversity after suitable genetic manipulations. Improved plants with improved states of health can be produced by tissue culture techniques. Tissue culture has been also exploited to increase the number of desirable germplasms available to the plant breeder. Summation of tissue culture with molecular techniques is useful to incorporate the desired gene (trait) and study its behavior in specific germplasms. In tissue culture the haploid production technique is more often used to create the new genetic variations from the protoplast, anther, microspore, ovule, and embryo cultures. These variations are sometimes called somaclonal and gametoclonal variants, having extreme crop-improvement potential. Somaclonal variation is the introduction of genetic variation in *in vitro* cultured cells and plants derived from such cells are called somaclones. Somaclones are the first choice because they have additional desired genetic character without the need to resort to hybridization. They are also utilized for producing agronomically useful cultivars with new genetic variability. But these new variations, such as polyploidy, aneuploidy, and mutations, sometimes result in the loss of desirable economic traits in the tissue-cultured products. Thus, genetic manipulation and stable transfer as well as expression of manipulated genes still require further attention to create more suitable and economically genetic diversity.

Genetic changes frequently associated with *in vitro* regenerated plants lead to stable, lasting modifications to the genome that are inherited in subsequent generations. Some of these molecular changes are associated with phenotypic differences and hence are referred to as somaclonal variations [92]. Epigenetic reprogramming of gene expression involves heritable, but potentially reversible, enzyme-mediated, chemical modifications to the DNA and associated proteins in the chromatin. The changes are called "epigenetic" because these variations are not "coded" by the DNA, but still can be transmitted to the next generation. Such types of changes often lead to the production of epigenetic marks or signatures [92]. Epigenetic regulation in plant cell cultures is arranged by DNA methylation and histones, chromatin remodeling, and small RNA-mediated regulation. The types of genetic variation and elements involved are listed in Table 5.7.

5.3.1.13 In vitro *Pollination*

One of the major advancements for hybrid embryo production in tissue culture science is *in vitro* pollination and fertilization under *in vitro* conditions, which replaces conventional methods of plant breeding. One of the major hurdles in plant breeding is sterility between the two plants, which originates from an incompatibility between the pollen of one plant and stigma of the other. *In vitro* pollination and fertilization are the two successful approaches to

TABLE 5.7 Types of Genetic Variation and the Elements that are Involved During Each Variation [92]

Elements	Types of genetic variation	Remarks
GENE EXPRESSION REGULATION OF DEVELOPMENTAL CELL FATE IN VITRO		
Protein kinases	• Binds with ligand, removes PO_4^{-2} from the nucleotide, and transfers to amino acids (serine or theorine) • Cellular signal transduction cascade • Modulates properties such as cell division • Altered transcription of array of genes	
Transcription factors	• Regulatory proteins that bind to specific DNA to induce or repress the transcription of genes and thereby regulate target gene expression • These are essential mediators of developmental transitions and cellular stress responses • They take part in morphogenesis	
Structural proteins and enzymes	• Gene identification for such proteins helps in cellular reprogramming in response to stress cues *in vitro*	
GENETIC CHANGES ASSOCIATED WITH TISSUE CULTURE		
Chromosomal level changes	• Ploidy level: number of chromosomes (monoploidy, diploidy, tetraploidy, polyploidy) • Aneuploidy: extra or missing chromosome state structural changes: deletion, duplication, inversion, translocation of specific chromosomal segments	Chromosomal structural changes are more frequent than chromosome number changes Cytokinins/auxins addition affects chromosome number and ploidy level
DNA sequence changes	• Single nucleotide substitution mutation (deamination of methylated cytosine thiamine)	
Gene amplification or gene transposition	• Elements that are more sensitive to stress condition and mutation are: – Ribosomal DNA repeats – Microsatellites (affects the gene expression of adjacent genes) – Transposable elements (ability to transpose to nonnative genomic locations)	Long-term repeated subcultures result in repeated copies of all these elements
EPIGENETIC REGULATION IN VITRO		
DNA methylation	• Involves the addition through covalent bonding of a methyl group to the cytosine base in the DNA at CpG, CpHpH, and CpHpG sites, where H denotes any nucleotide other than guanine	DNA methylation is promoted by growth regulators especially auxins
Chromatin methylation	• Chromatin (basic repeating unit, nucleosome) is the complex of DNA and proteins (histones), packed inside the cell; aids in DNA replication and gene expression • Euchromatin (transcriptionally active) and heterochromatin (transcriptionally inactive)	Posttransitional modification (methylation, phosphorylation, acetylation of amino acid of histone proteins)
Small RNA regulation	• Noncoding elements that typically mediate posttranscriptional gene silencing by mRNA degradation or by repression of translation • These originate from transposable elements and tandem repeats	RNA-dependent DNA methylation pathway

overcome this problem. Moreover, these two techniques bring hybridization of plants from different species (intergeneric and interspecific hybridization), of which hybridization occurs less frequently in nature. The common cause behind unsuccessful hybridization is the hindrance of the growth of pollen tube on the stigma or style by certain barriers. Techniques such as intraovarian pollination (the style or part of it can be excised and pollen grains are either placed on the cut surface of the ovary or transferred through a hole in the wall of the ovary, e.g., *Papaver somniferum*) can also be used as an alternative but due to several demerits it is currently not used [93,94]. Direct pollination of cultured ovules (*in vitro* ovular pollination) or excised ovule with placenta (*in vitro* placental pollination) overcomes this barrier to pollen tube growth and thus forms a successful approach of *in vitro* pollination (Fig. 5.8). This technique was developed at Delhi University to produce hybrids among species of *Papaveraceae* and *Solanaceae* [93,94]. The intraovarian pollination opens a gateway for subsequent development of test tube fertilization. In this technique ovules and pollen grains are excised and cultured in the same medium for the successful fertilization of pollen and ovules under *in vitro* conditions. This application of plant tissue culture successfully overcomes the incompatibility barriers existing at the sexual level. Therefore, tissue culture techniques developed several alternatives to overcome the problems found during plant breeding. These approaches are:

- Ovular pollination (application of pollen to excised ovule)
- Placental pollination (application of pollen to ovule attached to placenta)
- Stigmatic pollination (application of pollen to stigma)

Chromosomal constitution also affects the state of pollen in plants. During their study on pollen abortion in chromosomal types of *Datura* Blakeslee and Cartledge discovered that abnormal chromosomal distributions are more frequent in tetraploids but the imbalance of single chromosomes is less, which indicates that the pollen of tetraploids shows only a slightly more abortive state than diploids [95].

Applications of *in vitro* pollination are:

- To overcome the self-incompatibility (*Petunia axillaris* and *P. hybrida*)
- To overcome the cross-incompatibility
- To promote haploid production through parthenogenesis
- To stimulate the production of stress-tolerant plants
- To encourage the feasibility of intraspecific, interspecific, intergeneric, and interfamilial crosses

5.3.1.14 *Induction of Haploidy*

Haploids are sporophytes of higher plants with a gametophytic chromosomal constitution, that is, they possess a single set of chromosomes that forms the alternation of generation (haploid and diploid as mentioned in Fig. 5.9). These types of plants are obtained from androgenesis, gynogenesis, parthenogenesis, semigamy, and polyembryony. In 1922, Belling and Blakeslee identified the first haploids in flowering plants (*D. stramonium*) [96,97]. The first culture of haploid plants (immature anthers of *D. innoxia*) was successfully established by Guha and Maheswari in Delhi University, which attracted worldwide attention in the application of tissue culture to synthesize haploid plants [98]. Normally somatic cells of higher plants have a diploid chromosome number while reproductive cells are haploid. They are succeeded in raising haploid embryoids and plantlets from developed

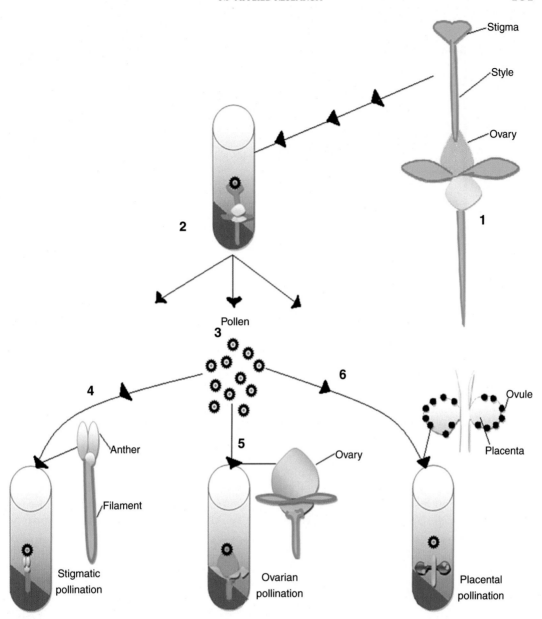

FIGURE 5.8 Diagrammatic representation of *in vitro* pollination.

culture (from microspores within the anthers). This opens the field of androgenesis. In the following year Bourgin and Nitsch confirmed the totipotency of pollen grains raising full haploid plants of tobacco, rice, and wheat [99]. Haploids by anther culture are now reported to have been raised in 247 species belonging to 34 families. Induction of haploid plants from pollinated ovaries and ovules (gynogenesis) is another recent advancement in plant

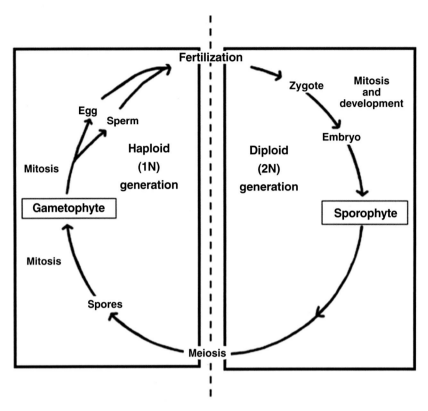

FIGURE 5.9   Plant life cycle alternation of generations.

tissue culture and experimental embryology. San Noeum reported her first result on *in vitro* culture of ovary isolated from *Hordeum vulgare* [100]. This demonstrates that not only the microspores but also the megaspores or female gametophytes of angiosperms can be triggered *in vitro* to saprophytic development, thus making way for an alternative approach to haploid plant breeding. It may be noted that anther culture has given rise to diploid, polyploid, and aneuploid plants. Thus, haploid induction or haploid represents significant applications for plant breeders and genetics in agriculture and plant tissue culture science.

5.3.1.15 Somatic Hybridization

Isolation, regeneration, and fusion of plant protoplast under *in vitro* conditions offer a new way to achieve successful breeding and genetic manipulation in plants. Somatic hybridization is an asexual hybridization method of producing somatic hybrids by the fusion of isolated somatic protoplasts. Unlike the sexual reproduction in which organelles are generally contributed by the maternal parent, somatic hybridization combines the cytoplasmic organelles of both parents. Products of fusion of two protoplasts (heterokaryons) could be cultured to regenerate a somatic hybrid plant of desired genotype. Carlson et al. obtained the first somatic hybrid by fusion of protoplasts isolated from *Nicotiana glauca* and *N. langsdorffii* [101].

This somatic hybridization is the approach by which sexually sterile and two different parental genomes can be recombined to produce hybrids.

5.3.1.16 Genetic Transformation

As discussed in Chapter 7, gene transfer techniques allow the successful transfer of specific traits (genes) in plants and hence contribute further applications in plant biotechnology. In simple terms gene transfer conveys a gene from one DNA molecule to another DNA molecule. There are various methods introduced for microbial or animal cell transfection such as lipid-mediated, calcium-phosphate-mediated, DEAE-dextran-mediated, electroporation, biolistics, viral vectors, polybrene, laser transfection, and gene transfection enhanced by elevated temperature [102]. These methods are broadly categorized under transfection by biochemical methods, transfection by physical methods, and virus-mediated transduction. The gene transfer results can be transient and stable transfection. Genetic transformation can be transient or stable, and transformed cells may or may not give rise to gametes that pass genetic material on to subsequent generations. In transient transfection, the transfected DNA is not integrated into host chromosome. DNA is transferred into a recipient cell in order to obtain a temporary but high level of expression of the target gene. Stable transfection is also called permanent transfection. By stable transfection, the transferred DNA is integrated (inserted) into chromosomal DNA and the genetics of recipient cells is permanent changed. There are only few techniques available for gene transfer in plants such as:

- Use of *Agrobacterium tumefaciens* as a vector
- Direct DNA uptake facilitated by polyethylene glycol or electroporation
- Microinjection of DNA into cells with a particle gun
- Microinjection
- Silicon carbide crystals

During genetic transformation, bacteria transfer its genetic information to plant cells in form of plasmid.

Genetic transformation of plants occurs naturally [103].

Agrobacterium-mediated transfer is one of the most rapidly used methods among all other gene transfer methods for plants. *Agrobacterium* has a further two strains *A. rhizogene* and *A. tumefaciens*. Cultures infected with *A. rhizogene* give a hairy root culture and *A. tumefaciens* induces crown or gall diseases in plants. Hairy root culture does not require hormone supplementation for its growth irrespective of normal culture, which requires hormones. On the another hand, crown's disease leads to an increase in cellular mass, which may lead to an increase in secondary metabolites and other useful compounds, which can be isolated later.

There are several plant transformation methods that avoid tissue culture or regeneration. Utilization of these methods allows direct targeting of viable meristems or other tissues that will finally give rise to gametes [104,105]. In this nontissue culture-based method, *Agrobacterium* or tungsten particles have been used in a number of species to transform cells in or around the apical meristems that are subsequently allowed to grow into plants and produce seeds [104,105]. A disadvantage of this method is that transformed traits usually do not persist into gametes at desirable frequencies and the methods have been difficult to reproduce [105]. Zhou et al. reported the transformed progeny by direct injection of naked DNA into ovaries [106]. Modifications of this method and "pollen tube pathway" delivery of DNA are still practiced in China [107]. In addition to *Agrobacterium* and biolistics, electroporation-mediated gene transfer into intact meristems in planta and a variety of pollen transformation procedures have also been reported [108,109]. All these methods have been difficult to reproduce, and therefore have not gained widespread attention. However, in tissue culture-based transformation methods, explants are transformed and then carried through tissue culture to regenerate shoots or roots, for example, corn, rice, wheat, and soybean, which target young apical meristems for transformation [104].

With the development in recombinant DNA technology it is also possible to transfer the manipulated gene through these vectors for their successful expression in plants so that plants will act as biofactories (manufacturing the desired compound). Useful genes like herbicide, pathogen, and antibiotic resistance can be transferred in cultures of GM plants for crop improvement (resistance to weeds and plant disease or in the study of mechanisms of gene action). Plant tissue culture is currently finding increased applications in studies of GM crops (corn, potato, soybean, cotton, and conola). Production additives (enzymes from genetically engineered microorganisms) for use in processed products like soft drinks, cakes, cheese, bread, meat, fish, etc. account for 90% of foodstuffs likely to contain GM components in the United States [110].

5.3.1.17 Metabolic Engineering

Metabolic engineering involves the targeted and purposeful alteration of metabolic pathways found in an organism. This is done to achieve better understanding and use of cellular pathways for chemical transformation, energy transduction, and supramolecular assembly [111]. Application of this technique to plants allows endogenous biochemical pathways to be manipulated. This manipulation resulted in generation of transgenic crops in which quality of plants' existing natural products is improved to provide beneficial commercial, agronomic, and/or postharvest processing characteristics [112]. From very early times *in vitro* propagation methods have been intensively investigated as a possible tool for the production of commercial plant secondary metabolites, including fine chemicals such as pharmaceuticals, agrochemicals, flavors, insecticides, fragrances, and cosmetics [113]. After much research in the field of *in vitro* production of phytochemicals, only a few industrial processes have been developed, involving only a limited number of secondary products, such as shikonin, berberine, ginsenosides, and paclitaxel [114].

Availability of extreme knowledge regarding complete genomes of several plants, biosynthetic pathways (precursors to intermediate to secondary metabolites), genes involved in these pathways, and several techniques (rDNA, gene transfer, etc.) led to the development a new branch called metabolic engineering. It is a powerful complement to classical chemical synthesis for the production of specialized pharmaceuticals and industrial compounds. The genetic simplicity and low cost of growing plants make them ideal systems for metabolic engineering. In general terms metabolic engineering is defined as the branch that deals with the study of genes that are employed to provide improved productivity in plant cell cultures, plant tissue cultures, or intact plants. In 1991, Bailey defined metabolic engineering as:

> The improvement of cellular activities by manipulation of enzymatic, transport, and regulatory functions of the cell with the use of recombinant DNA technologies [115].

Plant metabolic engineering saves the energy of the plants by focusing on a single pathway for the production of the desired compound. This can be done by manipulation of existing metabolic pathways by instructing the genes or either increasing or diverting energy resources from undesired products to generate the chemical entities that are either present or not normally found in the respective plant system. Summation of several pathways in a single plant system for the production of a single metabolite is also known to be a good strategy to yield high value compounds in larger quantities. Metabolic engineering can provide various strategies to improve production of secondary metabolites such as:

- Decreasing catabolism
- Increasing the carbon flux through a biosynthetic pathway by overexpression of genes codifying for rate-limiting enzymes or blocking the mechanism of feedback inhibition and competitive pathways
- Increasing the number of producing cells

5.3.1.18 *Molecular Pharming*

Production of therapeutic and high value proteins from various hosts such as transgenic plants and animals, human beings, bacteria, plants, yeast, and many others is called molecular pharming. This term appeared in the literature in the 1980s when the first animal-based product was obtained. In other terms it is defined as the production of recombinant proteins (including pharmaceuticals and industrial proteins) and other secondary metabolites in plants. The whole process involves the growing, harvesting, transport, storage, and downstream processing of extraction and purification of the protein [116]. This technique is dependent on the genetic transformability of plants, which was first demonstrated in the 1980s [117]. Human growth hormone was the first recombinant plant-derived pharmaceutical protein produced in transgenic plants in 1986 [118]. In 1989 the first recombinant antibody was expressed in the progeny of the cross of two individual transgenic plants expressing single immunoglobulin gamma and kappa chains [119]. Again in 1997 the first recombinant protein, avidin (an egg protein), was expressed in transgenic maize for commercial purposes [120]. These achievements demonstrated that plants could be turned into biofactories for the large-scale production of recombinant proteins. Later reports explored the potential of plants to produce even more complex functional mammalian proteins with therapeutic activity, such as human serum proteins and growth regulators, antibodies, vaccines, hormones, cytokines, enzymes, and antibodies [121]. This has been possible owing to their potential to execute posttranslational modifications, which allow recombinant proteins to fold properly and maintain their structural and functional integrity. Due to genetic simplicity (such as haploid plant) plant systems act as the most suitable host for the production of pharmaceutically important and commercially valuable proteins in plants. Furthermore, plant cells combine the advantage of a full posttranslational modification potential with simple growth requirements and basically unlimited scalability of whole plants in the field. Plants and plant cells are versatile production systems, also allowing targeting of the recombinant proteins produced to different organs or subcellular compartments, thus permitting improved protection against proteolysis. Plants are not known to harbor human or zoonotic pathogens, making them a safe host for the production of biopharmaceuticals. Various biopharmaceuticals are listed in Table 5.8. The commercial market for these recombinant biopharmaceuticals accounted for about 10% of the pharmaceutical market in 2007 [122], and had been predicted to expand to US$100 billion in 2010 [123].

TABLE 5.8   Important Pharmaceutical Proteins that Have Been Produced in Plants [124,125]

Protein	Host plant	Applications
HUMAN BIOPHARMACEUTICALS		
Aprotinin	Maize	Human pharmaceutical protein produced in maize
Collagen	Tobacco	First human structural protein polymer produced in plant; correct modification achieved by cotransformation with modification enzyme
Enkephalins	*Arabidopsis*	Antihyperanalgesic by opiate activity
Epidermal growth	Tobacco	Wound repair and control of cell proliferation
Erythropoietin	Tobacco	First human protein produced in tobacco suspension cells/anemia
Granulocyte-macrophage colony-stimulating factor	Tobacco	Neutropenia
Growth hormone	Tobacco, sunflower	First human protein expressed in plants; initially expressed as fusion protein with *nos* gene in transgenic tobacco; later the first human protein expressed in chloroplasts, with expression levels ~7% of total leaf protein
Hirudin	Canola	Thrombin inhibitor
Human serum albumin	Tobacco, potato	First full size native human protein expressed in plants; low expression levels in transgenics (0.1% of total soluble protein) but high levels (11% of total leaf protein) in transformed chloroplasts/liver cirrhosis, burns, surgery
Human-secreted alkaline phosphatase	Tobacco	Produced by secretion from roots and leaves
Lactoferrin rice	Tomato	Antimicrobial activity
α1-Antitrypsin	Rice	First use of rice suspension cells for molecular farming
α-Interferon	Rice, turnip	First human pharmaceutical protein produced in rice
RECOMBINANT ANTIBODIES		
Cholera toxin B and A2 subunits, rotavirus enterotoxin	Potato	First example of oral feeding inducing protection in an animal
Cholera toxin B subunit	Tobacco, potato	First vaccine candidate expressed in chloroplasts
Diabetes autoantigen	Tobacco, potato	First plant-derived vaccine for an autoimmune disease
E. coli heat-labile enterotoxin	Tobacco, potato	First plant vaccine to reach clinical trials stage
Hepatitis B virus envelope protein	Tobacco	First vaccine candidate expressed in plants; third plant-derived vaccine to reach clinical trials stage

TABLE 5.8   Important Pharmaceutical Proteins that Have Been Produced in Plants [124,125] *(cont.)*

Protein	Host plant	Applications
Immunoglobulin G (herpes simplex virus)	Soybean	First pharmaceutical protein produced in soybean
Immunoglobulin G1	Tobacco	First antibody expressed in plants; full length serum IgG produced by crossing plants that expressed heavy and light chains
Immunoglobulin M	Tobacco	First IgM expressed in plants and protein targeted to chloroplasts for accumulation
Rabies virus glycoprotein	Tomato	First example of an "edible vaccine" expressed in edible plant tissue
Secretory immunoglobulin A protein	Tobacco	First secretory antibody expressed in plants by sequential crossing of four lines carrying individual components; at present the most advanced plant-derived pharmaceutical

5.3.1.19 Organogenesis

When organs like roots, shoots, and leaves (except embryo) are induced in plant tissue culture by stimulation caused by the nutrients of the medium, substances present in original explants and endogenous compounds are produced in the culture by a process called organogenesis. Organogenesis of embryos is not possible because it is an independent structure and thus does not have vascular supply; it is not supposed to be the plant organ [126]. Organogenesis simply means development of organs, which is mainly affected by manipulation of plant growth regulators, especially hormones (Fig. 5.10).

Organogenesis consists of many aspects such as perception of phytohormone, dedifferentiation (loss of specialized characteristics) of differentiated cells to acquire organogenic competence, reentry of quiescent cells (G_0 phase of the cells when cells are not dividing) into cell cycle, and association of cells to form specific organs [126]. Furthermore, identification of the certain molecular processes and genes involved in organ formation may also be helpful in stimulation of organogenesis. Organogenesis is helpful in regulation of cell division, cell expansion, cell and tissue type differentiation, understanding the mechanism of hormones and other plant growth regulators' action, patterning of the organ as a whole, and the study of how organs are initiated and how they develop (identification of organogenic pathways) [127].

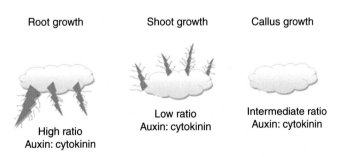

Root growth   Shoot growth   Callus growth

High ratio
Auxin: cytokinin

Low ratio
Auxin: cytokinin

Intermediate ratio
Auxin: cytokinin

FIGURE 5.10   **Effect of hormones on the root and shoot formation.**

5.3.1.20 Somatic Embryogenesis

In 1958, Steward et al. reported the first evidence of somatic embryogenesis with carrot (*Daucus carota*) cell suspension cultures, which had great similarities with zygotic embryogenesis [128]. Somatic embryogenesis is defined as the propagation of the embryo or plant from single or a group of vegetative cells. In plants there are two types of cells, vegetative, and germ cells. Somatic embryos are formed from vegetative cells that are not involved in the development of embryos. Nature has zygotic embryogenesis, which produces seeds, whereas somatic embryogenesis (only executed under *in vitro* conditions) produces callus initially (undifferentiated mass of cells) and somatic embryos later. Thus, this type of embryogenesis produces seeds without endosperm and an outer coat, which is called callus. Callus is defined as a group of cells derived from competent source tissue that is cultured under *in vitro* conditions to form an undifferentiated mass of cells. Plant growth regulators play an important role in the production and development of callus. Manipulation of PGR in tissue culture medium instructs the cells to form callus and further callus to form embryo. The proportionate quantity of different plant growth regulators required in inducing callus or embryo formation varies with the type of plant. There are enormous applications of somatic embryogenesis, for example, clonal propagation of genetically uniform plant material, elimination of viruses, provision of source tissue for genetic transformation, generation of whole plants from single cells called protoplasts, and development of synthetic seed technology. Moreover, somatic embryogenesis has served as a model to understand the physiological and biochemical events that occur during plant developmental processes as well as a component to biotechnological advancement.

5.3.2 Mutant Selection

Improvement of crops by mutant selection is the main use of cell culture. In cell culture several types of mutation with different frequencies are used with the help of mutagens. This may yield the most stable and high yielding live stocks [129]. In tissue culture millions of mutants have been selected and screened at the cellular level. There are various methods adopted for the selection of these mutants. Treatment with the toxic substance mutant cells is the most suitable and extensively used method for screening mutants at the cellular level. Using this method, cell lines resistant to herbicides, antibiotics, fungal toxins, amino acid analogs, etc. have actually been isolated [129].

5.3.3 Somaclonal Variation

When the *in vitro* cultured cells have gone through genetic variation it is then called somaclonal variation and the plants derived from such cells are called "somaclones." Somaclonal variation is always associated with chromosomal variations, which have been generally found in long-term callus, cell suspension culture, and plants regenerated from such cultures. This type of genetic variation generates various potential applications such as crop improvement, in the production of mutants and variants (e.g., disease resistance in potato). Larkin and Scowcroft coined the term "somaclones" for plant variants obtained from tissue cultures of somatic tissues. Similarly, if the somatic tissue-derived variants have a gametophytic origin such as pollen or egg cell, then it is known as "gametoclonal" variation [130]. Several causes of this type of variation are heterogeneity between the cells and explant tissue, spontaneous mutation and activation of culture environment of transposition of genetic materials. In 1980, Shepard and his coworkers screened 100 somaclones produced from leaf protoplasts of large white potato (Russet Burbank) [131]. They established that there was a significant amount of stable variation in compactness of growth habit, maturity, date, tuber uniformity, tuber skin color, and photoperiodic requirements. Among the various applications, plant breeding is the major application of somaclonal variations where the new traits with desired or improved characters are introduced into the plants.

5.3.3.1 *Advantages of Somaclonal Variation*

- Methodology of introducing somaclonal variations is simpler and easier as compared to recombinant DNA technology.
- This approach provides additional genetic variability.
- Suitable for breeding of higher plants.
- Large numbers of populations, for example, tens of thousands of cell lines, are screened simultaneously.
- Stable cell line can be preserved by cryopreservation.
- Somaclonal variation may alter the gene expression to increase the synthesis of secondary metabolites.
- This protoplast-based approach is widely used in agricultural science (crop improvement) for development and production of plants with disease resistance (e.g., rice, wheat, apple, tomato), abiotic stress resistance (e.g., aluminum tolerance in carrot, salt tolerance in tobacco and maize), herbicide resistance (e.g., tobacco resistant to sulfonylurea), and plants with improved quality of seeds (e.g., a new variety of *Lathyrus sativus* seeds with low content of neurotoxin). Some changes occur at a high frequency, for example, chromosomal rearrangement (translocation).
- Novel variants can also arise that are not possible through conventional methods.
- Somaclonal variation is stable and occurs at high frequencies.
- It is the only approach for the isolation of biochemical variants.
- Provides a platform to study the various genetic variants under *in vitro* conditions.
- It can be performed in all types of cells of vegetatively, sexually, and asexually propagated plants.
- Various alternatives were explored, for example: Bio-13, a somaclonal variant of *Citronella java* (with 37% more oil and 39% more citronellon); a medicinal plant has been released as Bio-13 for commercial cultivation by the Central Institute for Medicinal and Aromatic Plants (CIMAP), Lucknow, India; Supertomatoes: Heinz Co. and DNA plant Technology Laboratories (USA) developed Supertomatoes with a high solid component by screening somaclones, which helped in reducing the shipping and processing costs.

5.3.3.2 *Disadvantages of Somaclonal Variation*

- This technique is only limited to those plants that are having the power to regenerate into whole plants.
- Somaclones obtained are sometimes unstable and nonheritable.
- Somaclones more often come with undesirable features such as reduced fertility, growth rate, and overall performance of plant.

- Repeated selection is required to confirm the stability of the plant cell line.
- Plants obtained from somaclonal variation have often lost the power of regeneration.

5.3.4 Somatic Hybridization

Somatic hybridization is the *in vitro* fusion of isolated protoplasts to form a hybrid cell and its subsequent development to form a hybrid plant [132]. This process includes three main steps.

5.3.4.1 Fusion of Protoplasts

Various treatments have been introduced to achieve successive fusion of plant protoplasts. This is achieved by spontaneous, mechanical, or induced fusion methods [132]. Agents like polyethylene glycol, $NaNO_3$, high pH with high Ca^{2++} ion concentration, and electrofusion, responsible for protoplast fusion, are called fusogen. PEG treatment is the most widely used method for protoplast fusion as it has certain advantages over others [132]:

- It has low toxicity to the cell and results in a reproducible high frequency of heterokaryon formation.
- PEG fusion is nonspecific and therefore can be used for a wide range of plants.
- The formation of binucleate heterokaryons is low.

The mechanism of protoplast fusion involves three sequential steps: agglutination, plasma membrane fusion, and formation of heterokaryons. In the first step, two protoplasts come in contact and finally adhere to each other [132]. This type of fusion can be achieved by fusogen (PEG, high pH, and high Ca^{2+}). The second step includes the selection of specific fusogen. The localized site fusion of protoplast membranes results in the formation of cytoplasmic bridges between protoplasts. The surface charge of agglutinated protoplasts is neutralized under high pH and high Ca^{2+} ions, which allows closer contact and membrane fusion between. The last step leads to the formation of spherical homokaryon or heterokaryon from fused protoplasts [132].

5.3.4.2 Hybrid Selection and Identification

Selection of hybrids is the most crucial step and requires different techniques for different species to recover the most suitable hybrid and its callus tissue after the protoplast fusion. It is very difficult to identify the hybrid cells microscopically, thus various important selection procedures are discussed below.

5.3.4.2.1 AUXIN

In this method, parent cell or protoplast requires auxins for its growth whereas hybrid callus tissue does not require auxins for its growth because the cells are auxin autotrophic. Therefore, somatic hybrid cells can be isolated selectively by growth on auxin-free culture medium, for example, the selection of hybrids of *N. glauca* and *N. langsdorffii* is based on auxin autotrophy of the hybrid cells [133].

5.3.4.2.2 USE OF GENETIC COMPLEMENTATION

Chlorophyll deficiency genetic complementation was first used for hybrid selection of *N. tabacum*. When two plant species with different homozygous recessive mutations produce the same, which produces offspring with the wild-type phenotype when mated or crossed, it is called genetic complementation. This type of complementation test can be used to test whether the mutations in two strains are in different genes. In addition, morphological markers can also be used in combination with the genetic complementation [133].

5.3.4.2.3 USE OF UNCOMMON AMINO ACID

Certain uncommon amino acids, which are usually mitotic inhibitors, are also utilized as selective markers to form amino acid-resistant products, for example, legume-derived conavalin inhibits division of soybean and pea cells but sweet clover and alfalfa are unaffected. Heterokaryon obtained by the fusion of protoplast from soybean with those from any one of the resistant plants will divide in the presence of conavalin [133].

5.3.4.2.4 USE OF CELLS RESISTANT TO AMINO ACID ANALOG

Several amino acid analogs (e.g., 5-methyl tryptophan and S-2 amino ethyl-cysteine, both amino acid analogs for interspecific hybrids of *N. sylvestris*) are used for the selection of hybrid cells after protoplast fusion [133].

5.3.4.2.5 USE OF PHYTOTOXIN

Some fungal toxins (phytotoxin) may also be used in hybrid selection, for example, the protoplast of soybean cultured cells is resistant to HmT toxin produced by *Helminthosporium maydis*, whereas the leaf protoplasts of *Zea mays* are sensitive to this toxin. It has been observed that fusion product of soybean and *Z. mays* survive on toxin-containing medium [133].

5.3.4.2.6 USE OF ANTIBIOTIC

Traits exhibiting dominant features such as resistance to antibiotics, herbicides, amino acid analogs, and other toxic compounds (e.g., phytotoxin) are chosen as potential selectable markers for hybrid selection. The fusion of two protoplasts leads to the formation of hybrid protoplast in which the sensitivity trait of one parent is dominated by the resistance trait of the other parent plant. This will now grow on a medium containing both the metabolites because of the double resistance as compared to the single resistance, for example, actinomycin D has been used in the selection of somatic hybrids of two *Petunia* species. Similarly, a kanamycin-resistant cell line of *N. sylvestris* has been used as genetic marker to identify the fusion product of *N. sylvestris* and *N. knightiana*. Similarly, streptomycin-resistant mutants of *N. tabacum* are also used to recover interspecific hybrids with *N. sylvestris*. Cyclochexamide-resistant cells of *D. carota* can be used as a marker for fusion with the albino cell line of *D. carota* [133].

5.3.4.2.7 USE OF AUXOTROPHIC MUTANT

Auxotrophic mutants provide ideal material for physiological and genetic studies. They provide the useful genetic markers for the isolation of somatic hybrids through complementation. Auxotrophic mutants have been successfully used to isolate hybrid protoplast. The auxotrophic mutant selection method involves the auxotrophs, which are mutants that cannot grow on a minimal medium. Therefore, specific compounds are added to the medium. The regenerated hybrids are identified on the basis of morphology and karyotype [133].

5.3.4.2.8 USE OF METABOLIC MUTANTS

One of the way to screen the hybrids is to induce the mutation in such a manner so that product can be easily distinguished, for example, mutation in haploid cells of *N. tabacum* causes nitrate reductase deficiency, which is unable to grow on nitrate medium. Thus, cells that contain nitrate reductase will perform nitrate reduction. Similarly chlorophyll-deficient mutants have also been selected from haploid cells of *D. innoxia* after radiation treatment.

5.3.4.2.9 USING ISOENZYME ANALYSIS

Isozymes can also be used to verify the somatic hybrids. Isozymes are the various forms of enzymes that differ in amino acid sequence but catalyze the same reaction. They form the unique banding pattern in polyacrylamide gel electrophoresis. The pattern of all these enzymes, including the number of band and Rr value, remains constant and specific for each parental plant species. Hybrid callus is the summation of isoenzyme, which overall may help in hybrid cell selection.

5.3.4.2.10 HERBICIDES

Different plants possess different capacities to metabolize the herbicides. This property can form the basis for the selection of hybrids, for example, variation in the rate of propanil resistance among various rice plants.

5.3.4.2.11 CHROMOSOME ANALYSIS OF HYBRID CELL

Chromosome is the microscopic structure that contains all genetic information of an individual. In a coiled fashion, chromosomes contain DNA and various proteins. The DNA contains genetic information in the form of a genetic code, which is protected by proteins and allows the DNA to duplicate properly when the cell divides. Chromosome analysis of different cellular samples derived from their different protoplasts and karyotype assay clearly indicate the formation of hybrids.

5.3.4.3 Applications of Somatic Hybridization

Generally somatic hybridization is the sum of the chromosome number of both parental protoplasts, which is called symmetric hybridization and the hybrids formed are symmetric hybrids. On the contrary, wide variation in the chromosome number rather than the exact total of two species is called asymmetric hybridization and their products are asymmetric hybrids. These concepts lead to the germination of the first interspecific somatic hybrid (between *N. glauca* and *N. langsdorffii*) and the first intergenetic somatic hybrid (between *Solanum tuberosum* (potato) and *Lycopersicon esculentum* (tomato) [134–136]). The hybrids are known as "pomatoes or topatoes." Various prominent examples of interspecific and intergeneric hybrids are mentioned in Table 5.9.

TABLE 5.9 Various Examples of Interspecific and Intergeneric Hybrids

Interspecific hybrids	Intergeneric hybrids
In genus *Dacus* and its relatives and in genus *Nicotiana* and *Brassica*	• *Rice + Echnichola = Oryzochola* • *R. sativus + B. oleracea = Raphanobrassica* • *N. tabacum + L. esculentum = Solanopersicon* • *S. tuberosum + L. esculentum = Solanopersicon*

Various advantages of Somatic hybridization:

- Recombinants can be created in asexually propagated crops or sterile plants, for example, potato.
- The barrier of self-incompatibility can be overcome. For example, *N. tabacum* × *N. nesophila* (disease resistant)
- Cytoplasmic male sterility lines can be produced using cybridization method.
- Herbicide-tolerant plants (brassica) can be produced.
- Creation of hybrids with disease resistance. Many disease-resistant genes (e.g., tobacco mosaic virus, potato virus X, club rot disease) could be successfully transferred from one species to another, for example, resistance has been introduced in tomato against diseases such as TMV, spotted wilt virus, and insect pests.
- Environmental tolerance – using somatic hybridization the genes conferring tolerance for cold, frost, and salt were introduced in, for example, tomato.
- Quality characters – somatic hybrids with selective characteristics have been developed, for example, the production of high nicotine content.
- Somatic cell hybridization/parasexual hybridization or protoplast fusion offers an alternative method for obtaining distant hybrids with desirable traits significantly between species or genera, which cannot be made to cross by conventional the method of sexual hybridization.

5.3.4.4 *Limitations of Somatic Hybridization*
- Somatic hybridization does not guarantee that plants will produce fertile and visible seeds.
- There is genetic instability associated with protoplast culture.
- Some hybrid selection methods are not efficient, which makes limitations in the selection of hybrids. Somatic hybridization is suitable for haploid protoplasts because fusion between two diploids results in the formation of an amphidiploid, which is not favorable.
- Somatic hybridization does not guarantee the successful expression of a specific trait.
- Due to many reasons such as somaclonal variations, chromosomal elimination, organelle segregation, etc., the regenerated plants obtained from somatic hybridization sometimes show variation.
- Fusion of protoplast between different varieties of species/genus is easy, but the production of viable somatic hybrids is not always possible.

5.3.5 Cybrids

Cybridization is the fusion of the nucleus from one parent and the cytoplasm of both parents. The product formed is called a cybrid and the process is known as cybridization. In cybridization one protoplast contributes to the cytoplasm while the other contributes to the nucleus alone. In this process protoplasts are inactivated (nondividing) with either gamma rays, X-rays, or any metabolic inhibitors. By this method genetic traits in certain plants are cytoplasmically controlled [137–139]. Cybridization application covers the transfer of cytoplasmic male sterility and antibiotic and herbicide resistance in agriculturally useful plants, for example, male sterility (*Raphanus sativus*), *B. raphanus* that contains the nucleus of *B. napus* and atrazine-resistant *B. campestris* [137–139].

5.3.6 *In vitro* Plant Germplasm Conservation

Germplasm conservation is the most successful method to conserve the genetic traits of endangered and commercially valuable species. Germplasm is a live information source for all the genes present in the respective plant, which can be conserved for long periods and regenerated whenever it is required in the future. Different plants' genetic diversity is also preserved and this in turn creates a pool of different genes that acts as resource house (gene bank/library) for new or unidentified species [139]. This gene bank also assists the *in vitro* testing of germplasms for their genetic alterations (transgene) and to screen the elite germplasms among them. Genetic variation leads to the loss of genetic information of earlier generations, which makes germplasm conservation an important aspect to preserve this information regarding endangered, primitive, or even any existing species. The International Board of Plant Genetic Resources (IBPGR) is a global organization that has been recognized for germplasm conservation and provides essential support for collection, conservation, and utilization of plant genetic resources throughout the world [139]. Germplasm conservation includes:

- Breeding lines
- Cultivated species
- Commercial varieties
- Special genetic stocks
- Landraces
- Wild species (for direct use (crop species) and indirect use (as root stocks))

5.3.6.1 *Germplasm Preservation [139,140]*

5.3.6.1.1 *IN-SITU* CONSERVATION

On-site conservation is called as *in-situ* conservation, which means conservation of genetic resources in the form of natural populations by establishing biosphere reserves such as national parks and sanctuaries. Practices like horticulture and floriculture also preserve plants in a natural habitat.

5.3.6.1.2 *EX-SITU* CONSERVATION

Off-site conservation is called as *ex-situ* conservation, which deals with conservation of an endangered species outside its natural habitat. In this method genetic information of cultivated and wild plant species is preserved in the form of *in vitro* cultures and seeds, which are stored as gene banks for long-term use. This type of conservation creates a bank of genes/DNA, seeds, and germplasms and forms a genetic information library (e.g., common garden archives) for endangered, primitive, and commercially valuable species. It also includes certain preservation (cryopreservation) and gene transformation techniques for the incorporation of disease, pest and stress tolerance traits, and environmental restoration of endangered plant species.

Genetic resources are used for a variety of reasons such as genetic improvement, conservation of biodiversity, mechanistic studies of adaptation, systematics and taxonomy, environmental monitoring, epidemiology, and forensics. One of the main strategies behind germplasm conservation is to maintain the biological integrity and provide germplasms with validated phenotypic and genetic descriptions. Gene banks are represented as *in vivo* and *in vitro* gene banks. Banks in which genetic resources are preserved by conventional methods, for example, seeds, vegetative propagules, etc., are called *in vivo* gene banks, whereas banks in which the genetic resources are preserved by nonconventional methods such as cell and tissue culture methods are called *in vitro* gene banks. Both these ensure the availability of valuable germplasms to a breeder to develop new and improved varieties.

5.3.6.2 *Methods Involved in the in vitro Conservation of Germplasm*

5.3.6.2.1 CRYOPRESERVATION

In this technique (Greek *krayos*, meaning frost) the cells or tissues are preserved in a frozen state at very low temperatures using solid carbon dioxide (at –79°C), with low temperature deep freezers (at –80°C), using vapor nitrogen (at –150°C) and liquid nitrogen (at –196°C) [141,142]. This technique includes four stages freezing, thawing, and reculture (details are described in the next chapter). This freezing temperature inactivates the cell and thus can be preserved for a longer time. Any tissue from a plant can be used for cryopreservation, for example, meristems, embryos, endosperms, ovules, seeds, cultured plant cells, protoplasts, and calli. To prevent the damage caused to the cells (by freezing or thawing) various compounds like dimethylsulfoxide, glycerol, ethylene, propylene, sucrose, mannose, glucose, praline, acetamide, etc. are added during cryopreservation. These compounds are called cryoprotectants, which prevents the damage caused to cells by reducing the freezing point and super cooling point of water [141,142].

5.3.6.2.2 COLD STORAGE

This is a slow growth conservation method that conserves the germplasm at a low and nonfreezing temperature (1–9°C). The main advantage of this method over cryopreservation is that it slows down growth of the plant material at cold storage (1–9°C) in contrast to complete stoppage during cryopreservation, hence it protects the plants against cryogenic injuries. Moreover this method is simple, cost effective, and yields germplasms with better survival rates. Many outstanding examples of cold storage have recently been reported, for example, virus-free strawberry plants could be preserved at 10°C for about 6 years and several grape plants have been stored for over 15 years by using cold storage at temperature around 9°C (by transferring them in the fresh medium every year) [141,142].

5.3.6.2.3 LOW PRESSURE AND LOW OXYGEN STORAGE

In this method atmospheric pressure (below 50 mmHg reduces plant tissue growth) and oxygen concentration surrounded by plant material are reduced, which causes the reduced availability of O_2, reduced production of CO_2, and hence photosynthetic activity is reduced, which inhibits plant tissue growth and dimension. These conditions may lead to slow and reduced growth of the plant material, which assists in increasing the shelf-life of many fruits, vegetables, and flowers [141,142]. Therefore, conservation of germplasm by conventional methods has several limitations such as seed dormancy, short-lived seeds, seed-borne diseases, and high inputs of cost and labor. These modern techniques, like cryopreservation (freezing cells and tissues at –196°C) and cold storage, help to overcome these problems.

5.3.7 Plant-Made Pharmaceuticals (PMPs)

With the advent of plant tissue culture, techniques like genetic engineering especially rDNA technology have started paying more attention to the production of transgenic plants, which are having high potential in the production of biopharmaceuticals such as proteins and peptides. Production of biopharmaceuticals is dependent on the successful expression of genes (transgenes) in host (plant) cells. The first successful recombinant protein expressed in plants was human growth hormone [143–148]. This was followed by production of various other therapeutic proteins such as immunoglobulin-G1 antibody (tobacco plants), human serum albumin (tobacco and potato), human α-IF (rice), hirudin (seeds of oil seed rape), human protein C serum protease and glucocerebrosidase (tobacco), interleukin-2 and interleukin-4 (tobacco NT-1 suspension cell cultures), and interleukin-12 in tomato (Table 5.11). Planet Biotechnology Inc. was the first company to conduct a clinical trial for protein, CaroRx™ (IgA against *Streptococcus mutans*, causative agent of tooth decay) produced in tobacco [143–148]. In 2006, Dow Agro Sciences of Indianapolis introduced the first plant-based vaccine (chicken vaccine) against Newcastle disease virus in tobacco cell culture. Unfortunately it was not introduced into the market. Then for the treatment of the genetic lysosomal storage disorder (Gaucher's disease), Israel-based Protalix BioTherapeutics launched the first plant-made biopharmaceutical, recombinant protein (glucocerebrosidase), which is approved for parenteral human application [143–148].

Plant-made pharmaceuticals (PMPs) or biopharming is the sub-branch of biotechnology that is actively involved in the production of biopharmaceuticals such as therapeutic proteins, peptides, and secondary metabolites from genetically engineered plants [143–148] (Table 5.10). These biopharmaceuticals can be easily harvested and used to produce pharmaceuticals. One of the main reasons for their demand is their higher efficacy and fewer side effects than small organic molecules (which are often screened as potential drugs). Moreover selecting the plant as an ideal host system or biofactories for the production of these biopharmaceuticals decreases the cost of establishing a complex infrastructure (having expensive fermentation, purification, cold storage, transportation, and sterile delivery facilities) [143–148].

Secondary metabolites also cover the classification of PMPs as they are biologically active, safe, and economic molecules [143–148]. There are various strategies adopted in plant tissue culture to increase the yield of secondary metabolites. Engineering the transgenic plant for the better yield of secondary metabolites is one the successful strategies to combat the low yield-related problems. But this may be expensive. Thus, manipulation of media of the respective culture (parent plant) is the most economic and successful method to achieve the high yield of secondary metabolites. The first commercial product was shikonin, a naphthoquinone from *Lithospermum erythrorhizon* obtained from plant cell culture [143–148]. Subsequently various therapeutic products have been obtained. The best examples for the commercial application of plant tissue culture are ginseng, shikonin, and berberine. Moreover, the practice of *in vitro* propagation of plants to control their development stages yields elite species of high value secondary metabolites, which forms the basis of many practical applications in agriculture, horticulture, industrial chemistry, and pharmaceutical sciences, and is an essential requirement for plant genetic engineering [143–148].

5.3.8 Phytoremediation

Utilization of plants to eliminate the pollutants from the environment, especially from the pollutant-affected sites, is called phytoremedation. Pollutants are classified in two classes: organic and inorganic pollutants. Inorganic pollutants such as extremely toxic metal pollutants can be absorbed by the plants in their leaves where they can be disposed of easily, whereas organic pollutants are degraded by the plant by their respective metabolic activities [149,150].

TABLE 5.10   Prominent Secondary Metabolites Under PMPs Classification [143–148]

Plant name	Active ingredient	Culture type
Vinca faba *Mucuna* sp. *Baptisia* sp. *Lupinus* sp.	L-DOPA	Cell cultures Callus cultures
Taxus baccata, *T. cuspidata,* *T. brevifolia*	Taxol	Cell cultures Callus cultures Suspension cultures
S. laciniatum	Solasodine	Suspension
Salvia miltiorrhiza	Tanshinones	Plant cell Organ culture Hairy root cultures
Rauwolfia serpentina	Reserpine	Suspension
Podophyllum peltatum *P. hexandrum*	Podophyllotoxin	Cell cultures Suspension cultures
P. somniferum	Morphine Codeine	Callus Suspension cultures
Panax ginseng	Ginsenosides	Root callus
N. tabacum	Nicotine	suspension
D. deltoidea *D. doryphora*	Diosgenin	Cell suspension culture
Coptis japonica *Phellodendron amurense* *Thalictrum minus*	Berberine	Cell cultures
C. arabica	Caffeine	Callus
C. roseus	Vinblastine Vincristine	Hairy root cultures
C. frutescens	Capsaicin	Cell cultures
Camptotheca acuminata *Nothapodytes foetida*	Camptothecin	Cell cultures

Plant–microbial symbiotic association may also be helpful to remedy contaminated soils, sediments, and groundwater against hazardous pollutants, for example, bacterial action on plant roots. Phytoremediation is a detoxification of environmental contaminants such as toxic metals and synthetic organic compounds in a growth matrix (e.g., water and soil). Phytoremediation efficiency of plants can be significantly improved by using a tissue culture technique. A tissue culture technique increases the detoxification efficiency of normal plants several fold. Tissue culture allows the genetic study of plants under *in vitro* conditions, which can further assist in their genetic manipulations to form transgenic plants. Overexpression of genes responsible for metal uptake, transport, and sequestration or activation of enzymes responsible for degradation of organic compounds opens new opportunities for phytoremediation. Plant tissue culture provides a model system for *in vitro* testing of the plant to interact with hazardous

TABLE 5.11 Biopharmaceuticals from Transgenic Plants

Plant host	Protein	Applications
HUMAN PROTEIN		
Tobacco, tomato	Angiotensin-converting enzyme	Hypertension
Tobacco	Protein C	Anticoagulant
Tobacco	Granulocyte-macrophage colony-stimulating factor	Neutropenia
Tobacco	Somatropin, chloroplast	Growth hormone
Tobacco	Erythropoietin	Anemia
Tobacco	Epidermal growth	Wound repair and control of cell proliferation
Tobacco	Serum albumin	Liver cirrhosis, burns, surgery
Tobacco	Hemoglobin α, β	Blood constituent
Tobacco	Homotrimeric collagen	Collagen
Tobacco	α-Trichosanthin from TMV-U1 subgenomic coat protein	HIV therapies
Tobacco	Glucocerebrosidase	Gaucher's disease
Rice, turnip, tobacco	Interferon-α Interferon-β	Hepatitis B and C
Rice	α-1 antitrypsin	Cystic fibrosis, liver disease
Potato	Lactoferrin	Antimicrobial
Potato		
NONHUMAN PROTEIN		
Canola	Hirudin	Thrombin inhibitor
Arabidopsis	Enkephalins	Antihyperalgesic activity

pollutants in the form of cultures such as organ, callus, cell suspension, hairy root, and shoot multiplication cultures [149,150]. There are different types of mechanisms and processes present in plants for degradation of organic and inorganic pollutants such as accumulation, complexation, and volatilization. The role of plant tissue culture in phytoremediation of organic and inorganic pollutants is demonstrated in Fig. 5.11.

5.3.8.1 Phytoremediation is Broadly Classified in Two Parts

5.3.8.1.1 METALS (HAIRY ROOT CULTURE)

Naturally plants (roots) have their intrinsic potential to detoxify some heavy toxic metals from the soil. Tissue culture conveys the concept of hairy root culture, which can hyperaccumulate the pollutants in larger concentration than natural ones [149,150]. Furthermore, harvesting them can be an economical method to remove metal in an ecologically friendly manner.

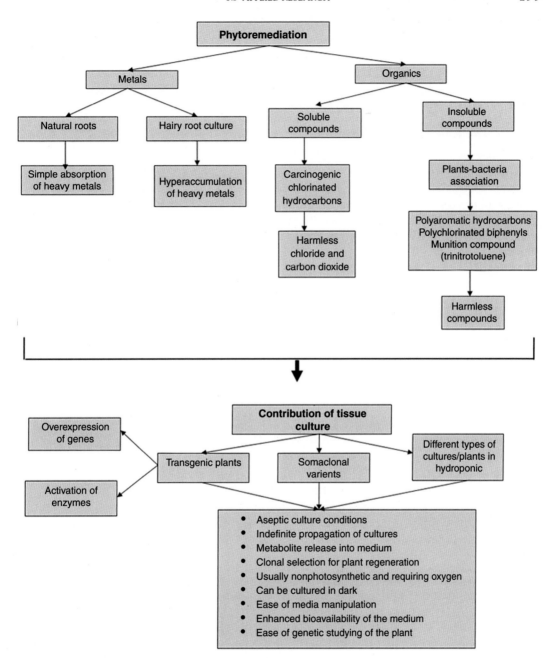

FIGURE 5.11   Role of plant tissue culture in phytoremediation of organic and inorganic pollutants.

5.3.8.1.2 ORGANICS

Soluble Compounds One of the popular examples of soluble compounds is the conversion of cancer-causing chlorinated hydrocarbons in groundwater into harmless products.

Insoluble Compounds With the help of microorganisms plants degrade certain toxic insoluble chemicals such as polyaromatic hydrocarbons, polychlorinated biphenyls, and munition compounds (trinitrotoluene), to perform the phytoremediation process.

5.3.8.2 The Role of Tissue Culture in Preserving Threatened and Endangered Plant Species

5.3.8.2.1 GLOBAL STATUS

Plant species that are either few in number or at risk of becoming extinct due to sudden change in environmental conditions are called endangered species. There are several factors that can affect the environmental conditions. One of the major factors is exploitation of natural resources by human beings. At the world level there is one organization that used to monitor the percentage of endangered species, the International Union for Conservation of Nature (IUCN). In spite of the various conservation attempts the percentage of endangered species is still rising. IUCN estimated about 12.5% of the world's vascular plants (34,000 species) are under different degrees of threat. They also categorize the level of extinction of species: extinct, extinct in the wild, critically endangered, endangered, vulnerable, near threatened, least concern, data deficient, and not evaluated.

5.3.8.2.2 NATIONAL STATUS

IUCN have included 560 plant species of India, some of which come under the category of endangered plants of India, highlighted in Table 5.12.

The IUCN has marked 319 terrestrial plant species of Indian origin and having known medicinal value in its 'Red List of Threatened Species' (Vinson Kurian, The Hindu Businessline; Monday, Nov 04, 2002).

5.3.8.2.3 ROLE OF *IN VITRO* PROPAGATION

The wide contribution of *in vitro* propagation in conserving rare and endangered plants is done to increase biomass and conserve germplasms especially when population numbers are low in the wild. Conserving natural diversity both *in situ* and *ex situ* is the most rapid and suitable method. The tissue culture technique provides better alternatives for those plants:

- Plants that are not grown or difficult to regenerate by conventional methods
- Where population number is rare or decreased due to overexploitation or any climatic change
- Where there is a need to grow similar (monotype) plants having uniform elite features
- When species are frequently utilized for medicine, food, or fragrance
- Where genetic manipulation is required to achieve either high biomass or high yield of secondary metabolites
- To produce dihaploid and polyploid plants
- To overcome the problems faced during *in vitro* pollination

TABLE 5.12 *In vitro* Propagation of Some Rare and Threatened Plant Species of India [151]

Botanical name	Family	Explant used
Syzygium travancoricum[CR]	Myrtaceae	Node
Sternbergia fischeriana[R]	Amaryllidaceae	Bulb scale
Saussurea obvallata[En]	Asteraceae	Root, hypocotyl, cotyledon, leaf
Rheum emodi[En]	Polygonaceae	Shoot tips
Pittosporum napaulensis[R]	Pittosporaceae	Node
Pimpinella tirupatiensis[En]	Apiaceae	Hypocotyl
Nepenthes khasiana[En]	Nepenthaceae	Node
Nardostachys jatamansi[CR]	Valerianaceae	Petiole
Meconopsis simplicifolia[En]	Papaveraceae	Hypocotyl, cotyledon
Kaempferia galanga[En]	Zingiberaceae	Rhizome
Geodorum densiflorum[En]	Orchidaceae	Rhizome
Gentiana kurroo Royle[CR]	Gentianaceae	Shoot tips, nodes
Dendrobium moschatum[En]	Orchidaceae	Stem
Celastrus paniculatus[En]	Celastraceae	Stem
Adhatoda beddomei[En]	Acanthaceae	Node

CR, Critically endangered; En, Endangered; R, Rare.

5.3.9 Other Applications

- Trends for using synthetic seeds were started by plant tissue culture, which is now widely used for crop improvement. Tissue culture comprises certain techniques like artificial seed and cryopreservation, which can be helpful in preservation of embryos/germplasms.
- Tissue culture provides certain classes of chemicals and mutagens, which are extensively used in breeding programs (to achieve homozygous lines), for example, colchicine treatment causes doubling of the chromosome number to furnish the homozygous dihaploid plant.
- Tissue culture eases the pollination between distantly related species. Protoplast fusion is known to be the most popular technique to cross distantly related species to regenerate novel hybrids.
- Techniques like meristem tip culture can be used to produce virus-free plants from virused stock, for example, potatoes and many species of soft fruit.
- Plant tissue culture produces many valuable compounds such as *edible vaccines*, which are of great interest currently.
- Plant tissue culture also overcomes certain problems such as self-sterility and dormancy.
- Plant tissue culture is widely used for the production of somatic hybrids/GM crops. Certain monotype (having similar traits) plants/clones/identical sterile hybrid species can also be obtained by using the plant tissue culture technique.

- Plant biotechnology manifests various applications in plant basic and applied science. These applications furnish selective breeds of mutant, which carry selective traits, for example, resistance to disease, pesticide, mineral ions, herbicide, amino acids, and analogs, and tolerance to abiotics stressors.
- Micropropagation is widely used in forestry, floriculture, horticulture, and agricultural science.
- Micropropagation can also be used to conserve rare or endangered plant species.
- It also decreases the workload in screening the large number of hybrid plants, that is, instead of screening plants for their elite traits a plant breeder may use tissue culture to screen cells for their superior characteristics.
- *In vitro* micropropagation provides wide scope for the production and *in vitro* testing of GM/transgenic plants. It also allows *in vitro* testing of gene constructs (transgene) using gene transformation techniques.
- *In vitro* micropropagation can be scaled up (bioreactors) for large-scale production of valuable compounds, like plant-derived secondary metabolites and recombinant proteins, which are used as biopharmaceuticals. Cultures like plant cell suspension and hairy root culture give better yields of secondary metabolites than can be achieved in nature (intact plant).

References

[1] Haberlandt G. Culturversuche mit isolierten Pflanzenzellen. Sitz-Ber Mat Nat Kl Kais Akad Wiss Wien 1902;111:69–92.

[2] Skoog F, Miller CO. Chemical regulation of growth and organ formation in plant tissue cultured *in vitro*. Symp Soc Exp Biol 1957;XI:118–31.

[3] Ball E. Development in sterile culture of stem tips and adjacent regions of *Tropaeolum majus* L. and of *Lupin albus* L. Am J Bot 1946;33:301–18.

[4] Morel G. La culture *in vitro* du meristema apical de certaines orchidees. CR Hebd Seances Acad Sci 1963;256:4955–7.

[5] Murashige T. Principle of rapid propagation. In: Hughes KW, editor. Propagation of higher plants through tissue culture. Washinghton, DC: US Deptt. of Energy; 1978. p. 14–24.

[6] Gaspar T. Selenieted forms of indolylacetic acid: new powerful synthetic auxins. Across Organics Acta 1995;1:65–6.

[7] Nomura K, Komamine A. Physiological and biochemical aspects of somatic embryogenesis. In: Thorpe TA, editor. *In vitro* embryogenesis in plants. Dordrecht: Kluwer Academic; 1995. p. 249–66.

[8] Komamine A, Ito M, Kawahara R. Cell culture systems as useful tools for investigation of developmental biology in higher plants: analysis of mechanisms of the cell cycle and differentiation using plant cell cultures. In: Soh WY, Liu JR, Komamine A, editors. Advances in developmental biology and biotechnology of higher plants. Korea: The Korean Society of Plant Tissue Culture; 1993. p. 289–310.

[9] Kaeppler SM, Phillips RL. Tissue culture-induced DNA methylation variation in maize. Proc Natl Acad Sci USA 1993;90:8773–6.

[10] Thorpe TA. Organogenesis *in vitro*: Structural, physiological and biochemical aspects. int Rev Cytol Suppl 1980;11A:71–111.

[11] Charles LA. Regeneration of plants from somatic cell cultures: applications for *in vitro* genetic manipulation. The Maize Handbook. New York: Springer Lab Manuals; 1994. pp. 663–671.

[12] Leal F, Loureiro J, Rodriguez E, Pais MS, Santos C, Pinto-Carnide O. Nuclear DNA content of *Vitis vinifera* cultivars and ploidy level analyses of somatic embryo-derived plants obtained from anther culture. Plant Cell Rep 2006;25:978–85.

[13] Jin S, Mushke R, Zhu H, Tu L, Lin Z, Zhang Y, Zhang X. Detection of somaclonal variation of cotton (*Gossypium hirsutum*) using cytogenetics, flow cytometry and molecular markers. Plant Cell Rep 2008;27:1303–16.

[14] Rezaei M, Arzani A, Sayed-Tabatabaei BE. Meiotic behaviour of tetraploid wheats (*Triticum turgidum* L.) and their synthetic hexaploid wheat derivates influenced by meiotic restitution and heat stress. J Genet 2010;89(4):401–7.

[15] Bento MJ, Gustafson P, Viegas W, Silva M. Size matters in Triticeae polyploids: larger genomes have higher remodeling. Genome 2011;54:175–83.

[16] Dermen H. Colchicine polyploidy and technique. Bot Rev 1940;6(11):599–635.

[17] Zeng SH, Chen C, Hong L, Liu J, Deng XX. *In vitro* induction, regeneration and analysis of autotetraploids derived from protoplasts and callus treated with colchicine in Citrus. Plant Cell Tiss Org Cult 2006;87(1):85–93.

[18] Rowson JM. Increased alkaloid contents of induced polyploid of *Datura*. Nature 1949;154:81–2.

[19] Maluszynski M, Ahloowalia BS, Sigurbjörnsson B. Application of *in vivo* and *in vitro* mutation techniques for crop improvement. Euphytica 1995;85(1–3):303–15.

[20] Libbert E, Wichner S, Schiewer U, Risch H, Kaiser W. The influence of epiphytic bacteria on auxin metabolism. Planta 1966;68:327–34.

[21] Maheshwari R. Applications of plant tissue and cell culture in the study of physiology of parasitism. Proc Indian Acad Sci. – Section B 1969;69(3):152–72.

[22] Ardanov P, Sessitsch A, Häggman H, Kozyrovska N, Pirttilä AM. Methylobacterium-induced endophyte community changes correspond with protection of plants against pathogen attack. PLoS ONE 2012;7(10):e46802.

[23] Yadeta KA, Thomma Bart PHJ. The xylem as battleground for plant hosts and vascular wilt pathogens. Front Plant Sci 2013;4:97.

[24] Gelvin SB. Agrobacterium-mediated plant transformation: the biology behind the "gene-jockeying" tool. Microbiol Mol Biol Rev Mar 2003;67(1):16–37.

[25] Michael G, Hahn, Alan G, Darvil P, Albersheim P. Host-pathogen interactions – the endogenous elicitor, a fragment of a plant cell wall polysaccharide that elicits phytoalexin accumulation in soybeans. Plant Physiol November 1981;68(5):1161–9.

[26] Wang M-B, Bian X-Y, F Wu L-M, Liu L-X, Smith NA, Isenegger D, Wu R-M, Masuta C, Vance VB, Watson JM, Rezaian A, Dennis ES, Waterhouse PM. On the role of RNA silencing in the pathogenicity and evolution of viroids and viral satellites. Proc Natl Acad Sci 2004;101(9):3275–80.

[27] Zenk M.H. The impact of cell culture on industry. In: Thorpe TA, editor. Frontiers of plant tissue culture. Calgary, Canada :University of Calgary; 1978. p. 1–13.

[28] O'Dowd NA, McCauley PG, Richardson DHS, Wilson G. Callus production, suspension culture and *in vitro* alkaloid of Ephedra. Plant Cell Tiss Org Cult 1993;34:149–55.

[29] Ishimaru K, Sudo H, Salake M, Malsugama Y, Hasagewa Y, Takamoto S, Shimomura K. Amarogentin and amaroswertin and four xanthones from hairy root cultures of *Swertia japonica*. Phytochemistry 1990;29:1563–5.

[30] Qu JG, Yu XJ, Zhang W, Jin MF. Significantly improved anthocyanins biosynthesis in suspension cultures of *Vitis vinifera* by process intensification. Sheng Wu Gong Cheng Xae Bae 2006;22:299–305.

[31] Nazif NM, Rady MR, Seif MM. Stimulation of anthraquinone production in suspension cultures of *Cassia acutifolia* by salt stress. Fitoterapia 2000;71:34–40.

[32] Rao KV, Venkanna N, Lakshmi NM. Agrobacterium rhizogenes mediated transformation of *Artemisia annua*. J Sci Ind Res 1998;57:773–6.

[33] Kim OT, Bang KH, Shin YS, Lee MJ, Jang SJ, Hyun DY, Kim YC, Senong NS, Cha SW, Hwang B. Enhanced production of asiaticoside from hairy root cultures of *Centella asitica* (L.) Urban elicited by methyl jasmonate. Plant Cell Rep 2007;26:1914–49.

[34] Sujanya S, Poornasri DB, Sai I. *In vitro* production of azadirachtin from cell suspension cultures of *Azadirachta indica*. J Biosci 2008;33:113–20.

[35] Nair AJ, Sudhakaran PR, MAdhusudanan JR, Ramakrishna SU. Berberine synthesis by callus and cells suspension cultures of *Coscinium fenustratum*. Plant Cell Tiss Org Cult 1992;29:7–10.

[36] Sakuta M, Takagi T, Komamine A. Effects of sucrose on betacyanin accumulation and growth in suspension cultures of *Phytolacca americana*. Physiol Plantarum 1987;71(4):455–8.

[37] Waller GR, Mac Vean CD, Suzuki T. High production of caffeine and related enzyme activities in callus cultures of *Coffea arabica* L. Plant Cell Rep 1983;2:109–12.

[38] Vineesh VR, Fijesh PV, Jelly LC, Jaimsha VK, Padikkala J. *In vitro* production of camptothecin (an anticancer drug) through albino plants of *Ophiorrhiza rugosa var. decumbens*. Curr Sci 2007;92:1216–9.

[39] Johnson T, Ravishankar GA, Venkataraman L.V. *In vitro* capsaicin production by immobilized cells and placental tissue of *Capsicum annuum* L. grown in liquid medium. Plant Sci 1990;70:223–9.

[40] Hagimori M, Matsumoto T, Obi Y. Studies on the production of Digitalis cardenolides by plant tissue culture. II. Effect of light and plant growth substances on digitoxin formation by undifferentiated cells and shoot-forming cultures of *Digitalis purpurea* L. grown in liquid media. Plant Physiol 1982;69:653–6.

[41] Farzami MS, Ghorbant M. Formation of catechin in callus cultures and micropropagation of *Rheum ribes* L. Pak J Biol Sci 2005;8:1346–50.

[42] Ramani S, Jayabaskaran C. Enhanced catharanthine and vindoline production in suspension cultures of *Catharanthus roseus* by ultraviolet-B light. J Mol Signal 2008;3:9–14.

[43] Wagiah ME, Alam G, Wiryowidagdo S, Attia K. Improved production of the indole alkaloid cathin-6-one from cell suspension cultures of *Brucea javanica* (L.). Merr Ind J Sci Technol 2008;1:1–6.

[44] Williams RD, Ellis BE. Alkaloids from *Agrobacterium rhizogenes* transformed *Papaver somniferum* cultures. Phytochemistry 1992;32:719–23.

[45] Venkateswara RM, Sankara Rao K, Vaidyanathan CS. Cryptosin – a new cardenolide in tissue culture and intact plant of *Cryptolepis buchanani* Roem and Schult. Plant Cell Rep 1987;6:291–3.

[46] Heble MR, Staba EJ. Diosgenin synthesis in shoot cultures of *Dioscorea sylvatica* (Kunth) Eckl. MSc thesis, Pietermaritzburg: University of Natal ; 1980.

[47] Shohael AM, Murthy HN, Hahn EJ, Paek KY. Methyl jasmonate induced overproduction of eleutherosides in somatic embryos of *Eleutherococcus senticosus* cultured in bioreactors. Elect J Biotechnol 2007;10:633–7.

[48] Sasaki K, Udagava A, Ishimaru H, Hayashi T, Alfermann AW, Nakanishi F, Shimomura K. High forskolin production in hairy roots of *Coleus forskohlii*. Plant Cell Rep 1998;17:457–9.

[49] Mehrotra S, Kukreja AK, Khanuja SPS, Mishra BN. Genetic transformation studies and scale up of hairy root culture of *Glycyrrhiza glabra* in bioreactor 2008;11:717–28.

[50] Gopi C, Vatsala TM. *In vitro* studies on effects of plant growth regulators on callus and suspension culture biomass yield from *Gymnema sylvestre* R. Br Afr J Biotechnol 2006;5:1215–9.

[51] Hilton MG, Rhodes MJC. Factors affecting the growth and hyoscyamine production during batch culture of transformed roots of *Datura stramonium*. Planta Med 1993;59:340–4.

[52] Kornfeld A, Kaufman PB, Lu CR, Gibson DM, Bolling SF, Warber SL, Chang SC, Kirakosyan A. The production of hypericins in two selected *Hypericum perforatum* shoot cultures is related to differences in black gland culture. Plant Physiol Biochem 2007;45:24–32.

[53] Tallevi SG, Dicosmo F. Stimulation of indole alkaloid content in vanadium treated *Catharanthus roseus* suspension cultures. Planta Med 1998;54:149–52.

[54] Shinde AN, Malpathak N, Fulzele DP. Induced high frequency shoot regeneration and enhanced isoflavones production in *Psoralea corylifolia*. Rec Nat Prod 2009;3:38–45.

[55] Oostdam A, Mol JNM, Vanderplas LHW. Establishment of hairy root cultures of *Linum flavum* producing the lignan 5-methoxy podophyllotoxin. Plant Cell Rep 1993;12:474–7.

[56] Misra N, Misra P, Datta SK, Mehrotra S. *In vitro* biosynthesis of antioxidants from *Hemidesmus indicus* R. Br Cult in vitro Dev Biol Plant 2005;41:285–90.

[57] Komaraiah P, Ramakrishna SV, Reddanna P, Kavikishore PB. Enhanced production of plumbagin in immobilized cells of *Plumbago rosea* by elicitation and *in situ* adsorption. J Biotechnol 2003;10:181–7.

[58] Arya D, Patn V, Kant U. *In vitro* propagation and quercetin quantification in callus cultures of Rasna (*Pluchea lanceolata* Oliver & Hiern.). Ind J Biotechnol 2008;7:383–7.

[59] Kuch JSH, Mac Kenzie IA, Pattenden G. Production of chrysanthemic acid and pyrethrins by tissue cultures of *Chrysanthemum cinerariaefolium*. Plant Cell Rep 1985;4:118–9.

[60] Nurchgani N, Solichatun S, Anggarwulan E. The reserpine production and callus growth of Indian snake root (*Rauvolfia serpentina* (L.) Benth. ex Kurz.) cultured by addition of Cu^{2+}. Biodiversitas 2008;9:177–179.

[61] Kin N, Kunter B. The effect of callus age, VU radiation and incubation time on trans-resveratrol production in grapevine callus culture. Tarim Bilimleri Dergisi 2009;15:9–13.

[62] Lee SY, Cho SJ, Park MH, Kim YK, Choi JI, Park SU. Growth and rutin production in hairy root culture of buck weed (*Fagopyruum esculentum*). Prep Biochem Biotechnol 2007;37:239–46.

[63] Fukui H, Feroj HAFM, Ueoka T, Kyo M. Formation and secretion of a new benzoquinone by hairy root cultures of *Lithospermum erythrorhizon*. Phytochemistry 1998;47:1037–9.

[64] Rahnama H, Hasanloo T, Shams MR, Sepehrifar R. Silymarin production by hairy root culture of *Silybium marianum* (L.). Gaertn Iranian J Biotechnol 2008;6:113–8.

[65] Krolicka A, Kartanowicz R, Wosinskia S, Zpitter A, Kaminski M, Lojkowska E. Induction of secondary metabolite production in transformed callus of *Ammi majus* L. grown after electromagnetic treatment of the culture medium. Enzym Microb Technol 2006;39:1386–9.

[66] Granicher F, Cristen P, Kaptanidis I. Production of valepotriates by hairy root cultures of *Centranthes ruber* DC. Plant Cell Rep 1995;14:294–8.

[67] Lee-Parsons CWT, Rogce AJ. Precursor limitations in methyl jasmonate-induced *Catharanthus roseus* cell cultures. Plant Cell Rep 2006;25:607–12.

[68] Murthy HN, Dijkstra C, Anthony P, White DA, Davey MR, Powers JB, Hahn EJ, Paek KY. Establishment of *Withania somnifera* hairy root cultures for the production of withanolide A. J Integ Plant Biol 2008;50:915–81.

[69] White PR. Potentially unlimited growth of excised tomato root tips in a liquid medium. Plant Physiol 1934;9:585–600.

[70] Morel G, Martin C. Guerison de dahlias atteints d'ume Maladie a Virus. C R Acad Sci Paris 1952;235:1324–5.

[71] Mulwa RMS, Mwanza LM. Biotechnology approaches to developing herbicide tolerance/selectivity in crops. Afr J Biotechnol 2006;5(5):396–404.

[72] Barton K, Whiteley H, Yang NS. *Bacillus thuringiensis* dendotoxin in transgenic *Nicotiana tabacum* provides resistance to lepidopteran insects. Plant Physiol 1987;85:1103. 1109.

[73] Benedict JH, Sachs ES, Altman DW, Deaton DR, Kohel RJ, Ring DR, Berberich BA. Field performance of cotton expressing CryIA insecticidal crystal protein for resistance to *Heliothis virescens* and *Helicoverpa zea* (Lepidoptera: Noctuidae). J Econ Entomol 1996;89:230–8.

[74] Hu H, Xiong L. Genetic engineering and breeding of drought-resistant crops. Annu Rev Plant Biol 2014;65:715–41.

[75] Jackson MB, Ishizawa K, Osamu I. Evolution and mechanisms of plant tolerance to flooding stress. Ann Bot 2009;103(2):137–42.

[76] Zhu JK. Plant salt tolerance. Trends Plant Sci 2001;6(2).

[77] Kant S, Bi YM, Weretilnyk E, Barak S, Rothstein SJ. The Arabidopsis halophytic relative *Thellungiella halophila* tolerates nitrogen-limiting conditions by maintaining growth, nitrogen uptake, and assimilation. Plant Physiol July 2008;147(3):1168–80.

[78] Swaminathan MS. Genetic engineering and food security: ecological and livelihood issues. In: Persley GJ, Lantin MM, editors. Agricultural biotechnology and the rural poor. Washington DC, USA: Consultative Group on International Agricultural Research; 2000. p. 37–44.

[79] Liu Y, Wang G, Liu J, Peng X, Xie Y, Dai J, Guo S, Zhang F. Transfer of *E. coli* gutD gene into maize and regeneration of salt-tolerant transgenic plants. Life Sci 1999;42:90–5.

[80] Sharma KK, Lavanya M. Recent developments in transgenics for abiotic stress in legumes of the semi-arid tropics, in: Ivanaga, M. editor. Genetic engineering of crop plants for abiotic stress. Jap Int Res Cent Agric Sci Work Rep 2002;23:61–73.

[81] Borlaug NE. Ending world hunger. The promise of biotechnology and the threat of antiscience zealotry. Plant Physiol 2000;124(2):487–90.

[82] Prakash CS. The genetically modified crop debate in the context of agricultural evolution. Plant Physiol 2001;126(1):8–15.

[83] Signora L, Galtier N, Skot L, Lukas H, Foyer CH. Overexpression of phosphate synthase in *Arabidopsis thaliana* results in increased foliar sucrose/starch ratios and favors decreased foliar carbohydrate accumulation in plants after prolonged growth with CO_2 enrichment. J Exp Bot 1998;49:669–80.

[84] Amasino RM, Gan S. Transgenic plants with altered senescence characteristics. Patent Application EP 804,066, 1997.

[85] Sonnewald U, Willimitzer L. Plasmids for the production of plants that are modified in habit and yield. US Patent 5,492,820, 1996.

[86] Stoger E, Vaquero C, Torres E, Sack M, Nicholson L, Drossard J, Williams S, Keen D, Perrin Y, Christou P, Fischer R. Cereal crops as viable production and storage systems for pharmaceutical scFv antibodies. Plant Mol Biol 2000;42:583–90.

[87] Grula J.W, Hudspeth RL. Promoters derived from the maize phosphoenolpyruvate carboxylase gene involved in C4 photosynthesis. US Patent 5,856,177, 1999.

[88] Leaver CJ, Hill SA, Jenner HL, Winning BM. Transgenic plants having increased starch content. Patent Application WO 98/23,757, 1998.

[89] Williams ME, Levings CS III. Molecular biology of cytoplasmic male sterility. Plant Br Rev 1992;10:23–53.

[90] Savidan Y. Apomixis: genetics and breeding. Plant Br Rev 2000;18:13–86.

[91] Gelvin SB. Improving plant genetic engineering by manipulating the host. Trends Biotechnol 2003;21(3):95–8.

[92] Neelakandan AK, Wang K. Recent progress in the understanding of tissue culture-induced genome level changes in plants and potential applications. Plant Cell Rep 2012;31:597–620.

[93] Kanta K, Ranga Swamy NS, Maheshwari P. Test-tube fertilization in a flowering plant. Nature 1962;194:1214–7.

[94] Guha S, Maheshwari SC. *In vitro* production of embryos from anthers of Datura. Nature 1964;204:497.

[95] Blakeslee AF, Cartledge JL. Pollen abortion in chromosomal types of Datura. Proc Natl Acad Sci USA 1926;12(5):315–23.

[96] Anon. Zeitschrift für Induktive Abstammungs- und Vererbungslehre. J R Microscop Soc 1923;43:237–56.

[97] Belling J, Blakeslee AF. The assortment of chromosomes in Triploid Daturas. Zeitschrift für Induktive Abstammungs- und Vererbungslehre 1924;35(1):190.

[98] Guha S, Maheshwari SC. Cell division and differentiation of embryos in the pollen grains of Datura *in vitro*. Nature 1966;212:97–8.

[99] Bourgin JP, Nitsch JP. Obtention de Nicotiana haploïdes à partir d'etamines cultivées *in vitro*. Ann Physiol Veg 1967;9:377–82.

[100] San Noeum LH. Haploids d'ffordeum vulgare L. par culture *in vitro* d'ovaries non fecondes. Ann Amklior Plant (Paris) 1976;26:751–4.

[101] Carlson PS, Smith HH, Dearing RD. Parasexual interspecific plant hybridization. Proc Natl Acad Sci 1972;69:2292–4.

[102] Sambrook J, Russell DW. Molecular cloning: a laboratory manual. Cold Spring Harbor Laboratory Press, Cold Spring Harbor, NY, USA. 2001;3(16):16.1–16.62.

[103] Hooykaas PJJ, Schilperoort RA. Agrobacterium and plant genetic engineering. Plant Mol Biol 1992;19:15–38.

[104] Chee PP, Slighton JL. Transformation of soybean (Glycine max) via *Agrobacterium tumefaciens* and analysis of transformed plants. In: Gartland KMA, Davey MR, editors. Agrobacterium protocols: methods in molecular biology, vol. 44.Totowa, (NJ): Humana Press; 1995. p. 101–119.

[105] Birch RG. Plant transformation: problems and strategies for practical application. Annu Rev Plant Physiol Plant Mol Biol 1997;48:297–326.

[106] Zhou GY, Weng J, Zeng YS, Huang JG, Qian SY, Liu G.L. Introduction of exogenous DNA into cotton embryos. In: Wu R, Grossman L, Moldave K, editors. Methods in enzymology, vol. 101. New York: Academic Press; 1983. p. 433–481.

[107] Hu C-Y, Wang L. In planta transformation technologies developed in China: procedure, confirmation and field performance. *In Vitro* Cell Dev Biol-plant 1999;35:417–20.

[108] Chowrira GM, Akella V, Lurquin PF. Electroporation-mediated gene transfer into intact nodal meristems in planta: generating transgenic plants without *in vitro* tissue culture. Mol Biotechnol 1995;3:17–23.

[109] Touraev A, Stöger E, Voronin V, Heberle-Bors E. Plant male germ line transformation. Plant J 1997;12:949–56.

[110] Trigiano RN, Gray DJ, editors. Plant tissue culture concepts and laboratory exercises. 2nd ed. Boca Raton: CRC Press; 2000. p. 430 p.

[111] Lessard P. Metabolic engineering, the concept coalesces. Nat Biotechnol 1996;14:1654–5.

[112] Kinney AJ. Manipulating flux through plant metabolic pathways. Curr Opin Plant Biol 1998;1:173–8.

[113] Whitmer S, Van der Heijden R, Verpoorte R. In: Oksman-Caldentey KM, Barz WH, editors. Plant biotechnology, transgenic plants. Marcel & Dekker: New York-Basel; 2002. p. 373–405.

[114] Ramachandra SR, Ravishankar GA. Plant cell cultures: chemical factories of secondary metabolites. Biotechnol Adv 2002;20:101–53.

[115] Bailey JE. Toward a science of metabolic engineering. Science 1991;252(5013):1668–75.

[116] Wilde CD, Peeters K, Jacobs A, Peck I, Depicker A. Expression of antibodies and Fab. fragments in transgenic potato plants: a case study for bulk production in crop plants. Mol Breed 2002;9:271–82.

[117] Bevan MW, Flavell RB, Chilton MD. A chimaeric antibiotic resistance gene as a selectable marker for plant cell transformation. Nature 1983;304:184–7.

[118] Hiatt A, Cafferkey R, Bowdish K. Production of antibodies in transgenic plants. Nature 1989;342:76–8.

[119] Barta A, Sommengruber K, Thompson D, Hartmuth K, Matzke MA, Matzke AJM. The expression of a nopaline synthase human growth hormone chimeric gene in transformed tobacco and sunflower callus tissue. Plant Mol Biol 1986;6:347–57.

[120] Hood EE, Witcher DR, Maddock S, Meyer T, Baszczynski C, Bailey M, et al. Commercial production of avidin from transgenic maize: characterization of transformant, production, processing, extraction and purification. Mol Breed 1997;3:291–306.

[121] Liénard D, Sourrouille C, Gomord V, Faye L. Pharming and transgenic plants. Biotechnol Ann Rev 2007;13: 115–47.

[122] Lowe JA, Jones P. Biopharmaceuticals and the future of the pharmaceutical industry. Curr Opin Drug Discov Dev 2007;10:513–4.

[123] Knäblein J. Plant-based expression of biopharmaceuticals. In: Meyers RA, editor. Encyclopedia of molecular cell biology and molecular medicine. Weinheim: WileyVCH Verlag GmbH and Co. KGaA; 2005. p. 386–407.

[124] Ma JK-C, Drake PMW, Christou P. The production of recombinant pharmaceutical proteins in plants. Genetics 2003;4:794–805.

[125] Thomas BR, Van Deynze A, Bradford KJ. Production of therapeutic proteins in plants. Agricultural Biotechnology in California Series 8078; University of California-Davis, CA, 2002.

[126] Sugiyama M. Organogenesis *in vitro*. Curr Opin Plant Biol 1999;2:61–4.

[127] Irish VF. The Arabidopsis petal: a model for plant organogenesis. Trends Plant Sci 2008;13(8):430–6.

[128] Steward FC, Mapes MO, Smith J. Growth and organized development of cultured cells: I Growth and division of freely suspended cells. Am J Bot 1958;45:693–703.

[129] Bhojwani SS, Razdan MK. Plant Tissue Culture: Theory and Practice. Developments in Crop Science, Vol. 5. Amsterdam: Elsevier; 1983.

[130] Larkin PJ, Scowcroft WR. Somaclonal variation – a novel source of variability from cell cultures for plant improvement. Theor Appl Genet 1981;60:197–214.

[131] Shepard JF, Bidney D, Shahin E. Potato protoplasts in crop improvement. Science 1980;208:17–24.

[132] Chawla HS. Introduction to plant biotechnology. Oxford and IBH Publishing; New Delhi, India 2009. 112–115.

[133] Narayanaswamy S. Plant cell and tissue culture. New Delhi: Tata McGraw-Hill Education; 1994. 423–427.

[134] Melchers G, Sacristán MD, Holder SA. Somatic hybrid plants of potato and tomato regenerated from fused protoplasts. Carlsberg Res Comm 1978;43:203–8.

[135] Carlson PS, Smith HH, Dearing RD. Parasexual interspecific plant hybridization. Proc Natl Acad Sci 1972;69:2292–4.

[136] Navrátilová B. Protoplast cultures and protoplast fusion focused on Brassicaceae – a review. Hort Sci (Prague) 2004;4:140–57.

[137] Sakai T, Imamura J. Alteration of mitochondrial genomes containing atpA genes in the sexual progeny of cybrids between *Raphanus sativus* cms line and *Brassica napus* cv. Westar Theor Appl Genet 1992;84(7–8):923–9.

[138] Sakai T, Liu HJ, Iwabuchi M, Kohno-Murase J, Imamura J. Introduction of a gene from fertility restored radish (*Raphanus sativus*) into *Brassica napus* by fusion of X-irradiated protoplasts from a radish restorer line and iodacetoamide-treated protoplasts from a cytoplasmic male-sterile cybrid of *Brassica napus*. Theor Appl Genet 1996;93(3):373–9.

[139] Mathur S. Conservation of biodiversity through tissue culture. RRJMB 2013;2(3).

[140] Cruz-Cruz CA, González-Arnao MT, Engelman F. Biotechnology and conservation of plant biodiversity. Resources 2013;2:73–95.

[141] Kaczmarczyk A, Funnekotter B, Menon A, Phang PY, Al-Hanbali A, Bunn E, Mancera RL. Current issues in plant cryopreservation, Curr Front Cryobiol, In: Prof. Igor Katkov, editor. 2012, Available from: http://www.intechopen.com/books/currentfrontiers-in-cryobiology/current-issues-in-plant-cryopreservat.

[142] Kaviani B. Conservation of plant genetic resources by cryopreservation. Aust J Crop Sci 2011;5(6):778–800.

[143] Paul M, Ma JK. Plant-made pharmaceuticals: leading products and production platforms. Biotechnol Appl Biochem 2011 Jan-Feb;58(1):58–67.

[144] Thomas DR, Penney CA, Majumder A, Walmsley AM. Evolution of plant-made pharmaceuticals. Int J Mol Sci 2011;12(5):3220–36.

[145] Goldstein DA1, Thomas JA. Biopharmaceuticals derived from genetically modified plants. Q J Med 2004;97(11):705–16.

[146] Giddings G, Allison G, Brooks D, Carter A. Transgenic plants as factories for biopharmaceuticals. Nat Biotechnol 2000;18(11):1151–5.

[147] Fischer R, Stoger E, Schillberg S, Christou P, Twyman RM. Plant-based production of biopharmaceuticals. Curr Opin Plant Biol 2004;7(2):152–8.

[148] Twyman RM, Schillberg S, Fischer R. Transgenic plants in the biopharmaceutical market. Expert Opin Emerg Drugs 2005;10(1):185–218.

[149] Cherian S, Oliveira MM. Transgenic plants in phytoremediation: recent advances and new possibilities. Environ Sci Technol 2005;39(24):9377–90.

[150] Doran PM. Application of plant tissue cultures in phytoremediation research: incentives and limitations. Biotechnol Bioeng 2009;103(1):60–76.

[151] Kapaia VY, Kapoora P, Rao IU. *In vitro* propagation for conservation of rare and threatened plants of India – a review. Department of Botany, University of Delhi, Delhi, India.

Somatic Embryogenesis and Organogenesis

Saurabh Bhatia, Tanmoy Bera

Modern Applications of Plant Biotechnology in Pharmaceutical Sciences. http://dx.doi.org/10.1016/B978-0-12-802221-4.00006-6

6.1 INTRODUCTION

Plant regeneration is the major outcome of plant tissue culture, which is based on the principle of totipotency. Plant regeneration can be achieved by organogenesis and somatic embryogenesis (Fig. 6.1). Organogenesis means formation of organs from the cultured explants. The shoot buds or monopolar structures are formed by manipulating the ratio of cytokinin

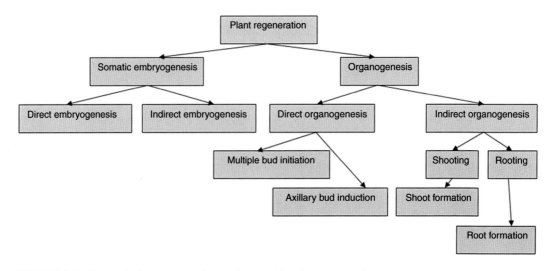

FIGURE 6.1   Types of plant regeneration system used in micropropagation.

to auxin in the cultures. In somatic embryogenesis, the totipotent cells may undergo embryogenic pathway to form somatic embryos, which are grown to regenerate whole plants. It was first established in carrots (*Daucus carota*), where bipolar embryos developed from single cells. The somatic embryogenesis is influenced by herbal extracts, phytohormones, and the physiological state of calli.

6.2 SOMATIC EMBRYOGENESIS

Generally, embryogenesis is the process of formation and development of embryo and occurs both in plants and animals. Zygotic embryogenesis is the result of normal pollination and fertilization whereas somatic embryogenesis is the result of the formation of embryos from sporophytic cells (cultured), which means that in this process embryos arise indirectly. Various stages of zygotic embryogenesis are highlighted in Fig. 6.2.

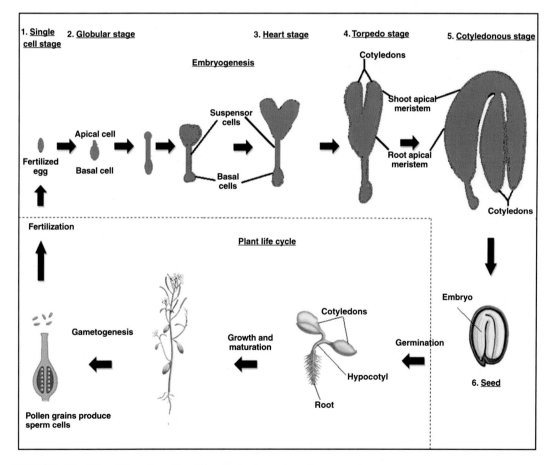

FIGURE 6.2   Plant life cycle with a closer look at zygotic embryogenesis.

Somatic embryogenesis is defined as a process in which embryo-like structures are formed from somatic tissues and developed into a whole plant. Somatic embryogenesis is a useful regeneration pathway for many monocots and dicots, but is especially useful for grasses. In this process composition of the culture medium controls the whole process. Various chief characteristics of somatic embryogenesis are mentioned below:

- Auxin plays a vital role in the development of somatic embryogenesis. Addition of auxin causes induction and formation of embryogenic clumps or proembryogenic callus (induction medium), whereas their deletion from the medium leads to the formation of mature embryos (maturation medium).
- During the development of somatic embryos the early cell division stage does not follow a fixed pattern, unlike with zygotic embryogenesis. But their later stages are very similar to zygotic embryogenesis (dicot pattern), for example, globular stage (multicellular), heart-shaped stage (bilateral symmetry), and bipolarity and torpedo-shaped stage (consists of initial cells for the shoot/ root meristem).

6.2.1 Types of Somatic Embryogenesis

6.2.1.1 Direct Somatic Embryogenesis

In direct somatic embryogenesis embryos are formed directly from a cell or small group of cells such as the nucellus, styles, or pollen without the production of an intervening callus. Direct somatic embryogenesis is generally rare.

6.2.1.2 Indirect Somatic Embryogenesis

In this process callus is first produced from the explant and then embryos are produced from the callus tissue or from a cell suspension culture (Fig. 6.3).

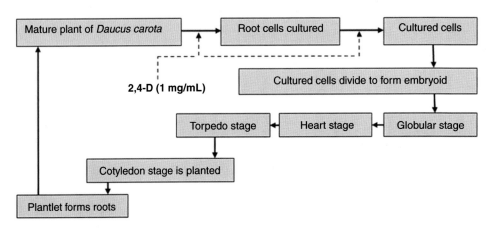

FIGURE 6.3   Indirect embryogenesis in carrot (*D. carota*).

6.2.2 Advantages of Somatic Embryogenesis

Large-scale production of plants through the multiplication of embryogenic cell lines is the most commercially attractive application of somatic embryogenesis [1]. This application can be widely applicable in the area of agricultural crops. In this respect it has many advantages over conventional micropropagation:

- It permits the culture of large numbers of somatic embryos, with up to 1.35 million somatic embryos capable of being regenerated per liter of the medium.
- Simultaneous production of root and shoot from such a plant regeneration system eliminates the need for a root induction phase as in conventional micropropagation.
- The mode of culture permits easy scale-up and subculture with low labor inputs.
- Cultures can be manipulated so that embryo formation and germination can be synchronized.
- Maximizing plant output can be achieved with minimum labor costs.
- As with zygotic embryos, somatic embryo dormancy can be induced, hence long-term storage is possible.

6.2.3 Limitations of Somatic Embryogenesis

Apart from various applications somatic embryogenesis carries certain limitations in micropropagation. First, the development of somatic embryos tends to be nonsynchronous [2,3]; therefore, embryos of all stages can be present in one culture system. However, Fujimura and Komamine demonstrated that the development of carrot somatic embryos could be synchronized by grouping cell aggregates of similar size and density from suspension cultures. This was accomplished by using sieving and density gradient centrifugation methods [4]. Synchronization of somatic embryos can be achieved using these strategies but it appears that the percentage of somatic embryos regenerated is affected by the size of cell aggregates. Chee and Cantliff pointed out that a decrease in the size of cell aggregates led to a reduction in the percentage of somatic embryo formation in sweet potato [5]. The strategy of selecting highly regenerable portions can be a more efficient propagation system than conventional micropropagation. For example, the rate of somatic embryo formation in banana suspension cultures can be over 100,000 mL^{-1} of cells [6]. Thus, selection of a subgroup of cells and discarding the remainder would provide the highly regenerable cell line for producing large numbers of plants *in vitro*. The second limitation and the most common is the stability of cell lines. Over a period of time, the proportion of cells that enter or complete embryogenesis decreases so that, eventually, regeneration may become impossible. Factors that limit the regeneration more often promote the mutation. This could be a certain advantage as delayed time in culture can lead to the accumulation of mutations (somaclonal variations), which can cause morphological abnormalities such as pluricotyledony, multiplex apex formation and fused cotyledons [7]. Thus, forcing the initiation of new cultures (as old ones lose regenerability) may reduce the chances of somaclonal variations. Perhaps this may be linked with increasing mutations associated with an inability to regenerate. While working with suspension cultures of carrot, Evans et al. showed that frequently initiating new cultures and maintaining the cultures for less than 1 year resulted in the regeneration of phenotypically normal somatic embryos and plants [7]. Apparently, somaclonal variation also occurs with conventional micropropagation, hence new cultures are also initiated on a regular basis. It should be noted, however, that somaclonal variation could have tremendous potential for producing novel and useful varieties.

6.2.4 Factors Affecting Somatic Embryogenesis in Modern Plant Breeding

6.2.4.1 Role of Plant Growth Regulators (PGRs) in the Development of Somatic Embryos

- *Auxins*: Supplementation of auxin promotes callus proliferation and inhibits differentiation while the removal or decrease in auxin allows progress in the development of somatic embryo. Auxins are also responsible for the establishment of cell polarity (apical basal axis). It was reported that auxin-mediated polar transport in early globular embryos is required for the establishment of bilateral symmetry during plant embryogenesis [8]. Relatively high levels of endogenous free indole-3-acetic acid (IAA) may be required for the induction of the process leading to polarity. Nevertheless, once induction has occurred, those high levels of IAA must be reduced to allow the establishment of the auxin gradient. If the levels are too low or high or do not diminish after the induction, the gradient cannot be formed and thus somatic embryogenesis cannot progress [1]. Recently it has been proposed that auxin (2,4-D) may initiate somatic embryogenesis by inducing a stress response in plant cells [9]. Expression of stress-related genes has been found in the early stages of embryogenesis, thus it has been proposed that this is an extreme stress response in cultured plant cells [9].
- *Cytokinins*: Cytokinin and its derivatives are also suitable candidates for induction of somatic embryogenesis, for example, in some cases thidiazuron (TDZ) has stimulated *in vitro* shoot regeneration and somatic embryogenesis [10–13]. It has been suggested that TDZ is more effective than other cytokinins used for somatic embryogenesis

6.2.4.2 Effect of Nature of Explant, Explant Genotype, and Culture Conditions on Somatic Embryogenesis

Several explants can be utilized; however, the correct development stage of explant determines the progress in initiation of embryogenic callus. In particular, young or juvenile explants yield more somatic embryos than older explants [14,15]. One of the difficulties encountered during selection of explants is that the different explant tissues from the same mother plant produced embryogenic callus at different frequencies [16] and required different concentration of growth regulators for the induction of somatic embryos. Thus, the type and age of explants has an impact on somatic embryogenesis. Generally young, dividing, and possibly less differentiated cells are preferred for embryogenic pathway than older cells. Apart from explant nature, its genotype plays an important role in determining somatic embryogenic competence. For example, out of the five cultivars of hybrid tea roses (*Rosa hybrida* L.) investigated, somatic embryogenesis could only be induced in two [17]. Furthermore, media modifications such as manipulations of the concentrations of inorganic salts and vitamins can have a significant effect on somatic embryogenesis possibly through altering the osmotic potential of the medium.

6.2.4.3 *The Effect of Light and Activated Charcoal*

Browning of the plant tissue due to oxidation caused by certain compounds (like polyphenol oxidases) under the influence of a phenolic-rich environment *in vivo* causes severe darkening of the tissue. Such oxidation-dependent darkening may also inhibit the activity of various proteins, which may have an inhibitory effect on somatic embryogenesis [7]. This can be justified by a report that confirmed the inhibition of somatic embryogenesis of carrot under continuous light unless activated charcoal filter papers were used [18]. White light-induced growth enhances the production of phenolic compounds and increased level of abscisic acid [7]. Activated charcoal absorbs the inhibitors of embryogenesis (phenylacetic acid, benzoic acid derivatives, and other colorless toxic compounds) and efficiently removes them from the growing culture [19,20]. In addition, it also has the capacity to remove an inhibitor (5-hydroxymethylfurfural), formed by the degradation of sucrose during autoclaving, as well as a considerable amount of auxins and cytokinins by absorption. Apart from its action of absorbing toxic inhibitors, which may hinder growth *in vitro*, it may also adsorb and reduce the levels of growth regulators that are essentially required for callus initiation, growth, and proliferation. Consequently, it has been always preferred that cultures should be preserved under reduced light intensity or in darkness, as this will decrease the production of inhibitory compounds from tissues in the culture medium [7]. Furthermore, this will also reduce or counteract the interference of activated charcoal in the medium, therefore ensuring that the potential effects of the growth regulators present in the medium will not be compromised.

6.2.4.4 *The Effect of Other Biochemical Factors on Somatic Embryogenesis*

Some biochemicals such as amino acids, glutamine, proline, tryptophan, and polyamines (putrescine) have been reported for their profound effects on somatic embryogenesis in some species. They are also known to be the enhancers of somatic embryogenesis. The potential of these compounds has been attributed to their diverse role in cellular processes such as precursor molecules for certain growth regulators [21–24], cell signaling process improvement during various signal transduction pathways [20], and DNA synthesis regulation [25,26]. In addition, several species do not require supplementation of these additives. It has been also reported that addition of complex organic extracts (coconut water, taro extract, potato extract, corn extract, and papaya extract) are essential for somatic embryogenesis in some species [27,28]. In addition, some researchers also proposed that supplementation of extracts does not cause mutation or less mutation than conventional growth regulators and inclusion of such extracts in the media may reduce the chances of somaclonal variations [29]. Nevertheless owing to the undefined composition of organic extracts it is not possible to determine the component that is responsible for somatic embryogenesis and it is always obligatory to prepare the fresh composition to maintain consistency in the actual extract.

6.2.4.5 *Somatic Embryo Maturation*

The sequential steps followed during embryogenesis are: embryogenic callus initiation from vegetative cells or tissues, maintenance and development of embryogenic cell lines, somatic embryo formation, and maturation and ultimately conversion (germination) of somatic embryos into viable plantlets [30]. Since the high rate of plant recovery from mature embryos, maturation is regarded as a crucial stage of embryogenesis. Maturation of embryo proceeds with carbohydrates, lipids, and protein reserves accumulation, and a decrease in cellular respiration and embryo dehydration [31]. Consequently, maturation is known to be a preliminary stage for embryo development, which is essentially required for effective germination. Etienne et al. stated that maturation is a temporary but essential stage between embryo development and embryo germination phases, therefore bypassing the maturation phase will result in fast germination of embryos causing a considerable reduction in viability of plantlets.

Water loss was assumed to be critical for maturation [32]. It was studied that supplementation of osmoticum restricts water uptake, supports development, and prevents precocious germination of plant embryos [32–34]. Penetration of osmoticum (e.g., sucrose) reduces the water potential of the culture medium, which ultimately leads to water stress, thereby promoting embryo development during *in vitro* culture. Osmotic recovery achieved after osmotic inclusion in the prolonged culture of plant cells was also studied [33]. In addition, nonpermeating osmoticum (e.g., polyethylene glycol-4000) continuously limits water uptake and thus offers longer-term drought stress during embryo development. Furthermore, the effect of desiccation rate on the germination and conversion of somatic embryos into plantlets is also reported, for example, germination capacity of *Hevea* was improved with rapid desiccation but limits its further growth into plantlets. Slow desiccation promotes considerable accumulation of starch and protein reserves required for continued development of immature embryo, resulting in enhancement of germination. Therefore, desiccation could be used for the effective stimulation of embryo (when the embryo approaches physiological maturity) into plantlets [32]. Furthermore, drying of embryo minimizes production expenses and promotes its storage to increase its availability throughout the year [33]. Such storage provides a platform for the synchronization of embryos according to the uniform age and size for planting during a favorable growing season.

It has been also discovered that exogenous supplementation of abscisic acid promotes the maturation of hybrid larch somatic embryos. Therefore, absence of abscisic acid causes the poor and nonsynchronous development of somatic embryos exhibiting abnormal morphology and precocious germination [34]. Such somatic embryos had the lowest potential for germination and plantlet development. In comparison large quantities of high quality and well-developed somatic embryos are obtained in the presence of abscisic acid in the maturation medium. These somatic embryos germinated and developed into plantlets at a high frequency under suitable conditions. Rather dependent on high-frequency embryo formation, the practical approach of somatic embryogenesis is more dependent on the capability of embryos in developing into normal plantlets [35].

6.2.5 Uses of Somatic Embryogenesis in Crop Improvement

6.2.5.1 Cell Selection

Selection of the cell is based on the regeneration of plant from cell populations, and therefore selection of desirable genetic characteristics of these regenerated plants [36]. To prevent the production of genetic chimeras it is obligatory to utilize a plant regeneration system able to regenerate plants from single selected cells. Somatic embryogenesis prevents the production of genetic chimeras by allowing the regeneration of whole plants from single cells [37], making possible its use in cell selection programs.

6.2.5.2 Regeneration of Genetically Transformed Plants

Gene transfer technologies are an essential part of modern plant tissue culture science. Uniform transformation of plant cells under *in vitro* conditions is required for the stable expression of genes. However, plant transformation techniques do not transform all cells. In addition, plants that are regenerated from transformed tissue (organogenesis) are often chimeras [38]. Development of somatic embryos provides a solution for such problems. Since they arise from single cells, they reduce the chances of chimera formation [37]. Moreover, somatic embryogenesis provides fewer rates of somaclonal variation when compared with organogenesis [39]. This method carries an advantage for plants that lack an efficient regeneration method. Such plants could be grown through somatic embryogenesis, for example, coffee [40]. From these evidences it has been proven that somatic embryos are the best candidates for genetic transformation. The following are various strategies that have been employed during the regeneration of transformed plants using somatic embryogenesis (Fig. 6.4).

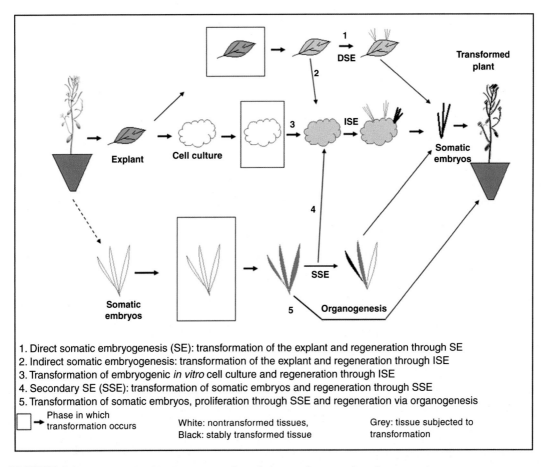

1. Direct somatic embryogenesis (SE): transformation of the explant and regeneration through SE
2. Indirect somatic embryogenesis: transformation of the explant and regeneration through ISE
3. Transformation of embryogenic *in vitro* cell culture and regeneration through ISE
4. Secondary SE (SSE): transformation of somatic embryos and regeneration through SSE
5. Transformation of somatic embryos, proliferation through SSE and regeneration via organogenesis

☐→ Phase in which transformation occurs

White: nontransformed tissues, Black: stably transformed tissue

Grey: tissue subjected to transformation

FIGURE 6.4 Steps involved in the regeneration of plants using somatic embryogenesis.

6.2.5.2.1 TRANSFORMATION OF THE EXPLANT AND REGENERATION VIA DIRECT SOMATIC EMBRYOGENESIS

Genetic transformation and then regeneration through direct somatic embryogenesis is fast, simple, and avoids the chances of somaclonal variation. Utilization of this methodology allows the successful transformation of some recalcitrant species for which plant regeneration has been reported only through direct somatic embryogenesis [41]. Apart from these advantages direct somatic embryogenesis has been reported in only a few plant species.

6.2.5.2.2 TRANSFORMATION OF THE EXPLANT AND REGENERATION VIA INDIRECT SOMATIC EMBRYOGENESIS

This method has been unsuccessful in eliminating somaclonal variation but can be used for a wide range of species.

6.2.5.2.3 TRANSFORMATION OF EMBRYOGENIC CELL CULTURE AND REGENERATION VIA INDIRECT SOMATIC EMBRYOGENESIS

Plant regeneration through this method is relatively fast and allows easier transformation of cultured cells.

6.2.5.2.4 TRANSFORMATION OF SOMATIC EMBRYOS AND REGENERATION THROUGH SECONDARY OR INDIRECT SOMATIC EMBRYOGENESIS

Somatic embryogenesis allows high rates of transformation than other methods. Transformed somatic embryos can be regenerated in many ways. Regeneration via secondary somatic embryogenesis and by producing embryogenic calli or cell cultures have been known for their high transformation efficiencies [42].

6.2.5.2.5 TRANSFORMATION OF SOMATIC EMBRYOS, PROLIFERATION THROUGH SECONDARY EMBRYOGENESIS, AND REGENERATION THROUGH ORGANOGENESIS

Secondary embryogenesis usually yields large numbers of easily transformed cells. However, screening for the transformation of somatic embryos in some species is difficult as these somatic embryos are very sensitive to the selective agents that are used to detect the transformed cell [43]. In 1996 Lie et al. introduced a method for the screening of somatic embryos by combining embryogenesis and organogenesis. In this study, embryos were transformed using *Agrobacterium* infection and regenerated through organogenesis after cycles of secondary somatic embryogenesis [44]. This and many other reports were based on the optimization of the methods using genes conferring resistance either to antibiotics or reporter genes. However, more practical research is required to utilize different types of transgenes, especially with disease resistance genes.

6.2.5.3 Somatic Hybrid Regeneration

Crosses between disease-resistant wild varieties and cultivated species of elite traits act as a potential source for plant genetic improvement [45]. However, resistance of some species toward crossing and regeneration limits this strategy. Introduction of the protoplast fusion technique overcomes these problems and allows a new combination of nuclear and organelle DNA. This technique requires a suitable plant regeneration system such as organogenesis or somatic embryogenesis, which can be employed to regenerate the fused protoplast. It has been reported that utilization of somatic embryogenesis is relatively more advantageous in regenerating plants from single cells. For this reason somatic embryogenesis is selected as the method of choice in many somatic hybridization projects.

6.2.5.4 *Homozygous and Polyploid Line Production*

Somatic embryogenesis potentially promotes polyploidy reactions in the presence of colchicine or the antimicrotubular drug amiprophos-methyl [46,47]. Increase in polyploidy reactions while regenerating via somatic embryogenesis was reported in the melon (*Cucumis melo*) and *Iochroma warscewiczii* [48,49]. It was also evidenced that somatic embryogenesis potentially regenerates triploid plants from the endosperm as explant. This was observed in *Prunus persica* [50], *Citrus* [51], and *Acacia nilotica* [52]. Regeneration of plants from microspores via somatic embryogenesis is possible but haploid regeneration from anthers (androgenesis) or ovules (gynogenesis) through embryo formation is not considered as somatic embryogenesis *sensu stricto* [53–55]. Haploid plant production is required to obtain homozygous cell line in a single generation. This can be achieved by using the chromosome doubling technique.

6.2.5.5 *Germplasm Preservation*

Procurement of seed at different dry and cold conditions is a reliable method for the long-term storage of the germplasm. However, the seeds of certain species cannot be stored at low temperature or cannot be desiccated. In addition, some plant species are only cultivated via vegetative a propagation method, which creates additional preservation problems. *In vitro* propagation provides a valuable solution to these problems. *In vitro* plant propagation allows maintenance of long-term embryogenic calli or cell-suspension cultures. However, expense, time consumption, and chances of contamination limit this strategy up to a certain extent. Additional problems induced by long-term cell cultures increase the chances of genetic changes by somaclonal variation, and reduces plant viability and regeneration capacity. Spontaneous initiation of new embryonic cell cultures can reduce these limitations. Furthermore, initiation of new cultures could be difficult in some species in which embryogenic cell cultures have proven to be complicated or in which the embryogenic explants are only available during short periods of the year.

6.2.5.6 *Virus Elimination*

Somatic embryogenesis under the influence of thermotherapy was proved to be an effective protocol in eliminating viruses. A developed vascular system of somatic embryos is not connected to the explant tissue, which makes possible the use of somatic embryogenesis as a method to eliminate viruses, combined or not with heat shock treatments [56,57]. The most popular examples of two viruses that were eliminated using somatic embryogenesis associated with thermotherapy are: grapevine GFLV (grapevine fanleaf virus) and 3-GLR viruses (grapevine leafroll-associated viruses) [57,58]. Calli produced from the infected tissue were exposed against heat shock (35°C) and somatic embryos were successfully produced. These somatic embryos were further converted into plants. Plants regenerated via this protocol were tested and the results indicated that plantlets obtained are completely virus free.

6.2.5.7 *Metabolite Production*

In conventional agricultural practices production of metabolites is based on the propagation of great quantities of plants, harvesting of organs or tissues that accumulate in the product, and various extraction procedures to extract the chemicals. Sometimes plant synthesizes secondary metabolites that are particularly organ specific (e.g., fruits, seeds, flowers, or embryos), and sometimes for extracting small quantities of metabolites very large quantities of plants are required. *In vitro* cell cultures for metabolite production have been proposed as an alternative for traditional methods. These techniques [59] successfully produced secondary metabolites but sometimes the undifferentiated cells or tissue lost the capacity to accumulate the metabolites or synthesize metabolites in very low quantities. Techniques like elicitation or precursor feeding can increase metabolite production [60,61], but not always. Organ culture and somatic embryogenesis are known to be the most successful methods to accumulate the products effectively. These alternative methods are influenced by several factors such as economics. Owing to the high cost of *in vitro* technology the metabolites obtained must be of high economic value. In 1993, Janick demonstrated that these metabolites are of high therapeutic value such as alkaloids and certain lipids, some flavor compounds and food additives, and pigments [62]. Some prominent examples are:

- Taxoids from *Taxus* species [63,64]
- Jojoba liquid wax from jojoba somatic embryos [65]
- Gamma-linolenic acid from borage (*Borago officinalis*) somatic embryos [66–68]
- Celery flavor compounds from celery somatic embryos
- Caffeine and theobromine from somatic embryos of cacao [69,70]

6.3 SYNTHETIC SEED TECHNOLOGY

Artificial or synthetic seed technology encapsulates somatic embryos in a protective coating. Artificial seed may often be referred to as synthetic seed. Synthetic seeds are artificially encapsulated somatic embryos, shoot buds, cell aggregates, or any other tissue that can be utilized for propagation as a seed. Synthetic seeds have the potential to convert into a plant under *in vitro* or *ex vitro* conditions and retain this potential after storage [71,72]. In earlier times synthetic seeds were only limited to somatic embryos that were of economic use in crop production. Recent research has introduced various other tissues such as bud shoot tips, organogenic or embryogenic calli, etc. that can also be employed in the production of synthetic seeds. Therefore, the concept of synthetic seeds is not only limited to somatic embryogenesis and its use (storage and sowing), but now is also linked with other techniques of micropropagation like organogenesis and the enhanced axillary bud proliferation system [71,72]. Axillary bud proliferation, somatic embryogenesis, and organogenesis are the efficient techniques for large-scale *in vitro* multiplication of elite and desirable plant species. These regeneration protocols yield a large number of somatic embryos or shoot buds that are potentially used for plant regeneration either after minor treatment or without any treatment with growth regulator(s). These naked structures, which are useful in synthetic seed production, are sensitive to desiccation and/or pathogens when exposed against the natural environment. Therefore, it was proposed that for large-scale planting and to improve the success of plant delivery to the field or greenhouse, these micropropagules would essentially require some protective coatings.

Shielding or encapsulation of propagules is reported to be the best method to provide protection and to convert the *in vitro* derived propagules into "synthetic seeds" or "synseeds" or "artificial seeds." Synthetic seed technology has been applied to produce synthetic seeds of a wide range of plant species belonging to angiosperms and gymnosperms. However, there are only few reports available on synseeds in comparison to the total number of plant species in which *in vitro* regeneration has been established [71,72]. Limitation of somatic embryos for utilization in

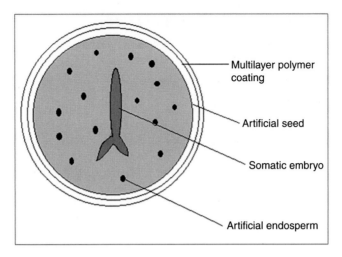

FIGURE 6.5 **Basic features of artificial seed.**

synthetic seed technology is based on the fact that they lack endosperm and protective coatings that make them inconvenient to store and handle. In addition, they usually lack a quiescent resting phase and are incapable of undergoing dehydration. One of the primary objectives of synthetic seed is to furnish somatic embryos that resemble more closely the seed embryos' storage and handling characteristics. Such seeds once developed can be utilized as a unit for clonal plant propagation and germplasm conservation. Encapsulation or protective shielding of viable tissues capable of regenerating plants such as embryos or axillary buds evolved as the first major step for production of synthetic seeds. It was later discovered that in addition to encapsulation, viable tissue also requires other supplementary nutritive material for its future growth and development. These may include growth nutrients, plant growth promoting microorganisms (e.g., mycorrhizae), and/or other biological components necessary for optimal embryo-to-plant development [71,72]. The basic features of artificial seed are mentioned in Fig. 6.5. The various differences between artificial seed technology and other propagation systems are highlighted in Table 6.1.

TABLE 6.1 Characteristics of Clonal Propagation System

Artificial seed	Micropropagation	Greenhouse cutting
• High volume, large-scale propagation method	• Low volume, small-scale propagation method	• Low volume, small-scale propagation method
• Maintains genetic uniformity of plants	• Maintains genetic uniformity of plants	• Maintains genetic uniformity of plants
• Low cost per plant	• High cost per plant	• High cost per plant
• Rapid multiplication of plants	• Relatively low multiplication rate	• Multiplication rate is limited by mother plant size
• Direct delivery of the propagules to the field	• Acclimatization of plantlets required prior to field planting	• Rooting of plantlets required prior to field planting

6.3.1 Need for Artificial Seed Technology [71,72]

- This technology is required to incorporate desired characters or to produce new embryos with improved characteristics that can be preserved for longer periods.
- Naked micropropagules are sensitive to desiccation and/or pathogens when exposed to the natural environment and hence necessarily require protective coatings. Encapsulation is expected to be the best method to provide protection and to convert the *in vitro* derived propagules into "synthetic seeds" or "synseeds" or "artificial seeds."
- *In vivo* vegetative propagation is a time consuming and expensive process.
- Due to various reasons such as heterozygosity of seed, minute seed size, presence of reduced endosperm, and the requirement of the mycorrhizal fungi association for germination (e.g., orchids) also in some seedless varieties of crop plants such as grapes, some plants lack seed propagation or successful propagation of seeds does not occur.
- Development of such techniques will provide an abundant supply of the desired plant species.

6.3.2 Advantages of Synthetic or Artificial Seed Over Somatic Embryos

- Serves as a channel for new plant lines produced through biotechnological advances to be delivered directly to the greenhouse or field
- Maintains the clonal nature of the resulting plants
- Has potential for long-term storage without losing viability
- Easy to transport
- Ease of handling while in storage
- Allows economical mass propagation of elite plant varieties

6.3.3 Disadvantages

Synthetic seed technology seems promising for propagating a number of plant species, though practical implementation of the technology is constrained due to the following main reasons:

- Even apparently normally matured somatic embryos and other micropropagules are poorly converted into plantlets, which limits the value of the synthetic seeds and ultimately the technology itself.
- Production of viable micropropagules useful in synthetic seed production is limited.
- There is a lack of dormancy and stress tolerance in somatic embryos, which limits the storage of synthetic seeds.
- The improper maturation of the somatic embryos makes them inefficient for germination and conversion into normal plants.
- For commercial applications, somatic embryos must germinate rapidly and should be able to develop into plants at least at rates and frequencies more or less similar if not superior to true seeds.
- Development of artificial seeds requires sufficient control of somatic embryogeny from the explants to embryo production, embryo development, and their maturation as well.

The mature somatic embryos must be capable of germinating out of the capsule or coating to form vigorous normal plants.

- Somatic embryos are subject to anomalous and asynchronous development.
- The concentration of the coating material is also an important limiting factor for the synthetic seed technology. The coat must contain nutrients, growth regulator(s), and other components necessary for germination and conversion and it should be transplantable using the existing farm machinery. Though many coating materials have been tried for encapsulation of somatic embryos, sodium alginate obtained from brown algae is considered the best and is being popularly used at present. Alginate has been chosen for ease of capsule formation as well as for its low toxicity to the embryo. The rigidity of the gel beads protects the fragile embryo during handling.
- The coating material may also limit success of the synthetic seed technology, and at present none of the embryo encapsulation methods described earlier is completely satisfactory. The hydrated capsules are more difficult to store because of the requirement of embryo respiration. A second problem is that capsules dry out quickly unless kept in a humid environment or coated with a hydrophobic membrane. Calcium alginate capsules are also difficult to handle because they are very wet and tend to stick together slightly. In addition, calcium alginate capsules lose water rapidly and dry down to a hard pellet within a few hours when exposed to the ambient atmosphere.
- In many plant species the somatic embryos have been found to be sensitive to desiccation.
- In an *in vitro* culture system the somatic embryos show great diversity in their morphology and accordingly in their response, which greatly limits the use of synthetic seed technology.

6.3.4 Types of Synthetic or Artificial Seed

Based on the technology established so far, two types of synthetic seeds are known.

6.3.4.1 Desiccated

Seeds that are obtained from somatic embryos either naked or encapsulated in polyoxyethylene glycol (Polyox™) followed by their desiccation are known as desiccated synthetic seeds [71,72]. Desiccation can be achieved either slowly over a period of 1 or 2 weeks sequentially using chambers of decreasing relative humidity, or rapidly by unsealing the Petri dishes and leaving them on the bench overnight to dry. Such types of synseeds are produced only in plant species whose somatic embryos are desiccation tolerant.

6.3.4.2 Hydrated

On the contrary, hydrated synthetic seeds are produced in those plant species where the somatic embryos are recalcitrant and sensitive to desiccation. Hydrated synthetic seeds are produced by encapsulating the somatic embryos in hydrogel capsules [71,72]. The production of synthetic seeds for the first time by Kitto and Janick involved encapsulation of carrot somatic embryos followed by their desiccation [73,74]. Of the various compounds tested for encapsulation of celery embryos, Kitto and Janick selected polyoxyethylene, which is readily soluble in water and dries to form a thin film, does not support the growth of microorganisms, and is nontoxic to the embryo.

6.3.5 Types of Tissues Chosen for the Production of Artificial Seed

6.3.5.1 Somatic Embryos

Somatic embryos have a bipolar structure with both apical and basal meristem regions, which are capable of forming shoot and root, respectively. A plant derived from somatic embryos is called an embling. Somatic embryos differ from zygotic embryos in that they develop from vegetative or somatic cells instead of zygotes (fusion product of male and female gamete) and thus potentially can be used to produce duplicates of a single genotype. Since natural seed develops as a result of sexual recombination, it is not genetically identical to their one single parent. Therefore, somatic embryogenesis not only allows clonal propagation but also induces the specific, defined, and well-directed changes into desirable elite individuals by inserting gene sequences into the somatic cells. Therefore, this process bypasses genetic recombination and can be potentially used as a clonal propagation system. Various micropropagules have been considered for synthetic seed production; the somatic embryos have been largely favored as these structures possess the radicle and plumule that are able to develop into root and shoot in one step, usually without any specific treatment [71,72].

6.3.5.2 Axillary Shoot Buds and Apical Shoot Tips

In many plant species the unipolar axillary shoot buds and/or apical shoot tips, which do not have root meristem, have also been encapsulated to produce synthetic seeds. Since these structures do not have root meristems they should be induced to regenerate roots before encapsulation.

6.3.5.3 Embryogenic Masses

Stable and regenerative embryogenic masses make an attractive tool for the production of clonal plants and for studies of genetic transformation. However, long-term maintenance of embryogenic masses in culture tubes or mechanically stirred bioreactors requires frequent transfer of tissue to fresh media, which is both labor-intensive and costly.

6.3.5.4 Protocorms or Protocorm-Like Bodies

In orchids such as *Cymbidium giganteum*, *Dendrobium wardianum*, *Geodorum densiflorum*, *Phaius tankervilleae*, and *Spathoglottis plicata* synthetic seeds have been produced by encapsulating the protocorm or protocorm-like bodies (PLBs) in sodium alginate gel. Corrie and Tandon have reported that the encapsulated protocorms of *C. giganteum* gave rise to healthy plantlets upon transferring either to nutrient medium or directly to sterile sand and soil.

6.3.6 Basic Components of Artificial Seed [71,72]

6.3.6.1 Gelling Agents

Gelling agents such as agar, aliginate, carrageenan, carboxymethy cellulose, guar gum, sodium pectate, gum tragacanth, and various others were tested for synthetic seed production. Due to quick gelation, moderate viscosity, low spin ability of the alginate solution, enhanced capsule formation, biocompatibility, and low cost characteristics alginate is found to be more suitable for synthetic seed production than other hydrogels. Alginate for orchids is one of the most common examples of alginate-based synthetic seed. Agar is also reported as a cheap alternative for encapsulation but alginate still provides better protection than agar.

6.3.6.2 Artificial Endosperm

Somatic embryos lack seed coat (testa) and endosperm that provide protection and nutrition for zygotic embryos in developing seeds. To augment these deficiencies addition of nutrients and growth regulators to the encapsulation matrix is desired, which serves as an artificial endosperm. Addition of nutrients and growth regulators to the encapsulation matrix results in increase in efficiency of the germination and viability of the encapsulated somatic embryos. These synthetic seeds can be stored for longer periods of time, even up to 6 months without losing viability especially when stored at 4°C.

6.3.6.3 Adjuvant

To prevent the desiccation, microbial attack, and mechanical injury-like problems various adjuvants are added to prevent any type of damage to embryos. Various adjuvants like nutrients, fungicides, insecticides, pesticides, and microorganisms (e.g., rhizobia) can be incorporated into the matrix. Addition of activated charcoal improves the conversion and vigor (physical strength) of the encapsulated somatic embryos. It has been suggested that charcoal breaks up the alginate and thus increases the respiration of somatic embryos. In addition, charcoal retains in the nutrients within the capsule and slowly releases them to the growing medium.

6.3.7 Production of Artificial/Synthetic Seed [71,72]

Aliginate is a straight chain, hydrophilic, colloidal polyuronic acid composed primarily of hydro-β-D-mannuronic acid residues with 1–4 glycosidic linkages. The major step (Fig. 6.6) involved in the alginate encapsulation process is that the sodium alginate droplets containing the somatic embryos when dropped into the calcium chloride solution ($CaCl_2 \cdot 2H_2O$) solution form round and firm beads due to the ion exchange between sodium in sodium aliginate with calcium ions in $CaCl_2 \cdot 2H_2O$ solution. The hardness or rigidity depends on the number of sodium ions exchanged. Hence, the concentration of the two gelling agents, i.e., sodium aliginate and $CaCl_2 \cdot 2H_2O$ solution, and the complexing time should be optimized for the formation of the capsule with optimum bead hardness and rigidity. In general 3% sodium aliginate upon complexation with 75 mM $CaCl_2 \cdot 2H_2O$ for half an hour gives optimum bead hardness and rigidity for the production of viable synthetic seeds.

6.3.8 Potential Uses of Artificial Seed and its Production Technology

- Pathogen-free propagules can be transported.
- Somatic embryogenesis is a potential tool in genetic engineering of plants.
- Multiplication of elite plats that are selected in plant breeding programs via somatic embryos avoids genetic recombination, which saves a considerable amount of time and other resources used in screening.
- In plants that are regenerated from somatic embryos from a transgenic cell, the progeny will not be chimeric.

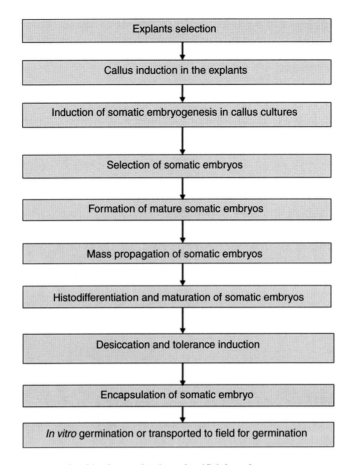

FIGURE 6.6 **Major steps involved in the production of artificial seed.**

- Cryopreserved artificial seed can also be used for germplasm preservation particularly in the recalcitrant seeds (seeds that do not survive drying and freezing during *ex situ* conservation) such as mango and coconut.
- Can be used for the multiplication of nonseed producing plants, ornamental hybrids, or the propagation of elite plant with elite characteristics.
- Can also be employed in the propagation of male or female sterile plants for hybrid seed production.

6.3.9 Applications of Synthetic Seeds

- While producing the synthetic seed encapsulation herbicides can be added to the formulation; these herbicides will provide extra protection to the explants against pests and diseases.
- This technology improves food production and also produces environmentally friendly plantation.

- Synthetic seeds can be transported from one country to another without obligations from the quarantine department.
- Synthetic seeds can be directly used in fields.
- Synthetic seeds are small, therefore they are easy to handle.
- Synthetic seed transportation is easy as the seeds do not contain any disease causing agents.
- Synthetic seed production is cost effective when compared to traditional methods.
- Synthetic seed plantation can be done by using sowing farm machinery.
- Synthetic seed encapsulation provides aseptic conditions to the plant material or explant, which is present inside the capsule.
- Synthetic seed crops are easy to maintain because of uniform genetic constituents.
- Hybrid plants can be easily propagated using synthetic seed technology.
- Genetically modified plants or crops can be propagated using synthetic seed technology.
- Genetic uniformity is maintained by using synthetic seed technology.
- Endangered species can be propagated using synthetic seed technology.
- Elite genotype can be preserved and propagated using artificial seed technology.
- Cereals, fruits, and medicinal plants can be studied anywhere in the world using synthetic seeds.
- Synthetic seeds can also be produced by using sterile plant materials using plant tissue culture techniques using plant tissue culture techniques.

6.4 ORGANOGENESIS

Organogenesis is the formation of organs, either shoots or roots. Organogenesis *in vitro* depends on the balance of auxin and cytokinins and the ability of the tissue to respond to phytohormones during culture. Organogenesis takes place in three phases. In the first phase the cells become competent; next, they differentiate. In the third phase, morphogenesis proceeds independently of the exogenous phytohormones [71,72]. Organogenesis *in vitro* can be divided into two types.

6.4.1 Indirect Organogenesis

Formation of organs directly through the callus is called indirect organogenesis. Induction of plants using this technique does not ensure clonal fidelity, but it could be an ideal system for selecting somaclonal variants of desired characteristics and also for mass multiplication. Induction of plants through the callus phase has been used for the production of transgenic plants in which the callus is transformed and the plant regenerated, or the initial explant is transformed and the callus and shoots are developed from the explants.

6.4.2 Direct Organogenesis

The production of direct buds or shoots from a tissue with no intervening callus stage is called direct organogenesis. Plants have been propagated by direct organogenesis for improved multiplication rates, production of transgenic plants, and most importantly for clonal propagation. Typically indirect organogenesis is more important for transgenic plant production. The axillary bud induction/multiple bud initiation technique is the most common means of micropropagation since it ensures the production of uniform planting material without genetic variation. Axillary shoots are formed directly from preformed meristems at nodes, and the chances of the organized shoot meristem undergoing mutation are relatively low. This technique is referred to as multiple bud induction. Many economically important plants have been propagated using this method.

References

[1] Jiménez VM. Regulation of *in vitro* somatic embryogenesis with emphasis on to the role of endogenous hormones. R Bras Fisiol Veg 2001;13:196–223.

[2] Zimmerman JL. Somatic embryogenesis: a model for early development in higher plants. Plant Cell 1993;5(10):1411–23.

[3] Zegzouti R, Arnold MF, Favre JM. Histological investigation of the multiplication steps in secondary somatic embryogenesis of *Quercus robur* L. Ann For Sci 2001;88:681–90.

[4] Fujimura T, Komamine A. Synchronization of somatic embryogenesis in a carrot cell suspension culture. Plant Physiol 1979;64:162–4.

[5] Chee RP, Cantliffe DJ. Composition of embryogenic suspension cultures of *Ipomoea batatas* Poir. and production of individualized embryos. Plant Cell Tiss Org Cult 1989;17:39–52.

[6] Cote FX, Domergue R, Monmarson S, Schwendiman J, Teisson C, Escalant JV. Embryogenic cell suspensions from the male flower of *Musa* AAA cv. Grand nain. Physiol Plant 1996;97:285–90.

[7] Evans DA, Sharp WR, Ammirato PV, Yamada Y. Handbook of plant cell culture: techniques for propagation and breeding, 1. New York: Macmillan Publishing Company; 1983.

[8] Liu CM, Xu ZH, Chua NH. Auxin polar transport is essential for the establishment of bilateral symmetry during early plant embryogenesis. Plant Cell 1993;5:621–30.

[9] Pasternak TP, Prinsen E, Ayaydin F, Miskolczi P, Potters G, Asard H, et al. The role of auxin, pH and stress in the activation of embryogenic cell division in leaf protoplast-derived cells of alfalfa. Plant Physiol 2002;129:1807–9.

[10] Thinh NT. Cryopreservation of germplasm of vegetatively propagated tropical monocots by vitrification. Doctoral Dissertation. Kobe University; 1997.

[11] Mithila J, Hall J, Victor JMR, Saxena P. Thidiazuron induces shoot organogenesis at low concentrations and somatic embryogenesis at high concentrations on leaf and petiole explants of African violet (*Saintpaulia ionantha* Wend I.). Plant Cell Rep 2003;21:408–14.

[12] Lin CS, Lin CC, Chang WC. Effect of thidiazuron on vegetative tissue-derived somatic embryogenesis and flowering of bamboo *Bambusa edulis*. Plant Cell Tiss Org Cult 2004;76:75–82.

[13] Srangsam A, Kanchanapoom K. Thidiazuron induced plant regeneration in callus culture of triploid banana (*Musa* spp.) "Gros Michel", AAA group. Songklanakarin J Sci Technol 2003;25:689–96.

[14] Woodward B, Puonti KJ. Somatic embryogenesis from floral tissue of cassava (*Manihot esculenta* Crantz). Euphytica 2001;120:1–6.

[15] Panaia M, Senaratma T, Dixon KW, Sivasithamparam K. The role of cytokinins and thidiazuron in the stimulation of somatic embryogenesis in key members of the Restionaceae. Aust J Bot 2004;52:257–65.

[16] Zhang BH, Feng R, Liu F, Wang Q. High frequency somatic embryogenesis and plant regeneration of an elite Chinese cotton variety. Bot Bull Acad Sin 2001;42:9–16.

[17] Kim YJ, Park T, Kim HS, Park HK, Chon SU, Yun SJ. Factors affecting somatic embryogenesis from immature cotyledon of soybean. J Plant Biotechnol 2004;6:45–50.

[18] Smith DL, Krikorian AD. Release of somatic embryogenic potential from excised zygotic embryos of carrot and maintenance of proembryonic cultures in hormone free medium. Am J Bot 1989;76:1832–43.

[19] Drew RLK. Effect of activated charcoal on embryogenesis and regeneration of plantlets from suspension cultures of carrot (*Daucus carota* L.). Ann Bot 1972;44:387–9.

[20] Lakshmanan P, Taji A. Somatic embryogenesis in leguminous plants. Plant Biol 2000;2:136–48.

[21] Siriwardana S, Nabors MW. Tryptophan enhancement of somatic embryogenesis in rice. Plant Physiol 1983;73:142–6.

[22] Ribnicky DM, Ilić N, Cohen JD, Cooke TJ. The effects of exogenous auxins on endogenous indole-3-acetic acid metabolism. Plant Physiol 1996;112:549–58.

[23] Jiménez VM, Bangerth F. Endogenous hormone levels in explants and in embryogenic and non-embryogenic cultures of carrot. Physiol Plant 2001;111:389–95.

[24] Jiménez VM, Bangerth F. Hormonal status of maize initial explants and of the embryogenic and non-embryogenic callus cultures derived from them as related to morphogenesis *in vitro*. Plant Sci Lett 2001;160:247–52.

[25] Kevers C, Gal NL, Monteiro M, Dommes J, Gaspar T. Somatic embryogenesis of *Panax ginseng* in liquid cultures: a role for polyamines and their metabolic pathways. Plant Growth Reg 2000;31:209–14.

[26] Astarita LV, Handro W, Floh ES. Changes in polyamine content associated with zygotic embryogenesis in the Brazilian pine, *Araucaria angustifolia* (Bert.) O. Ktze Revista Brazil Bot 2003;26:163–8.

[27] Ichihashi S, Islam MO. Effects of complex organic additives on callus growth in three orchid genera, *Phalaenopsis, Doritaenopsis* and Neofinetia. J Jpn Soc Hort Sci 1999;68:269–74.

[28] Islam MO, Rahman ARMM, Matsui S, Prodhan AKMA. Effects of complex organic extracts on callus growth and PLB regeneration through embryogenesis in the *Doritaenopsis* orchid. Jpn Agric Res Quarter 2003;37:229–35.

[29] Rahman ARMM, Islam MO, Prodhan AKMA, Ichihashi S. Effects of complex organic extracts on plantlet regeneration from PLBs and plantlet growth in the *Doritaenopsis* orchid. Jpn Agric Res Quarter 2004;37:229–35.

[30] Zegzouti R, Arnold MF, Favre J-M. Histological investigation of the multiplication steps in secondary somatic embryogenesis of *Quercus robur* L. Ann For Sci 2001;88:681–90.

[31] Trigiano RN, Gray DJ. Plant tissue culture concepts and laboratory exercises. New York: CRC Press, Inc.; 1996.

[32] Etienne H, Montoro P, Michaux-Ferriere N, Carron MP. Effects of desiccation, medium osmolarity and abscisic acid on the maturation of *Hevea brasiliensis* somatic embryos. J Exp Bot 1993;44:1613–9.

[33] Attree SM, Pomeroy MK, Fowke LC. Development of white spruce (*Picea glauca* (Moench.) Voss) somatic embryos during culture with abscisic acid and osmoticum and their tolerance to drying and frozen storage. J Exp Bot 1995;46:433–9.

[34] Gutmann M, von Aderkas P, Label P, Lelu MA. Effects of abscisic acid on somatic embryo maturation of *Hybrid larch*. J Exp Bot 1996;47:1905–17.

[35] Venkatachalam P, Geetha N, Khandelwal A, Shaila MS, Sita GL. Induction of direct somatic embryogenesis and plant regeneration from mature cotyledon explants of *Arachis hypogaea* L. Curr Sci 1999;77:269–73.

[36] Jacobs M, Negrutiu I, Dirks R, Cammaerts D. Selection programmes for isolation and analysis of mutants in plant cell cultures. In: Green CE, Somers DA, Hackett WP, Biesboer DD, editors. Plant tissue and cell culture. New York: Alan R. Liss; 1987. p. 243–64.

[37] Toonen MAJ, de Vries SC. Initiation of somatic embryos from single cells. In: Wang TL, Cuming A, editors. Embryogenesis: the generation of a plant. Oxford: Bios Scientific Publishers; 1996. p. 173–89.

[38] Krastanova S, Perrin M, Barbier P, Demangeat P, Cornuet N, Bardonnet L, et al. Transformation of grapevine rootstocks with the coat protein gene of grapevine fanleaf nepovirus. Plant Cell Rep 1995;13:357–60.

[39] Heinze B, Schmidt J. Monitoring genetic fidelity vs somaclonal variation in Norway spruce (*Picea abies*) somatic embryogenesis by RAPD analysis. Euphytica 1995;85:341–5.

[40] Spiral J, Thierry C, Paillard M, Petiard V. Regeneration of plantlets of *Coffee canephora* Pierre (Robusta) transformed by *Agrobacterium rhizogenes*. C R Acad des Sci Série III 1993;316:1–6.

[41] Tetu T, Sangwan RS, Sangwan-Norreel BS. Direct somatic embryogenesis and organogenesis in cultured immature zygotic embryos of *Pisum sativum* L. J Plant Physiol 1990;137:102–9.

[42] Been CG, Kim BD. Transformation through somatic embryo of *Oenanthe stolonifera* with Agrobacterium. J Korean Soc Hort Sci 1995;36:792–8.

[43] Schöpke C, Franche C, Bogusz D, Chavarriaga P, Fauquet CM, Beachy RN. Transformation in cassava (*Manihot esculenta* Crantz). In: Bajaj YPS, editor. Biotechnology in agriculture and forestry. Berlin: Springer–Verlag; 1993. p. 273–89.

[44] Li HQ, Sautter C, Potrykus I, Puonti-Kaerlas J. Genetic transformation of cassava (*Manihot esculenta* Crantz). Nat Biotechnol 1996;14:736–40.

[45] Glimelius K, Fahlesson J, Landgren M, Sjödin C, Sundberg E. Gene transfer via somatic hybridisation in plants. Trends Biotechnol 1991;9:24–30.

[46] Gmitter FG, Ling XB, Deng XX. Induction of triploid citrus plants from endosperm calli *in vitro*. Theor Appl Genet 1990;80:785–90.

[47] Binarova P, Dolezel J. Effect of anti-microtubular drug amiprophos-methyl on somatic embryogenesis and DNA ploidy levels in alfalfa and carrot cell suspension cultures. Biol Plant 1993;35:329–39.

[48] Canhoto JM, Ludovina M, Gimaraes S, Cruz GS. *In vitro* induction of haploid, diploid and triploid plantlets by anther culture of *Iochroma warscewiczii* Regel. Plant Cell Tiss Org Cult 1990;21:171–7.

[49] Ezura H, Oozawa K. Ploidy of somatic embryos and the ability to regenerate plantlets in melon (*Cucumis melo* L.). Plant Cell Rep 1994;14:107–11.

[50] Liu SQ, Liu JQ. Callus induction and embryo formation in endosperm culture of *Prunnus persica*. Acta Bot Sin 1980;22:198–9.

[51] Gmitter FG, Ling XB, Cai CY, Grosser JW. Colchicine-induced polyploidy in citrus embryogenic cultures, somatic embryos, and regenerated plantlets. Plant Sci 1991;74:135–41.

[52] Garg L, Bhandari NN, Rani V, Bhojwani SS. Somatic embryogenesis and regeneration of triploid plants in endosperm cultures of *Acacia nilotica*. Plant Cell Rep 1996;15:855–8.

[53] Raghavan V. Biochemistry of somatic embryogenesis. In: Evans DA, Sharp WR, Ammirato PV, Yamada Y, editors. Handbook of plant cell culture: techniques for propagation and breeding, 1. New York: Macmillan; 1983. p. 655–71.

[54] Gudu S, Procunier JD, Ziauddin A, Kasha KJ. Anther culture derived homozygous lines in *Hordeum bulbosum*. Plant Breed 1993;110:109–15.

[55] Zhao JP, Simmonds DH. Application of trifluralin to embryogenic microspore cultures to generate doubled haploid plants in *Brassica napus*. Physiol Plant 1995;95:304–9.

[56] Newton DJ, Goussard PG. The ontogeny of somatic embryos from *in vitro* cultured grapevine anthers. South Afr J Enol Viticult 1990;11:70–5.

[57] Goussard PG, Wiid J. The elimination of fanleaf virus from grapevines using *in vitro* somatic embryogenesis combined with heat therapy. South Afr J Enol Viticult 1992;13:81–3.

[58] Goussard PG, Wiid J, Kasdorf GGF. The effectiveness of *in vitro* somatic embryogenesis in eliminating fanleaf virus and leafroll associated viruses from grapevines. South Afr J Enol Viticult 1991;12:77–81.

[59] Fujita Y, Tabata M. Secondary metabolites from plant cells. Pharmaceutical applications and progress in commercial production. In: Green CE, Somers DA, Hackett WP, Biesboer DD, editors. Plant tissue and cell culture. New York: Alan R. Liss; 1987. p. 169–85.

[60] Luckner M, Diettrich B. Biosynthesis of cardenolides in cell cultures of *Digitalis lanata*. The result of a new strategy. In: Green CE, Somers DA, Hackett WP, Biesboer DD, editors. Plant tissue and cell culture. New York: Alan R. Liss; 1987. p. 187–97.

[61] Eilert U, Kurz WGW, Constabel F. Alkaloid accumulation in plant cell cultures upon treatment with elicitors. In: Green CE, Somers DA, Hackett WP, Biesboer DD, editors. Plant tissue and cell culture. New York: Alan R. Liss; 1987. p. 213–9.

[62] Janick J. Agricultural uses of somatic embryos. Acta Hort 1993;136:207–15.

[63] Lee BS, Son SH. A method for producing taxol and taxanes from embryo cultures of *Taxus* species. WO Patent No. 95/02063; 1995.

[64] Wann SR, Goldner WR. Induction of somatic embryogenesis in *Taxus*, and the production of taxane-ring containing alkaloids theys from. WO Patent No. 93/19585; 1994.

[65] Gabr MF. *In vitro* production of jojoba liquid wax from somatic embryos proliferated via vegetative tissues. Egyptian J Hort 1993;20:135–44.

[66] Janick J, Simon JE, Whipkey A. *In vitro* propagation of borage. HortScience 1987;22:493–5.

[67] Whipkey A, Simon JE, Janick J. *In vivo* and *in vitro* lipid accumulation in *Borago officinalis* L. J Am Oil Chem Soc 1988;65:979–84.

[68] Quinn J, Simon JE, Janick J. Recovery of gamma-linolenic acid from somatic embryos of borage. J Am Soc Hort Sci 1989;114:511–5.

[69] Janick J, Wright DC, Hasewaga PM. *In vitro* production of cacao seed lipids. J Am Soc Hort Sci 1982;107:919–22.

[70] Paiva M, Janick J. *In vivo* and *in vitro* production of alkaloids in *Theobroma cacao* L. Acta Hort 1983;131:249–73.

[71] Saiprasad GVS. Artificial seeds and their applications. Resonance May 2001;6(5):39–47.

[72] Ara H, Jaiswal U, Jaiswal VS. Synthetic seed: prospects and limitations. Curr Sci 2000;78:12.

[73] Kitto SK, Janick J. Polyox as an artificial seed coat for asexual embryos. Hort Sci 1982;17:488–90.

[74] Kitto SL, Janick J. Production of synthetic seeds by encapsulating asexual plant embryos of carrot. J. American Soc. Hort. Sci. 1985;110:277–82.

Classical and Nonclassical Techniques for Secondary Metabolite Production in Plant Cell Culture

Saurabh Bhatia, Tanmoy Bera

Modern Applications of Plant Biotechnology in Pharmaceutical Sciences. http://dx.doi.org/10.1016/B978-0-12-802221-4.00007-8

7.1 INTRODUCTION

In vitro experimentation on plant physiology gives a wide range of secondary metabolites that are used as therapeutics, flavors, fragrances, colors, and food additives. Development in *in vitro* technology allows easier access toward the cellular machinery of plant cells and tissues, assisting the convenient utilization of plant cells for the production of natural or recombinant compounds of commercial interest. For increasing the entire biomass and production of high amounts of secondary metabolites, plant cells and tissues are produced from explant and regularly maintained in the form of cell suspension, callus, tissues, and somatic embryos under aseptic conditions. Currently, secondary metabolites represent an important source of pharmaceuticals. Secondary metabolites control the defense mechanism of plants and are also responsible for the adaptation of plants according to environmental conditions. Summation of all biochemical reactions represents the whole metabolism of organisms. Biochemical reactions are broadly divided into primary and secondary metabolic pathways. Primary metabolism yields very few end products whereas secondary metabolism yields large amount of products. The study of both pathways and their end products is called metabolomics. During 1985, 3500 new chemical structures and 2600 chemical structures from higher plants were identified. Various traditional and conventional methods have been adopted to extract and further isolate these secondary metabolites. Nevertheless the constant deforestation of plants has posed a major warning to the plight of plant species over the years. In addition, dependency of plant cell secondary metabolites production on environmental conditions restricts its utilization as pharmaceuticals. These conditions require the development of *in vitro* plant science, which generates considerable interest in the use of plant cells for the production of therapeutic compounds.

Plant cell and tissue culture technology has provided an alternative source for useful secondary metabolites for about the last two decades. In tissue culture practice, cell, tissue, or organ is cultivated under optimum *in vitro* conditions, which promotes secondary metabolite production in less time than when cultivated in its natural habitat and ultimately the desired amount of product is extracted from the cultured cells. Current developments in plant tissue culture concepts and technologies have shown significant outcomes to improve the yield by many folds. Therapeutic compound production by plant tissue culture proposes various advantages such as:

- Supply control of product is independent of the availability of the plant itself.
- Controlled and optimized conditions are offered for the growth of the cell or tissue.
- Strain improvements are available with programs analogous to those used for microbial systems.
- Harmful herbicides and pesticides are not required.
- Supplementation of analogous to natural substrates increases the chances of production of novel synthetic compounds that are not present in nature.
- Plant tissue culture is not dependent on climate, geographical location, etc.

Practices such as strain improvement, methods for the selection of elite or high-producing cell lines, and medium optimizations are adopted to increase secondary metabolite production. However, in most of the tissue culture practices plant cell cultures fail to produce the desired products. Therefore, various strategies and techniques to improve the production of secondary metabolites must be considered. On the basis of their foundation these techniques are broadly divided into classical and contemporary techniques (Fig. 7.1). The usual problem faced while adopting such techniques is the lack of basic information regarding biosynthetic pathways, their enzymes, intermediates, and mechanisms responsible for plant secondary metabolite production. Productivity of metabolites is also influenced by lack of particular precursors and improper knowledge regarding biotransformation, genetic manipulation, and metabolic engineering. Metabolic intermediate or enzyme inhibition or inhibition of membrane transport elements can be prevented by the synthesized product's accumulation in a second phase, supplemented into the aqueous medium. Influence of the various types of cultures over the production of secondary metabolites can also be studied. Localized production of metabolites in organ cultures is widely studied nowadays. Thus, identification of cellular mechanics and the compartments that are responsible for site-specific production and storage of secondary metabolites facilitates its collection during the isolation process. Studying the plant metabolite production capacity *in vitro* against different amplitudes of biotic and abiotic stress is a good means of optimizing the yield of metabolites. This process of activating plant defense mechanisms by triggering the formation of secondary metabolites under abiotic or biotic stress is called elicitation. Various biotic elicitors include polysaccharides (e.g., pectin and chitosan), which are also used in the immobilization and permeabilization of plant cells. Plant cell immobilization offers several advantages over other techniques in enhancing the yield of secondary metabolites. Several scale-up techniques for biomass production of plant cells are preferred for obtaining the desirable amount of secondary metabolites in significantly less time. This chapter highlights classical and nonclassical methods used in the production of valuable secondary metabolites *in vitro*.

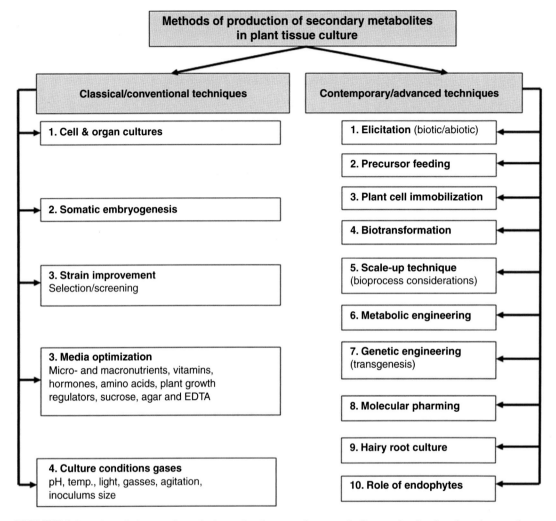

FIGURE 7.1   **A broad view on the techniques for the secondary metabolite production by plant tissue culture.**

7.2 CONVENTIONAL METHODS

7.2.1 Plant Cell Culture

As already discussed in Chapter 2, plant cell cultures are the potential source for the production of high-value secondary metabolites. The totipotent nature of culturing cells preserves their genetic information and is thus capable of producing a large number of biochemicals found in the parent plant. Some of the earlier development events of plant cell culture are highlighted in Table 7.1. Apart from plant cell culture-mediated metabolite production, there is also the opportunity to identify cell lines that can produce amounts of compounds equal or even higher than those in the plant. In addition, certain compounds that are not present/

TABLE 7.1 Development in Plant Cell Culture in Secondary Metabolites Production [1–3]

Year	Events/contribution in plant tissue culture toward the production of secondary metabolites
1939–1940	Plant tissue cultures were first established
1956	The first patent for the production of metabolites by mass cell cultures was filed (Pfizer Inc.)
Late 1960s	Potential of plant cell cultures to produce useful compounds, especially for drug development
Kaul and Staba (1967) and Heble et al. (1968)	Isolated visnagin and diosgenin, respectively from cell cultures
Zenk and his coworkers (1976) (Munich)	Demonstrated the outstanding metabolic capacities of plant cells and highlighted the spontaneous variability of plant cell biosynthetic capacity
Late 1970s	High increase in the number of patent applications filed, especially by the scientific and corporate sectors in the Federal Republic of Germany and Japan
1983	For the first time, a dye, shikonin, with anti-inflammatory and antibacterial properties, was produced by plant cell cultures on an industrial scale by Mitsui Petrochemical Industries Ltd
1990	Up to this period, shikonin was produced at a large level by cell culture
Present	Any substance of plant origin (alkaloids, flavonoids, terpenes, steroids, glycosides, etc.) can be produced by cell cultures

synthesized in plants can be produced by cell cultures. Therefore, by this technology plant cells can generate natural or artificial compounds, through an array of reactions such as isomerization, dehydrogenation, hydrogenation, hydroxylation, glycosylation, opening of a ring, and addition of carbon atoms. A quality check of the products produced from plant tissue culture is required for their regular production without dependence on climatic variations. Screening, selection, stabilization, and isolation of a high producing cell line, culturing conditions, scale-up technique, mass cultivation in bioreactors, and downstream processing, i.e., extraction and purification of the compounds, affects the end product or yield obtained after sequential stages or developments of plant cell culture. The general protocol for the production of secondary metabolites from the cell is illustrated in Fig. 7.2.

Several advantages of this technology over the conventional agricultural production are as follows:

- Rapid production.
- Production of new compounds from cheap precursors.
- Represents a production system that ensures the constant supply of products with uniform quality and yield.
- Several new compounds can be produced via cell cultures that are not normally found in the parent plant.
- Independent of political interference.
- Independent of climatic variations and various environmental factors.
- Plant cell allows stereo- and regiospecific biotransformation for the efficient downstream recovery and product.

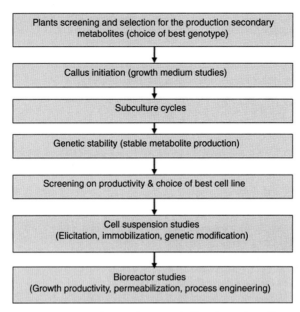

FIGURE 7.2 **Protocol for the production of secondary metabolites from the cell.**

Various reports are available for plant cell cultures producing a higher amount of secondary metabolites than in intact plants (Table 7.2), though plant tissue culture-based industries are still facing problems in the production of metabolites by cell cultures resulting from the instability of cell lines, low yields, slow growth, and scale-up problems. Different classes of secondary metabolites isolated from the tissue and suspension culture of plants are highlighted in Fig. 7.3.

TABLE 7.2   High Yields of Secondary Products

Product	Plant species	Yield (% D.W.)
Shikonin	*Lithospermum erythrorhizon*	12.4
Serpentine	*Catharanthus roseus*	2.2
Sanguinarine	*Papaver somniferum*	2.5
Rosmarinic acid	*Salvia officinalis*	36.0
Rosmarinic acid	*Coleus blumei*	21.0
Jatrorrhizine	*Berberis wilsoniae*	10.0
Diosgenin	*Dioscorea deltoidea*	3.8
Berberine	*Thalictrum minus*	10.6
Berberine	*Coptis japonica*	7.5
Anthraquinones	*Morinda citrifolia*	18.0
Anthocyanins	*Perilla frutescens*	8.9

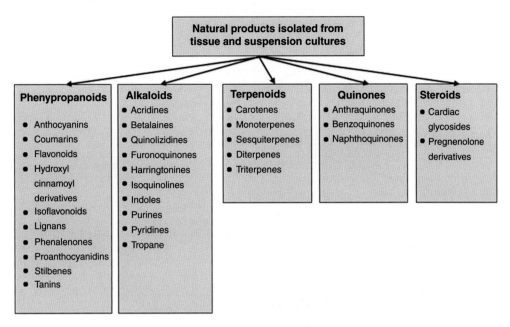

FIGURE 7.3 Various natural products isolated from tissue and suspension cultures of higher plants.

7.2.2 Organ Cultures for Secondary Metabolite Production

Organ culture and its various developments are described in Chapter 2. Attempts on organ culture were started from 1902. During this period, Hannig for the first time isolated embryos of crucifers and successfully grew on mineral salts and sugar solutions [4]. Subsequently, large calli, buds, and roots were cultured on indole-3-acetic acid-rich medium by Simon [5]. After these attempts inclination toward production of secondary metabolites from localized compartments (organs) of plants has been raised. Organ-mediated secondary metabolite production research has become more intensified since Skoog and Miller's achievements [6]. Supplementation of optimum ratio of hormones for directing the growth (either shoot or root or callus) results in proliferation of specified cells. Such localized proliferation efficiency of hormones in developing whole organ or compartment can also be utilized in localized production of secondary metabolites. It was later discovered that the production of secondary metabolites is generally higher in differentiated tissue. Owing to the increased stability and potential in retaining secondary metabolites in specified compartments than other cultures, organ cultures are widely studied in the form of shoot and root cultures. Shoot cultures are preferred for secondary metabolite production where the root of higher plants normally shows slower growth and difficulty to harvest. To increase the biomass of cell and secondary metabolites, root cultures can be transformed into hairy roots. This can be achieved by infecting with *Agrobacterium rhizogenes* (Fig. 7.4). Similarly shoot cultures can also be infected with *A. tumefaciens* to form transgenics or tetratomas (Fig. 7.4). Both organ cultures (shoot and root) have some comparable features of genetic stability and good capacities for secondary metabolite production.

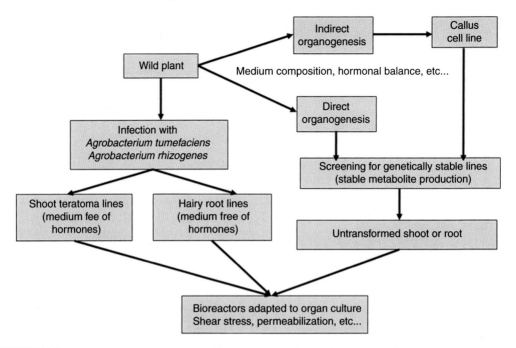

FIGURE 7.4   Procedure for the production of secondary metabolites from organ culture.

There are various reports that support the high secondary metabolite production by using *in vitro* organ culture. Alkaloidal content and other microelements in the cultured bulbs of *Fritillaria unibracteata* on Murashige and Skoog (MS) media supplemented with appropriate concentration of benzyladenine (BA) and indole-3-butyric acid were found to be higher than in the wild bulb. In addition, growth rate was 30–50 times higher than that under natural wild growth conditions [7]. *In vitro* shoot multiplication of *Frangula alnus* on woody plant medium with indole-3-acetic acid and 6-benzylaminopurine (BAP) showed highest metabolite production (1731 mg/100 g) of total anthraquinone. Similarly, highest metabolite production of total anthraquinone was found in the shoots of *F. rupestris* when cultured on medium with 2,4-dichlorophenoxyacetic acid (2,4-D) and BAP. These examples established a novel protocol to produce this natural plant drug in future studies and achieve scale-up for industrial production. In contrast there are some reports available where *in vitro* organ culture fails to enhance secondary metabolite production. Shoot cultures of *Gentianella austriaca* on MS medium supplemented with BA and naphthalene acetic acid produce secondary metabolites (xanthones) with no significance than those obtained from nature. In fact the concentration of demethylbellidifolin, demethylbellidifolin-8-O-glucoside, and bellidifolin-8-O-glucoside was found to be two times lower than in samples from nature. It was also discovered that secondary metabolite production was strongly affected by the presence of BA in the medium [8]. Organ culture carries certain advantages over conventional methods for propagation of whole plants, e.g., plant cells under *in vitro* conditions produce varied quantities of secondary metabolites. This system is more manageable and reliable.

- Useful compound production under controlled physical and chemical conditions is always independent of climatic changes or soil conditions.
- At present any plant can be cultivated under *in vitro* conditions to produce their specific metabolites.
- Scale-up technology using automated and robust techniques allows convenient production of secondary metabolites with improved productivity and reduced labor costs.
- *In vitro* organ, tissue, and cell cultures may provide defined sources of standard phytochemicals in ample amounts.
- Diseases, pathogens, and the insect-free nature of organ, tissue, and cell culture allow more uniform amounts of secondary metabolites.
- These cultures can be procured for longer periods.
- Organ, tissue, and cell cultures allow the screening of high secondary metabolite yielding cells.
- Organ cultures offer the platform to execute strategies like elicitation, cell immobilization, etc., and to study their affect on secondary metabolite production.

7.2.3 Somatic Embryogenesis for the Production of Secondary Metabolites

One of the usual strategies to generate high yielding secondary metabolite cell lines *in vitro* is by somatic embryogenesis induction. This process plays an essential role in the production of secondary metabolites. Recently, it has been found that accumulation of large amounts of secondary metabolites is more in somatic embryos than in zygotic embryos. Various secondary metabolites, which are isolated from somatic embryos and have shown better yield than its native state, are mentioned in Table 7.3. Several advantages and applications of somatic embryogenesis are described in Chapter 6.

TABLE 7.3   Various Examples of Secondary Metabolite Produced From Somatic Embryogenesis

Sr. no.	Plant	Plant	Type of culture
1	Flavonoids	Alfalfa (*Medicago sativa*)	Somatic embryogenic callus
2	Solasodine	*Solanum khasianum*	Somatic embryogenic callus
3	Santalols, phenolics, and arabinogalactan proteins	*Santalum album*	Somatic embryogenic callus
4	Eleutheroside	*Eleutherococcus senticosus*	Somatic embryogenic callus
5	Camptothecin	*Nothapodytes foetida*	Somatic embryogenic callus
6	Morphinan alkaloids	*P. somniferum, P. orientale*	Somatic embryogenic callus
7	Reserpine	*Rauwolfia serpentina*	Somatic embryogenic callus
8	Rosmarinic acid (RA)	*Ocimum sanctum* (L.)	Somatic embryogenic callus

7.2.4 Strain Improvement

Strategies implemented for the overproduction of microorganisms in microbiology can also be applied in plant tissue culture for an enhancement in secondary metabolite production within plant cells. Strain improvement is based on the selection of the plant with high contents of the desired products to obtain high producing cell lines. Such a selection procedure allows the proper screening of a heterogeneous population for variant cell clones containing the highest levels of desired product. A heterogeneous cell line shows variation in biochemical production capacity of the cell population existing in the cell line, to exploit only those cell lines that are highly productive in nature. Therefore, high producing plants acquire the potential to produce high producing cell lines, though the production capacity of such cell lines would not remain uniform under *in vitro* conditions.

There are various steps involved in the production of highly productive cell lines. First, the mass production of plant cell or tissue followed by the maintenance or storage of cell lines and ultimately selection and isolation of high production cell lines. This protocol often causes a major problem in the form of inherent genetic and epigenetic instability. Such instability problems are attributed to genetic variation by mutation in the culture, epigenetic changes (due to change in physiologic conditions), or somaclonal variation. During regeneration under *in vitro* conditions, a plant cell loses plasticity and changes its cellular machinery and cell-to-cell commutations, which often causes somaclonal or epigenetic changes. This variability often leads to a fall in productivity. These changes are usually observed during subculturing and can be reversed by changing the *in vitro* conditions as well as by screening for a desired cell population from the heterogeneous population. Understanding of physical and chemical factors regulating secondary metabolism is important for the selection of high producing cell lines in increasing the production of secondary metabolites. Factors like optimization of the hormone, media, and environmental conditions directly or indirectly affect the secondary metabolism, e.g., auxin in high concentration is good for cell growth but harmful to secondary metabolite production. Similarly, N-sources supplementation enhances the product accumulation in plant cells whereas reduced phosphate levels often stimulate product accumulation. Selection is more convenient if products are in the form of a pigment. An *in vitro* report on *Lithospermum erythrorhizon* demonstrated the growth stimulatory effect, and inhibitory effect on shikonin synthesis by ammonium ions clearly reflected the necessity of change in nitrate levels. Production can also be further enhanced by using clonal selection, visual screening, and various other techniques (HPLC and RIA to screen for high yielding cell lines), inducing mutation (to obtain overproducing cell lines) and use of selective (inhibitor/toxic/cytotoxic) agents (p-fluorophenylalanine to select high yielding cell lines with respect to phenolics). Various examples of clonal selection are shown in Table 7.4. Exposure of plant cells against toxic or any inhibitory stimuli (e.g., environmental stress) and selection of cells that have survived against that stimulus is a reliable strategy to select high yielding cell lines. Various chemical agents that are used to select high yielding cell lines are 5-methyltryptophan, glyphosate, and biotin.

7.2.5 Media Optimization

Numerous chemical and physical factors affecting the *in vitro* propagation have been extensively studied with various plant cells. These factors include nature of explant, type of culture,

TABLE 7.4 Efficiency of Cell Cloning to Produce Secondary Metabolites

Products	Plants	No. of times of secondary metabolites production
Ubiquinone-10	*Nicotiana tabacum*	15
Biotin	*Lavandula vera*	9
Berberine	*C. japonica*	2
Anthocyanins	*Vitis* hybrid	2.3–4
Anthocyanins	*Euphorbia milii*	7

media and their components, phytohormones (growth regulators), microenvironmental conditions, etc. Media optimization is known to be the most fundamental approach in plant cell culture technology. Cultural conditions optimization is achieved in order to improve growth rates of cells and/or higher yield of desirable products. Some of the prominent studies are discussed as follows.

Culture environment manipulation of certain constituents (e.g., nutrient levels, stress factors, light, and growth regulators) is the effective means to increase product accumulation. This manipulation often influences the expression of many secondary metabolite pathways. Some constituents of plant cell culture media significantly determine the growth and accumulation of secondary metabolites.

7.2.5.1 Sugar Levels

Plant cell cultures behave heterotrophically under *in vitro* conditions and thus essentially require sugar supplementation as carbon inorganic source. It has been found that the amount of sucrose affects the accumulation of secondary metabolite in various cultures (Table 7.5). Osmotic stress created by sucrose alone and with other osmotic agents also affects secondary metabolite production. It was also noticed that sucrose has a dual function (carbon source and osmotic agent) in some plants, e.g., *Solanum melongena*, *Vitis vinifera*, etc. [9].

TABLE 7.5 Effect of Sugar on Secondary Metabolite Production

Cell culture	Sucrose concentration (w/v)	Effect on secondary metabolite production	Yield obtained
Cell culture of *C. blumei*	2.5% and 7.5%	Increases rosmarinic acid accumulation	0.8 and 3.3 g/L yields
Cell culture of *C. roseus*	8%	Increases indole alkaloid accumulation	
Suspension cultures of *Eschscholtzia californica*	8%	Increase benzophenanthridine alkaloids accumulation	150 mg/L
Cell culture of *Aralia cordata*	5%	Reduces anthocyanin production	
Cell culture of *A. cordata*	3%	Favors anthocyanin production	
Cell suspension cultures of *V. vinifera*		Regulate anthocyanin production	

TABLE 7.6   Effect of Nitrogen Content on Secondary Metabolite Production

Name of culture	Level of nitrogen	Effect on secondary metabolite production
Plant tissue cultures	Reduced levels of NH_4^+ and increased levels of NO_3^-	Promotes the production of shikonin and betacyanins
Plant tissue cultures	Higher ratios of NH_4^+/NO_3^-	Increases the production of berberine and ubiquinone
Capsicum frutescens cultures	Reduced levels of total nitrogen	Improves the production of capsaicin
M. citrifolia cultures	Reduced levels of total nitrogen	Improves the production of anthraquinones
Vitis species cultures	Reduced levels of total nitrogen	Improves the production of anthocyanins
Chrysanthemum cinerariaefolium cultures	Complete elimination of nitrate	Induces two-fold increases in pyrethrin accumulation

7.2.5.2 *Nitrate Levels*

In cell suspension cultures, nitrogen supplementation chiefly influences the level of protein or amino acid products. Certain media, e.g., MS, LS, or B5, are known to be the rich sources of nitrogen as they contain relatively high amounts of nitrate and ammonium salts. Production of secondary metabolite is highly influenced by the ratio of ammonium/nitrate–nitrogen and overall levels of total nitrogen. Various examples of the effect of variation in nitrogen level are highlighted in Table 7.6.

7.2.5.3 *Phosphate Levels*

In addition to sugar and nitrogen, phosphate levels also markedly affect the production of secondary metabolites in plant cell cultures. It has been studied that the higher concentration of phosphate enhances cell growth and negatively influences secondary metabolism. Various examples reported by Sasse et al. show that decreasing phosphate concentration in medium stimulates or induces both the product and its associated enzymes that are responsible for its production (Table 7.7) [10].

TABLE 7.7   Effect of Nitrogen Content on Secondary Metabolite Production

Name of plant (culture)	Phosphate level	Effect on secondary metabolite production
C. roseus	Reduced phosphate levels	Induces the production of ajmalicine and phenolics
N. tabacum	Reduced phosphate levels	Induces the production of caffeoyl putrescines
Peganum harmala	Reduced phosphate levels	Induces the production of harman alkaloids
Beta vulgaris	Reduced phosphate levels	Induces the production of betacyanins
Digitalis purpurea	Increased phosphate	Stimulates the synthesis of digitoxin
Chenopodium rubrum	Increased phosphate	Stimulates the synthesis of betacyanin
Phytolacca americana	Increased phosphate	Stimulates the synthesis of betacyanin

TABLE 7.8   Effect of Nitrogen Content on Secondary Metabolite Production

Name of plant (culture)	Hormone level	Effect on secondary metabolite production
Suspensions of *Populus*	2,4-D removal or replacement by naphthalene acetic acid or indole acetic acid	Enhances the production of anthocyanins
Suspensions of *D. carota*	2,4-D removal or replacement by naphthalene acetic acid or indole acetic acid	Enhances the production of anthocyanins
Suspensions of *Portulaca*	2,4-D removal or replacement by naphthalene acetic acid or indole acetic acid	Enhances the production of betacyanins
Suspensions of *N. tabacum*	2,4-D removal or replacement by naphthalene acetic acid or indole acetic acid	Enhances the production of nicotine
Suspensions of *L. erythrorhizon*	2,4-D removal or replacement by naphthalene acetic acid or indole acetic acid	Enhances the production of shikonin
Suspensions of *M. citrifolia*	2,4-D removal or replacement by naphthalene acetic acid or indole acetic acid	Enhances the production of anthraquinones
Suspensions of *D. carota*	2,4-D	Stimulates carotenoid biosynthesis
Callus cultures of *Oxalis linearis*	2,4-D	Stimulates anthocyanin production
Suspensions of *Haplopappus gracilis*	Kinetin	Stimulates the production of anthocyanin
Populus cell cultures	Kinetin	Inhibited the formation of anthocyanins
Cultures of several plants	Gibberellic acid and abscisic acid	Suppresses production of anthocyanins

7.2.5.4 Growth Regulators

There are various critical reports available on the affects of growth regulators on secondary product accumulation. Synthesis and accumulation of secondary metabolites in various cultured plant cells are markedly affected by the type and concentration of auxin or cytokinin or the auxin/cytokinin ratio. It has been studied in various reports that 2,4-D restricts the accumulation of secondary metabolites (Table 7.8). In addition, the effects of cytokinins varied according to the desired type of plant species and metabolite (Table 7.8).

7.2.6 Culture Conditions

In addition to media components culture environmental conditions such as pH, oxygen, light humidity, temperature, type, and nature of medium have significant effects on secondary metabolite accumulation in several cultures (Table 7.9).

7.2.6.1 Temperature

The favorable temperature range for callus induction and growth of cultured cells was evidenced between 17°C and 25°C. Nevertheless growth of different plant species *in vitro* varies

TABLE 7.9　Effect of Cultural Conditions on Secondary Metabolite Production

Plant cell culture	Culture conditions	Secondary metabolite production
TEMPERATURE		
Cell cultures of *Digitalis lanata*	19°C	Biotransformation of digitoxin to digoxin is enhanced
Cell cultures of *D. lanata*	32°C	Purpureaglycoside A formation was enhanced
Tobacco cell cultures [11]	32°C	Enhanced production of ubiquinone when compared to either 24 or 28°C
Cell cultures of *C. roseus* [12]	16°C	12-fold higher production of crude alkaloids as compared to the normal 27°C
ILLUMINATION		
Cell cultures of *D. carota* and *Vitis* hybrids [13]	Illumination	Stimulation of anthocyanin accumulation
Matricaria chamomilla callus cultures	Illumination	Affects the composition of sesquiterpenes
Citrus limon callus cultures	Exclusion of light	Prompted the accumulation of monoterpenes
pH		
C. rubrum photoautotrophic cell suspension cultures	External pH shift from 4.5 to 6.3	Increased the cytosolic pH by 3.0 units and the vacuolar pH by about 1.3 units
AERATION AND AGITATION		
Kreis and Reinhard [14]	50% dissolved oxygen	Allowed an alkaloid yield of around 3-g/L culture in an airlift bioreactor
	Higher aeration rates	Remarkable decrease in alkaloid productivity. It is evident that airlift and stirred tank bioreactors can allow similar secondary product levels in cultured plant cells
Fruit suspension cultures (Muscat grape suspensions) [15]	Addition of carbon dioxide	Stimulated the production of volatile oil and induced the formation of (monoterpenes) linalool
Kobayashi et al. in suspension cultures of *T. minus* [16]	Use of carbon dioxide at the 2% level	Prevent cell browning and sustain berberine production in bubble column reactors

at different temperatures. In 1992, it was reported that decline in cultivation temperature markedly increased the amount of fatty acid per cell in dry weight [17] (Table 7.9).

7.2.6.2 Illumination

Like temperature, flux intensity, exclusion of light, and intervals of illumination considerably affect the accumulation of secondary metabolites (Table 7.9).

7.2.6.3 Medium pH

Medium pH plays a vital role in secondary metabolite production. In solid media, it controls the gelling strength of solidifying agent (agar) and hence controls the transport of nutrients from medium to cultures. The optimum pH range prior to autoclaving is usually adjusted between 5 and 6.

Extreme pH is avoided since it can directly affect the strength of medium. Depending upon the exchange of ions between the medium and cultivated culture and environmental conditions, medium pH (H⁺ concentration) keeps on changing during the development of the culture. Medium pH increases during nitrate uptake and decreases during ammonia assimilation (Table 7.9).

7.2.6.4 *Agitation and Aeration*

Parameters like aeration and agitation play a vital role in large-scale production of secondary metabolites. Thus, the design of bioreactor or microenvironment facilitating agitation and aeration considerably affects secondary metabolites production. Type and amount of gas perfuse in the culture environment and design of propeller for agitation regulate the production level (Table 7.9).

7.3 MODERN OR NONCLASSICAL METHODS FOR THE PRODUCTION OF SECONDARY METABOLITES

7.3.1 Elicitation

Plant tissue cultures are an ample source of valuable pharmaceuticals and therapeutic compounds. Under certain conditions these cultures produce considerable amounts of secondary metabolites over extended periods in comparison with those found in the parent plant. Strategies like manipulation of media, culture conditions, and hormonal concentration often failed to satisfy the commercial requirement of the market. Thus, in-depth knowledge of secondary metabolism is required for the desirable production of secondary metabolites. Such understanding may include the information related with various intermediates, precursor compounds, key enzymes and genes, targeted receptors, and other factors that influence the respective secondary metabolism. Before the concept of elicitation it was impractical to synthesize secondary metabolites frequently. After the introduction of several elicitors (substances, when introduced in small concentrations to a living cell system, initiate or improve the biosynthesis of specific compounds) it was practically possible to synthesize secondary metabolites frequently with improved quality and quantity. Exposing the plant physiology *in vitro* against trace amounts of elicitors for either inducing or enhancing biosynthesis of metabolites is called elicitation. Currently, it is the most valuable tool to improve the yield of these valuable metabolites.

Various substances or stimuli that increase the production of secondary metabolites in plant cultures have been reported. On the basis of their origin and structural characteristics these are categorized into two major classes, physical and chemical elicitors (Fig. 7.5). Physical and chemical elicitors are the two major classes of elicitors, whereas chemical elicitors are further divided into biotic and abiotic elicitors (Fig. 7.5). For understanding elicitation it is essential to understand the molecular pathways including intracellular transduction systems, which control the actions of elicitors, namely, elicitor receptors, GTP binding proteins, the Ca^{2+} messenger system, and the PI3K, PLC/IP3-DAG/PKC and adenylyl cyclase/cAMP/PKA pathways. This system ultimately acts through mitogen-activated protein

Elicitors						Reported effects on
Physical elicitors	Injury, thermal stress, osmotic stress, UV irradiation					P
Chemical elicitors	Abiotic	Sodium orthovanadate, vanadyl sulfate, metal ions (lanthanum, europium, calcium, silver, cadmium), oxalate				Pc
	Biotic	Complex composition	Yeast cell wall, mycelia cell wall, fungal spores			Pc ,F
		Defined composition	Carbohydrates	Polysaccharides	Alginate	Pc, F, B
					LBG	F
					Pectin	Pc, F
					Chitosan	Pc
					Guar gum	Pc
				Oligosaccharides	Mannuronate	F
					Guluronate	F
					Mannan	F
					Galacturonides	Pc
				Peptides	Glutathione	Pc
			Proteics	Proteins	Cellulase, Elicitins, Oligandrin	Pc
			Lipids		Lipopolysacch-aride	Pc
			Glycoproteins		Not characterized	Pc
			Volatiles		C6-C10	Pc

Abbreviations: P, plants; Pc, plant cell culture; B, bacterial cell culture; F, fungal cell culture.

FIGURE 7.5   **Broad classification of elicitors and its uses in plant tissue culture science [18–23].**

kinases (MAPKs) affecting the expression of genes related to the biosynthesis of secondary metabolites [18–21]. Specific response of the elicitor is always dependent on the elicitor/plant culture interaction. Elicitors obtained from natural origins and having defined (unique chemical identity) or complex composition (contains several molecular substances) are known as biotic elicitors. Biotic elicitors are either derived from the pathogen or from the plant itself. Plant-derived elicitors are occasionally called endogenous elicitors. In contrast elicitors derived from nonbiological origin and categorized in physical factors, having abolic regulation in cultured plant cells, are called abiotic elicitors. The classification described in Fig. 7.5 is based on the nature of the elicitor; however, elicitors may be also classified according to plant/elicitor interaction.

Plant/elicitor interaction can be divided into two groups: general elicitors and race-specific elicitors. As the name suggests general elicitors act broadly or nonspecifically to

TABLE 7.10   Carbohydrate Elicitors and Metabolites in Plant Cell Cultures

Elicitor name	Plant	Product
β-Linked glucopyranosyl	*Glycine max*	Phytoalexins
β-1,6-1,3 Glucan	*G. max*	Isoflavonoids
β-Glucan	*G. max*	H_2O_2
β-D-glucan	*N. tobaccum*	Desease resistance
α-1,4-Oligogalacturonide	*G. max*	Phytoalexins
Rhamsan, xanthan	*M. citrifolia*	Anthraquinones
Pectic oligomers	*C. limon*	Phytoalexins
Oligogalaturonides	*N. tabacum*	H_2O_2
N-Acetylchito-oligosaccharides	*Avena sativa*	Anthranilate
N-Acetylchitohexose	*Taxus canadensis*	Taxol
Mannan	*Hypericum perforatum*	Hypercins
Laminarin	*N. tabacum*	H_2O_2
Hepta-β-glucoside	*G. max*	Phytoalexins
Chitosan	*N. tabacum, E. californica*	Phytoalexins
Chitosan	*Polygonum tinctorium*	Indirubin
Chitosan	*Lupinus albus*	Isoflavonoids
Chitosan	*L. albus*	Genistein
Chitosan	*Rheum palmatum*	Anthracene
Chito-oligosaccharides	*Juniperus chinensis*	Podophyllotoxin
Chitin and chitosan oligosaccharides	*T. canadensis*	Taxol
Chitin	*P. somniferum*	Sanguinarine

trigger defense responses both in host and nonhost plants whereas race-specific elicitors only act on host plants leading to disease resistance cultivars. During host-pathogen interaction, a complementary pair of genes in a specific pathogen and a host cultivar decides gene-for-gene resistance. Therefore, race-specific elicitors are those elicitors that are encoded by or produced by the action of a virulence gene present in a particular race of pathogens. Such pathogens elicit the resistance only in a host plant variety carrying the corresponding resistance gene. The absence of either gene product will often result in disease. Various types of fungal, carbohydrate, and abiotic elicitors are highlighted in Tables 7.10–7.12.

7.3.1.1 Different Properties of Elicitors [18]

Owing to elicitation there are opportunities for the accumulation of antimicrobial compounds in plant cell cultures. These compounds are known as elicitation products or elicitation metabolites, which should not be confused with phytoalexins. Optimization of elicitor

TABLE 7.11   List of Various Fungal Elicitors Used in Plant Tissue Culture Science [18–23]

Fungal elicitors		
Elicitor name	**Plant**	**Product**
Yeast cell wall	Alfa cell cultures	Increase in enzymatic activity (S-adenosyl-L-methionine)
Verticillium dahliae	*Cephalotaxus harringtonia*	Alkaloid
Ustilaginoidea verens (mycelial homogenate)	*C. roseus*	Indole alkaloid
Rhodotorula glutinis, R. rubra, Panus conchatus, Coriolus versicolor	*Xanthophyllomyces dendrorhous*	Carotenoids, astaxanthin
Pythium aphanidermatum, Phytophthora parasitica	Witloof chicory	Coumarins
Pseudomonas lachrymans	Tobacco cell cultures	Caspidiol, lubimin, phytuberin, phytuberol, rishitin
Phytophthora species	Rose cell cutures	Increase in ion transport and H_2O_2 synthesis
Phytophthora megasperma	Soybean cells	Glyceollin
Mycelia of tuber *Aestivum vita*	*Ganoderma lucidum*	Ganoderic acid
Fungus isolated from bark of *T. chinensis*	*Taxus chinensis*	Taxol
Fungal spores	*Datura stramonium*	Lubimin
Fungal polysaccharide	*Phaseolus vulgaris*	Krevitone
Fungal polysaccharide	*Carthamus tinctorius*	Polyacetylenes
Fungal mycelia	*D. deltoidea*	Steroid (diosgenin)
Fungal elicitor	*G. max* seedlings	Increase in enzymatic activity (leipoxegenase)
Fungal elicitor	*M. sativa*	Phytoalexins
Fungal elicitor	*Petroselinum crispum*	Enzymes
Fungal elicitor	*Cupressus lusitanica*	Beta-thujaplicin
Fungal culture filtrate	*Bidens pilosa*	Phenylheptaryn
Ectomycorrhizal fungus	Pine cell cultures	Phenolics
Conidia from *Alternaria alternata*	*C. limon*	Umbelliferone, scoparone
Colletotrichum lindemuthianum	*P. vulgaris*	Increase in protein concentration
Chitosan	*Oryza sativa*	Increase in octadecanoid pathway
Chitosan	*N. tabacum, E. californica*	Alkaloids
Callulase	*C. annuum*	Capsidiol
Botrytis species	*P. somniferum*	Dihydrosanguinarine
Aspergillus niger, Rhizopus oryzae	*Arnebia euchroma*	Shikonin
A. fumigatus, A. flavus, a. ochraseus	*C. tinctorius*	Kinobeon A formation

TABLE 7.12   List of Various Abiotic Elicitors Used for the Secondary Metabolite Production [18–21]

Abiotic elicitors		
Elicitor name	**Plant**	**Product**
Methyl jasmonate	*L. erythrorhizon*	Rasmarinic acid
	Taxus sp.	Paclitaxel cephalomannines, taxanes, diterpenes
	Vaccinium pahlae	Anthocyanins
	G. max	Vegetative storage proteins
	O. sativa leaves	Putrescine
	C. blumei	Rosmarinic acid
	C. forskohlii	Forskolin
Sodium alginate	*Glycyrrhiza echinata*	Echinatin
Salicylic acid	*D. carota*	Chitinase
Colchicine	*Valeriana wallichii*	Valepotriates
Calcium chloride	*C. forskohlii*	Forskolin
Curdlan, xanthan	*Capsicum frutescens*	Capsaicin
Activated carbon	*L. erythrorhizon*	Benzoquinone
Metal ions		
Copper sulfate	*Hyoscyamus albus*	Phytoalexins with vetispyrane skeleton
	L. erythrorhizon	Shikonin
Silver nitrate	*Solanum tuberosum*	Free and conjugated polyamines
Vanadium sulfate	*C. roseus*	Catharanthine, ajmalicine
Cu^{2+}, Cd^{2+}	*Atropa belladonna*	Tropane alkaloids
Cu^{2+}, Mn^{2+}, Hg^{2+}	*Cicer arietinum*	Pterocarpenes
Al^{3+}, Cr^{3+}, Co^{2+}, Ni^{2+}	*D. stramonium*	Sesquiterpenoids
Arachidonic acid	*Capsicum annuum*	Capsidiol, rishitin

dose is essential to avoid the toxicity to plant tissue culture and to synthesize the optimum amount of secondary metabolites. Elicitor optimization is based on several conditions:

- Elicitor specificity
- Elicitor concentration
- Duration of elicitor contact
- Elicitor cell line (clones)
- Time course of elicitation
- Growth stage of culture
- Growth regulation and nutrient composition

7.3.1.1.1 ELICITOR SPECIFICITY

It was studied that a similar elicitor has the potential to trigger secondary metabolism in different cell cultures whereas certain plant cultures are stimulated by diverse elicitors. Exposing plant culture against different elicitors results in the synthesis of similar compounds. These elicitors are specific to each plant culture while secondary metabolism is generally influenced by many other factors such as plant species, the kinetics of induction, or accumulation levels. A report suggested the differences in the kinetics of the induction and levels of release of hyoscyamine and scopolamine, elicitated by biotic or abiotic compounds in hairy root cultures of *Brugmansia candida*. Various elicitors and their respective binding site characteristics are mentioned in Table 7.13.

7.3.1.1.2 ELICITOR CONCENTRATION

Concentration of elicitor plays a vital role in the elicitation process. Accumulation of higher concentrations of ajmalicine in *C. roseus* after treatment with higher concentration of elicitor extract (*Trichoderma viride, Aspergillus niger*, and *Fusarium moniliforme*) as compared to lower concentration was reported by Namdeo et al. [18]. On the other hand, further increase in the concentration adversely influenced the synthesis of ajmalicine. A higher concentration of elicitor reported stimulation of a hypersensitive response leading to cell death. This was further supported by Nef-Campa et al. and Rijhwani and Shanks. Therefore, optimum dose is required for induction.

7.3.1.1.3 DURATION OF ELICITOR EXPOSURE

Namdeo et al. reported the affect of duration of elicitor (extracts of *T. viride, A. niger*, and *F. moniliforme*) exposure on the cells of *C. roseus*. They found that *C. roseus* cells elicited with *T. viride* for 48 h showed three-fold increase in ajmalicine while cells elicited with *A. niger* and *F. moniliforme* showed two-fold increase. However, decrease in ajmalicine with further increasing exposure time was also reported. These results were further supported by Rijhwani and Shanks, Moreno and coworkers, and Negeral and Javelle.

TABLE 7.13　Various Elicitors and Their Respective Binding Site Characteristics [18–21]

Elicitors	Elicitor characteristics	Binding site characteristics	Plant species
AVR9	Peptide	Kd 0.07 nM	Tomato
Cryptogein	Glycoprotein	193 kD protein	Tobacco
Flagellin	Peptide	115 kD protein	Tomato, *Arabidopsis*
Harpins	Protein	115 kD protein	Tobacco, *Arabidopsis*
Pgt-glycoprotein	Glycoprotein	Kd 2 mM	Wheat
Syringolides	Glycolipid	Kd 8.7 nM 34 kD protein	Soybean
Systemin	Peptide	SR-160 protein	Tomato
Chitin oligosaccharide	N-acetyl chito-oligosaccharide	Kd 23 nM Kd 5.4 nM 75 kD protein	Tomato Rice

TABLE 7.14   Effect of Culture Conditions on Elicitation [18–21]

Type of cultured cell	Changes in conditions	Affect on elicitation
Cultured carrot cells	Without auxin	Do not respond to elicitation
Cell suspensions of *Morinda citrifolia*	Different growth regulators	Anthraquinone production is affected
H. perforatum L. cells	When incubated in the dark rather than under light	Jasmonic acid-induced hypericin production

7.3.1.1.4 AGE OF CULTURE

Subculture age plays a significant role in bioactive compounds production by elicitation. It was reported that 20-day-old *C. roseus* cultures showed higher yields (166 µg-1 DW) of ajmalicine on elicitation with extracts of *T. viride* [18]. This study was further supported by Rijhwani and Shanks and Ganapathi and Kargi.

7.3.1.1.5 NUTRIENT COMPOSITION AND CULTURE CONDITIONS

Elicitors are often supplemented according to medium composition so that none of the medium components interferes with its function. Sometime media are designed according to the nature of elicitors and vice versa. In particular, growth regulators in the medium markedly affect the elicitation of secondary metabolism. There is no permanent relation between culture conditions and elicitation as the optimization of medium composition and culture conditions is obligatory to accomplish any elicitation protocols. Several examples are mentioned in Table 7.14.

7.3.1.2 *Uses and Various Advantages of Elicitation [18–23]*

There are several advantages of using elicitor-induced resistance to disease in plants. This method provides native immunity to plants by activating the genes that provide systemic and prolonged protective effects. Multiple defense systems can also be introduced by exposing plant cells with different elicitors affecting cell signal transduction differentially to produce different types of metabolites against different pathogens at one time. This method can also induce nonspecific resistance to the number of fungi, bacteria, viruses, nematodes, etc. Various other uses are highlighted in Fig. 7.6.

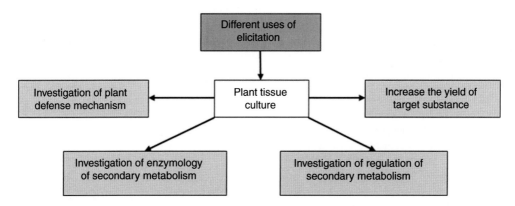

FIGURE 7.6   Stipulated MAP kinase-mediated biotic elicitation in plant cell [18–23].

7.3.1.3 *Mechanism of Elicitation in Plant Cells [18–23]*

Various efforts have been devoted to exploring the mechanism of elicitation in plants. Numerous reports on biotic elicitors such as carbohydrates on triggering secondary metabolites in plants were recently published but still the exact mechanics are poorly understood. Various theoretical mechanisms such as involvement of the key messenger Ca^{2+}, inhibition/activation of intracellular pathways, and changes in cell membrane and osmotic pressure are poorly understood. For understanding the plant-based elicitation the defense mechanism of animal cells was explored to hypothesize the role of plasma membrane-localized receptors, activated ion channels and protein kinases. Similarly, to regulate the defense mechanism, plant cells also carry plasma-membrane receptors. On exposure to biotic elicitors these receptors are activated and trigger an array of biochemical activities. These biochemical activities include:

- External biotic elicitor interaction with plasma membrane receptor is commenced by binding to a specific receptor. This interaction further begins a molecular reaction supporting the production of secondary metabolites. This binding may cause the change in ion fluxes across the plant cell membrane, i.e., Cl^- and K^+ efflux: Ca^{2+} influx. Ca^{2+} transport across the membrane further acts as a secondary messenger for an array of responses against external signals, including pathogens. This mechanism of elicitor responsive calcium channel was evidenced in parsley cells when exposed against a fungal elicitor. In addition to Ca^{2+} transport many more mechanisms were observed such as acidification of cytoplasm, depolarization of plasma membrane, and extracellular pH enhancement in elicitor-treated plant tissues. In addition, rapid alkalization of the apoplast and external medium of cultured plant cells signify the transport of protons from the apoplast into the cytosol. On the other hand, efflux of transient vacuolar protons causing cytoplasmic acidification was also reported in elicitor-treated cell cultures of *E. californica.*
- Among various mechanisms, enhancement of plant phospholipase activity after plasma membrane receptor/elicitor interaction was also reported in some cultured plants. This was further mediated by synthesis of secondary messengers (InsP3 and diacylglycerol). These secondary messengers further trigger the intracellular Ca^{2+} release, nitric oxide, and octadecanoid signaling pathway.

Elicitor treatment often induces the quick modification in protein phosporylation patterns in various cultures. It was stipulated that reversible phosphorylations play a vital role in the plant signal transfer during pathogen or stress defense and activation of proteins and transcription factors, and ultimately leads to secondary metabolite production. Various sequential steps involved in MAP kinase-mediated biotic elicitation are outlined in Fig 7.7.

- G-protein and nicotinamide adenine dinucleotide phosphate oxidase activation (responsible for active oxygen species and cytosol acidification), cytoskeleton reorganization, and production of active oxygen species reported in some plants.
- Synthesis of pathogenesis-related proteins (chitinases and glucanases, endopolygalacturonases, and protease inhibitors).
- Tissue necrosis at the infection site (hypersensitive response) and systemic acquired resistance. It has been reported that systemic necrosis is caused by transport of the elicitor within the tissue.

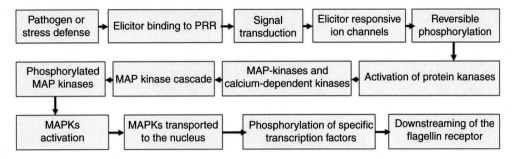

FIGURE 7.7   General mechanisms involved in fungal elicitation [18–23].

- Cell wall structural changes (lignifications of the cell wall, callus deposition).
- Transcriptional activation of the corresponding defense response genes.
- Accumulation of plant defense molecules such as tannins and phytoalexins after stimulation with the elicitor.
- Jasmonic and salicylic acids synthesis as secondary messengers.

Interconnection and orchestration between all these processes have not yet been established. Moreover, it is difficult to establish chronological order of these events as some of them are still under investigation. These sequences of events are not followed by all elicitors. Some peptides act through the periphery to induce the elicitation by generating several intermediate compounds during cascade of events, whereas some peptide elicitors act through plasma-membrane receptors reported to enter the cell and be transported to distal tissues acting themselves as messengers of the invasion signal.

7.3.1.4 Elicitation with Fungal Cell Wall Elicitors [18–23]

Plant cell cultures when elicited with fungal cell wall components result in the synthesis of low molecular weight compounds called phytoallexins and the process is called fungal elicitation. The cell wall polysaccharide of fungi triggers the calcium concentration in cytosol and potentiates various defense mechanisms leading to synthesis of low molecular weight antimicrobial compounds called phytoalexin. Fungal cell wall polysaccharide acts as a chemical messenger, which induces several pathways and cascades of events as illustrated in Figs 7.8 and 7.9. Several examples of fungal elicitors are highlighted in Table 7.15.

7.3.2   Precursor Feeding

Precursor feeding is the supplementation of biosynthesis initiator compounds or intermediates to increase the accumulation of secondary metabolites in the culture. On the basis of knowledge of biosynthetic pathways several organic compounds have been supplemented to the culture medium. These exogenous compounds are effective and improve the yield of secondary metabolites in many cases. Shikimic acid, jasmonic acid, malevonic acid, salicylic acid, ferrulic acid, cinnamic acid, cholesterol, various amino acids, etc. are the most common

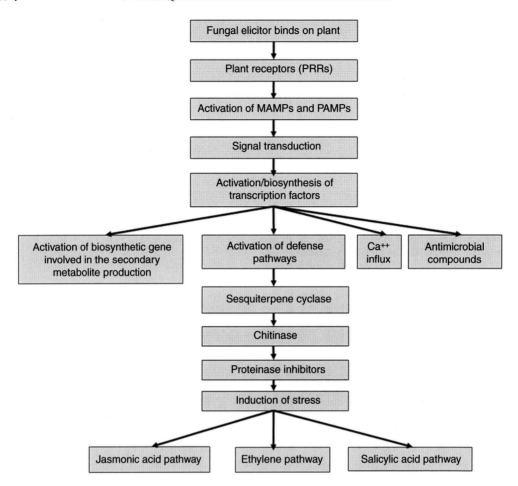

FIGURE 7.8 Cascade of events involved in the production of various secondary metabolites through acetate mevalonate and nonacetate mevalonate pathway during fungal elicitation [18–23].

examples that are frequently utilized in plant tissue culture [24]. Precursor feeding is the most economic strategy to enhance the secondary metabolite synthesis in the culture. For determining the type of precursor the exact knowledge of biosynthetic pathway with all the intermediates and the final compounds with their common origin point should be known. All these precursors are usually not complex as most of them form either a small moiety or unit of whole secondary metabolite. Some precursors go through lots of modifications and some are transformed with little modification into the final product. This would certainly be dependent on cascade of events or chain of intermediates. More the conversion or more the enzymes or reactants involved in this process, higher is the secondary metabolite production. Based on the physicochemical features of secondary metabolites, these precursors are supplemented during media preparation or sometime during the various intervals of growth periods [24]. Various examples are mentioned in Table 7.16.

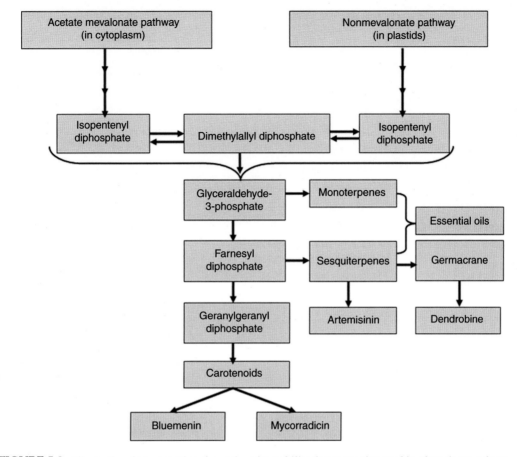

FIGURE 7.9   Illustration demonstrating the various immobilization strategies used in plant tissue culture.

TABLE 7.15   Fungal Elicitors and Their Secondary Metabolite Production [18–23]

Cell wall elicitors	Host	Secondary metabolites
Phytophthora cinnamon	–	Production and exudation of harmine/harmaline
Fusarium oxysporum (isolate Dzf17)	Cell suspension cultures of *Dioscorea zingiberensis*	Diosgenin accumulation was enhanced and jasmonic acid concentration was increased
Fungal polysaccharides	Cell suspensions of *Rubia tinctorum*	Enhanced anthraquinone content with high lucidin primveroside, ruberithic acid, and pseudopurpurin production

TABLE 7.16   Various Precursors and Their Responses on the Production of Secondary Metabolites in Various Commercial and Medicinally Active Plants [24]

Plant culture	Precursor	Product
Vanilla planifolia	Cinnamic acid	Vanillic acid
Taxus wallichiana	Phenylalanine	Taxol
T. cuspidata	Phenylalanine	Taxol
T. cuspidata	Carboxylic acid and amino acid	Taxol
T. chinesis	Phenylalanine	Taxol
Strawberry cells	L-Phenylalanine	Anthocyanin
Scopolia japonica	Tropic acid	Scopolamine
Ruta graveolens	4-Hydroxy 2-quinoline	Dictamine
Ricinus communis	Glycerol, succinic acid	Ricinine
Portulaca grandiflora	3,4-dihydroxyphenylalanine	Bexanthin
Podophyllum hexandrum	Phenylalanine	Podophyllotoxin
Papaver bracteatum	Tetrahydropalmatine	Benzazepine alkaloid
O. sativa	D-glucose	L-Ascorbic acid
N. tabacum	Nornicotine	Nicotine
M. citrifolia	O-Succinyl benzoic acid	Anthraquinons
Lunaria annua	Phenylalanine	Alkaloid lunarine
L. erythrorhizon	L-Phenylalanine	Rosmarinic acid
Holarrhena antidysenterica	Cholesterol	Conessine
Heimia salicifolia	Phenylalanine	Cryogenine
Ginkgo biloba	Terpenoid	Bilobalide
Duboisia leichhardtii	Phenylalanine	Tropane alkaloids
D. deltoidea	Cholesterol	Diosgenin
D. purpurea	Glucose	Digitoxose
D. lanata	Cholesterol	Pregnane derivatives
D. carota	Sinapic acid	Anthocyanin
Datura tabula	Tropic acid	Tropic acid
C. blumei	Phenylalanine	Rosmarinic acid
Cephaelis ipecacuanha	Phenylalanine, shikimic acid	Cephaeline
Celosia plumosa	Betanidin and betanin	Amaranthin
Ceanothus americanus	Amino acids	Macrocyclic alkaloids
C. roseus	Loganin	Ajmalicine
C. roseus	Tryptophan	Ajmalicine
C. roseus	Methyl jasmonate	Terpenoid indole alkaloid
C. annuum	Tyrosine DOPA	Capsaicin

TABLE 7.16 Various Precursors and Their Responses on the Production of Secondary Metabolites in Various Commercial and Medicinally Active Plants [24] *(cont.)*

Plant culture	Precursor	Product
Camptotheca acuminata	Tryptophan	Camptothecin
Azadirachta indica	Sodium acetate, Squalaine, IPP, GPP	Azadirachtin
A. belladonna	Tropic acid, tropinone and tropanoltropic acid, tropinone, tropanol	Tropane alkaloids
Allium cepa	S-alkenyl-cystein sulfoxides	Glutamyl peptides
Aesculus californica	Isoleucine	2-Amino-4-methylex-4-enoic acid

7.3.3 Biotransformation

Currently various chemicals including drugs, flavors, pigments, and agrochemicals are chiefly prepared from plant sources. Biotransformation is defined as the capability of the cultured plant cells to transform the exogenously supplied compounds. This may offer a potential and strategy toward modification of natural and synthetic chemicals. Bioconversions are preferred where the nature of some biochemical conversions in plant cells is complex and the type of reactions cannot be accomplished by synthetic routes. Owing to the presence of sufficient amounts of enzymes (biocatalyst), plant cell *in vitro* and organ cultures are the best platform to induce bioconversion reactions. Various compounds such as aromatics, steroids, alkaloids, coumarins, and terpenoids can undergo biotransformations using plant cells, organ cultures, and enzymes as suitable biocatalysts to perform these complex reactions [25]. This bioconversion is almost dependent on the enzymatic potential of cultured plant cells employed for bioconversion purposes. Enzymes of plant origin have the potential to catalyze regio- and stereospecific reactions and thus it can be applied for the production of desired substances. Types of reactions generally induced in plane cells *in vitro* are oxidations, reductions, hydroxylations, methylations, acetylations, isomerizations, glycosylations, and esterifications [25]. Molecular techniques involving site-directed mutagenesis and gene manipulation for substrate specificity can be used to improve biotransformation efficiency. In addition, genetic manipulation offers great potential to express heterologous genes and to clone and overexpress genes for key enzymes. Currently various types of plant cell cultures are used as model systems for the study of biosynthetic pathways. For achieving desirable product yields the desired product can be accumulated in a nonpolar organic phase or adsorbed by a resin or immobilized using a suitable polymer. Various examples are highlighted in Table 7.17.

7.3.4 Plant Cell Immobilization

Plant cell immobilization is a technique to immobilize plant cells in a suitable matrix. It is different from cell entrapment where immobilized cells can be entrapped but also the cells are absorbed onto support materials. The concept of cell immobilization was developed from enzyme immobilization, which now has many industrial applications. In terms of large-scale application microorganism immobilization is less developed; nevertheless it is widely used

TABLE 7.17 Various Examples of Biochemical Conversion in Plant Tissue Culture [25]

Sr. no.	Plant species	Reaction	Precursor	Product
1.	*R. graveolens*	Epoxidation	Hydroxyl coumarins	Furano coumarins
2.	*N. tabacum*	Reduction	Testosterone	Androsterone
3.	*Mentha* spp.	Reduction	(–) Menthone	(+) Neomenthone
4.	*D. lanata*	Glucosylation	Gitoxigenin	Gitoxin
5.	*Digitalis*	Hydroxylation	β-Methyldigoxin	β-Methyldigoxin
6.	*Datura* spp.	Esterification	Tropine	Acetyltropine
7.	*Datura innoxia*	β-D-glucosylation	Hydroxyquinone	Arbutin
8.	*Cannabis sativa*	Oxidation	Geraniol	Nerol
9.	*Anethum graveolens*	Hydroxylation	Agroclavine	C-8 compound

in the laboratory. Nowadays immobilization techniques are applied to plant cell cultures and suitable bioreactors are utilized for immobilizing cultures at a large scale.

Slow growth rate of plant cells, slower production of targeted compounds, and a tendency to become easily influenced by physical stress and various chemical signals lead to the development of the plant cell immobilization technique. Plant cell immobilization protects the plant cell from liquid shear forces and facilitates the importance of cellular cross-talk. This cross-talk establishes intercellular communication by the action of signaling molecules, which can enhance the biosynthesis of plant cells. It is well known that plant cells *in vitro* accumulate their secondary metabolites generally in the stationary phase of their growth cycle. Thus, immobilization of plant cells is one of the means to create a nongrowth condition or stationary condition under which the production of secondary metabolites may be improved [26]. Plant cell immobilization can also be employed to perform biotransformations and is reported to have higher production rates than freely suspended cells, e.g., supplementation of precursors in immobilized capsicum cultures accumulated more quantities of biotransformed compounds than freely suspended cultures [27,28]. Thus, immobilized plant cells can be used for various purposes, e.g., bioconversion, *de novo* synthesis, and synthesis from precursors. Various examples of immobilization in plant cells are highlighted in Tables 7.18 and 7.19.

7.3.4.1 Advantage and Disadvantage of Cell Immobilization

During immobilization, plant cell growth and production phases can be decoupled and controlled by various chemical and physical stress conditions, which allows the retention of cells in the bioreactor for extended periods. This may further facilitate the alternating rejuvenation/growth and secondary metabolite production cycles [30]. Bioprocess engineering complications may often develop from the aggregation of plant cells, which can block pipes and openings. This may also cause sedimentation of culture rapidly if it is not agitated continuously.

Owing to the shear sensitivity of culture, mechanical agitation is not preferred as it can be harmful to cells. In addition, these cultures cannot be transported using conventional pumps without significant loss of viability. Plant cell immobilization is a solution for all of these problems and provides a microenvironment protected from sustained shear [30]. Immobilization

TABLE 7.18 Various Examples of the Immobilization of Plant Cells [29]

Plant species	Support
Amaranthus tricolor	Chitosan
C. roseus	Polyurethane
Coffea arabica	Alginate
D. innoxia	Alginate
D. carota	Polyurethane
D. lanata	Alginate
G. echinata	Alginate
Mentha sp.	Polyacrylamide
M. citrifolia	Alginate
Mucuna sp.	Alginate
Nicotiana sp.	Polyacrylamide
P. somniferum	Alginate
S. tuberosum	Agarose
Taxus cuspidata	Glass fiber

TABLE 7.19 Application of the Immobilization in Biosynthesis and Biotransformation of Plant Cells [29]

Sr. no.	Plant species	Immobilization method	Product
BIOTRANSFORMATION			
1.	*D. lanata*	Alginate beads	β-Methyl digitoxin
2.	*Daucus carota*	Alginate beads	β-Methyl digitoxin
BIOSYNTHESIS			
1.	*Solanum aviculare*	Polyphenon oxide beads	Steroidal glycosides
2.	*P. somniferum*	Aliginate	Codeine
3.	*M. citrifolia*	Aliginate	Anthraquinones
4.	*Lavandula vera*	Aliginate	Blue pigments
5.	*C. roseus*	Alginate beads Alginate Acrylamide Xanthan-acrylamide	Ajmalicine
6.	*C. frutescens*	Nylon-polyurethane foam	Capsaicinoids

also allows separation of the cells that makes the easy exchange of medium for the purposes of metabolic control or nutrient replenishment. Thus, it would be quicker and easier to monitor immobilized culture conditions than other cultures. In addition end products can be easily collected continuously by adsorption on a suitable resin, or by other means [31]. Immobilization of horseradish decreases the activity of acid *invertase* and increases the availability of intracellular sucrose for glucosylation, hence producing glucosinolates in higher concentration than that of suspended cell cultures.

One of the main disadvantages of immobilization is that it can only be applied over the cell line that excretes the product of interest into the culture medium. Techniques to promote the excretion of end product usually retained by plant cells decrease cell viability to an undesirable extent. Among these techniques permeabilization is frequently utilized though in some cases reversible permeabilization is also utilized, e.g., reversible permeabilization of *C. roseus* using dimethyl sulfoxide has shown good results [30].

7.3.4.2 Methods of Immobilization

Various immobilization methods and their differentiated features are illustrated in Figs 7.10 and 7.11. Entrapment methods that are used with plant cell cultures can be divided as follows.

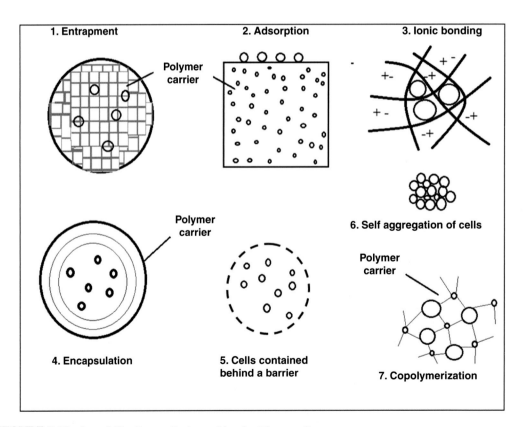

FIGURE 7.10   Immobilization methods used in plant tissue culture.

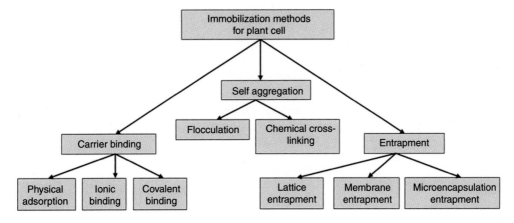

FIGURE 7.11   Gene transfer techniques used in plant tissue culture.

7.3.4.2.1 GEL ENTRAPMENT BY IONIC NETWORK FORMATION

Alginate beads-mediated plant cell entrapment by ionic network formation is the most widely used method. Alginate, which is commercially available as alginic acid, can be either water soluble or insoluble depending on the type of the associated salt. The salts of sodium, other alkali metals, and ammonia are soluble, whereas the salts of polyvalent cations, e.g., calcium are water insoluble, with the exception of magnesium. One of the most frequently used cations is calcium. Alginate is a biopolysaccharide having a strong yet firm skeleton that forms a stable gel in the presence of cations [30]. The alginate polymer itself is anionic (i.e., negatively charged) overall. In the process of gelation, the exchange of calcium ions for sodium ions is carried out under relatively mild conditions as follows:

$$2\,Na(Alginate) + Ca^{++} \rightarrow Ca(Alginate)_2 + 2Na^+$$

The gel formed is highly thermostable over the range of 0–100°C; therefore, heating will not be able to dissolve the gel. However, gel can be easily redissolved by immersing the alginate gel in a solution containing a high concentration of sodium, potassium, or magnesium. Alginate beads containing cells are prepared by dropping a cell suspension/sodium alginate solution mixture into a stirred calcium chloride solution.

Instead of alginate, κ-carrageenan can also be used in a similar manner using either calcium or potassium. In this method the gel can be reversible by adding ethylenediaminetetraacetic acid. Moreover, syneresis can happen in the presence of other calcium-chelating agent such as phosphates. So far various plant cells were successfully immobilized using this method, e.g., *M. citrifolia*, *C. roseus*, and *D. lanata* were immobilized with significant increase of metabolite and the stability of metabolic capacity was also extended [32].

7.3.4.2.2 GEL ENTRAPMENT BY PRECIPITATION

A matrix of biopolymer such as agar and agarose hydrogel can be used to entrap plant cells by precipitation. The polysaccharides form gel when a heated aqueous solution is cooled. Mixing of the warm gel with hydrophobic phase (e.g., olive oil) uniformly dispersed the particles into a matrix. After obtaining the desired particle size the whole mixture is cooled, which results in solidification. Gel entrapment by precipitation was observed in *C. roseus* when 5 g of wet weight cells were suspended in 5% agarose at 40°C.

7.3.4.2.3 GEL ENTRAPMENT BY POLYMERIZATION

The polyacrylamide-mediated gel entrapment method is the most common polymerization method used in plant tissue culture. However, initiator and cross-linking agents used in polymerization are toxic and sometimes cause death to plant cells. It was reported that *C. roseus* cells entrapped by polyacrylamide showed no growth at all [33].

7.3.4.2.4 ENTRAPMENT IN THE PREFORMED STRUCTURES

These structures are porous and have open network through which nutrient medium may pass. These structures can be constructed by using cotton fiber, fiberglass mats, reticulate polyurethane foam, and cloth nonwoven polyester short fibers. Among all, polyurethane foam has some advantages as a matrix such as being nontoxic to plant cells and no complicated operation causing microbial contamination is required. Immobilization of cells was achieved by their invasion into preformed polyurethane foam cut into blocks. It was studied that immobilized cells of *C. frutescens* cells in reticulate polyurethane foam produced more capsaicin than the free cells [34]. Owing to its inert nature, high surface free energy, and large surface area (for maximum adhesion), glassfiber material was shown to be an ideal substratum for immobilizing cultured *C. roseus*. This supports also the eradication of undefined physiological perturbation in gel systems caused by the high calcium content and the low phosphate level (essential to limit calcium ion chelation and the polysaccharide gel).

7.3.4.3 Factors Affecting Immobilization

7.3.4.3.1 CELL/MATRIX INTERACTION

While discussing this factor it is essential to acknowledge reticulated polyurethane foam, where the cells are reported to interact with the surface of polyurethane particles leading to intrusion of cells into the foam, simultaneous growth, coalescence of cells in the foam, and retention of cells in the foam [35].

7.3.4.3.2 MASS TRANSFER

Molecular diffusion of compounds through an immobilized cell matrix can be achieved through the microstructure of the immobilization matrix by adopting a mechanism such as capillary and active transport, e.g., reticulated foam, membrane, and fiber mat matrices [30]. The extent of resistance toward mass transfer determines the final yield of substance, i.e., increased resistance to lower transport of nutrient (increases stress factor) ultimately gives a higher yield of secondary metabolite. It was also investigated that mass transfer restriction can be reduced by surface immobilization (in layer form) where there is maximum contact between the surface of the immobilized cultures and the liquid phase [31].

7.3.4.3.3 AERATION OF IMMOBILIZED CELLS

So far no direct relation is established between concentration of dissolved oxygen and secondary metabolite production and growth. It has been reported that owing to insufficient supply of oxygen, alginate entrapped cells of *T. minus* failed to produce berberine [36]. On the other hand, it was also investigated that decline in the dissolved oxygen of the medium resulted in the production of capsaicin by polyurethane entrapped *C. frutescens* cells [37].

7.3.4.3.4 LIGHT

Periodic exposure to light can significantly influence the metabolism of cultures. In most cases light only penetrates the outer cell layers of the cultures and to some extent the immobilized matrix. Light penetration may be beneficial where some precursors are formed in light and some in dark, e.g., *Catharanthus* alkaloids. Supply of light to the cultures and matrix can be facilitated by the use of optical fibers.

7.3.4.3.5 HARVESTING IN IMMOBILIZED SYSTEM

During immobilization excretion of the product in medium can be harvested according to its rate of transport from the cell. Some plant cells are able to release their secondary metabolites spontaneously such as quinolines, quinolizidines, anthraquinones, phenolics, and terpenoids whereas in some cases the release of product is continuous. Plant cell culture facilitates the large-scale continuous harvesting of secondary metabolites that are excreted into the medium. Immobilization usually promotes spontaneous release of the products that are normally stored within the cells in suspension. This spontaneous release of metabolites into the medium can be enhanced by various methods such as permeabilization and *in situ* extraction. Electroporation and treatment with surface-active chemicals (dimethyl sulfoxide, phenetyl alcohol, chloroform, triton X-100, and hexadecyltrimethylammonium bromide) are the two most popular approaches used in permeabilization. Inert hydrophobic chemical-based various extraction and *in situ* adsorption procedures can be performed by adding inert hydrophobic chemicals those are having high adsorption capacity for the hydrophobic plant products [38].

7.3.4.4 Scaling-Up (Bioreactor)

For scaling up, immobilized plant cell bioreactors are preferred over the conventional stirred or fed batch bioreactors. Such bioreactors protect the cells from liquid shear forces, which enhance mixing speed and allow more efficient mass transfer. Due to the slow or retarded growth small cultured volumes can be maintained for an extended period. Using easily exchangeable growth and production media these bioreactors also allow the separation of growth and production phases [39]. There are various types of bioreactors used for immobilization (Table 7.20). These bioreactors are preferred as most of them are suitable for immobilization of plant cell.

7.3.5 Gene Transfer Techniques

Classical techniques such as organ, callus, and cell suspension culture are still known to be alternative strategies for secondary metabolite production in plant cells. However, utilization of these techniques is not sufficient to improve the yield of secondary metabolites. Gene introduction by using various gene transfer methods is the most reliable technique for introducing desirable or manipulated traits that naturally affect the secondary metabolites in plant cells. Genetic transformation is defined as the alteration of the genotype or genetic makeup by transferring DNA into an organism. The application of these techniques has considerable

TABLE 7.20   Bioreactors Used for the Immobilization of Plant cells [29]

Type of reactor	Immobilized cells	Immobilized medium	Production	Advantages/ Disadvantages	References
Packed bed reactors	*Pseudomonas* spp.	Alginate beads	L-Cysteine	Poor mass transfer characteristics and the beads may suffer from compression under their own static weights	[40]
Mechanically agitated and airlift reactors	*C. roseus* and *Thalictrum rugosum*	Alginate beads	Alkaloids	Mechanically agitated reactors cause more damage to beads or plant cells than airlift reactors (unsuitable for particles)	[31,41,42]
Bubble column reactor	*C. arabica*	Alginates	Alkaloids were not produced	Because of physical stress from thin film of bursting bubbles, cells were damaged at low aeration rate	[43,44]
Hollow fiber membrane reactors	*G. max, D. carota, Petunia hybrid, C. arabica* and *N. tabacum*	Cells were introduced into the shell side of the reactor		Good control of fluid dynamic and flow distribution, improved protection against contamination but expensive, liable to fouling, having problems with gas transfer and difficult to inoculate	[30,45]
Flat bed reactors	*C. frutescens*	Sheets of foam were suspended as vertical baffles in a stirred reactor		Immobilized cells are in direct contact with the nutrient medium; there is no permeability barrier	[30,34]

significance in the production of major food crops and overproduction of valuable plant secondary metabolites. Plant genetic transformation is carried out by physical, chemical, and biological agents. Hairy root culture, microinjection, electroporation, polyethylene glycol (PEG)-mediated gene transfer, virus-mediated gene transfer, and biolistics are the most common gene transfer methods used in plant tissue culture (Table 7.21) (Figs 7.12 and 7.13). Bacterial infection to plant cells is a natural phenomenon where bacteria exchange their genetic information through conjugation, thereby passing new genetic information to subsequent generations. One of the main benefits of using bacteria relates to their unicellular nature. Unlike multicellular organisms, in bacteria only a single cell is required to be altered in order to integrate the new genetic information and allow for its transmission to the next generation.

TABLE 7.21 Various Plant Transformation Techniques Used in Plant Tissue Culture

Gene transfer methods	Brief introduction
Agrobacterium-mediated gene transfer	Transfer of DNA from bacteria to plants
Biolistics	Rapidly propelled tungsten or gold microprojectiles coated with DNA are blasted into cells
Viral transformation method	DNA/RNA viruses of both types can be used for transformation
Polyethylene glycol-mediated gene transfer	Plant cell protoplasts treated with PEG are momentarily permeable, allowing uptake of DNA from the surrounding solution
Microinjection	Injection of DNA directly into the cell nucleus using an ultrafine needle
Electroporation	Electrical impulses are used to increase membrane and cell wall permeability to DNA contained in the surrounding solution

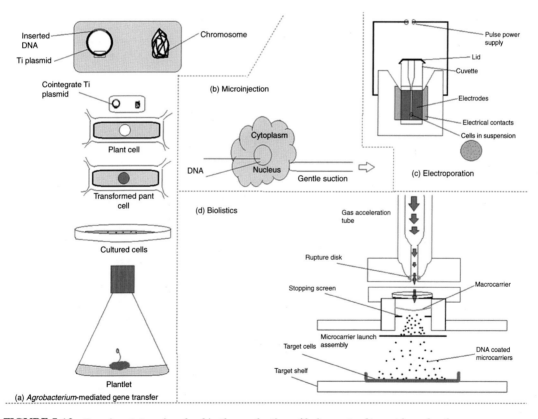

FIGURE 7.12 **Prominent steps involved in the production of hairy root culture at large level.**

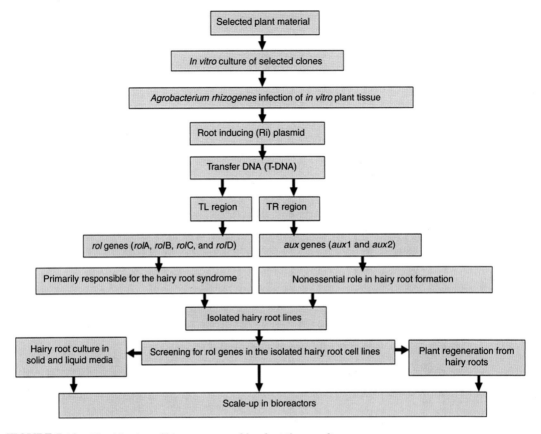

FIGURE 7.13   Classification of bioreactors used in plant tissue culture.

This type of natural genetic transformation often enhances the capacity of organisms to adapt to their environment. In most cases transformation is more difficult with multicellular organisms (e.g., plant) in order to fully integrate the new genetic information in each cell of tissue. Owing to the pluripotent nature of plant cells whole plants can grow from a single cell. Therefore, transformation to an individual plant cell and then regeneration into a whole organism is a better strategy for stable and uniform transformation throughout the organism. Among all these hairy root culture is currently the most successful and frequently utilized technique.

7.3.5.1 Agrobacterium-Mediated Genetic Transformation in Plant

In nature, infection through microbial sources causes significant transformation of genetic information to plants and other organisms. This is usually carried out by various types of bacteria. *A. tumefaciens* (a tumor inducing bacterial species) and *A. rhizogenes* (root inducing bacteria) are the soil bacteria that cause natural transformation in plant cells. In plants these bacteria cause transformation in the form of crown gall disease and hairy root syndrome (Fig. 7.12). Commercial significance of transgenic hairy root culture system in production of secondary metabolites is highlighted in Table 7.22.

TABLE 7.22 Commercial Production of Pharmaceutically Important Compounds Using Transgenic Hairy Root Culture System [46–48]

Strain	Sources of gene	Host pant with respective gene of interest	Affect on secondary metabolite production
A. rhizogenes	Soybean	*Brassica napus* with glutamine synthase gene	Three-fold increase in enzyme activity
A. rhizogenes	*C. roseus*	*P. harmala* with tryptophane decarboxylase gene	Serotonin
A. rhizogenes	Yeast	*Nicotiana rustica* with ornithine decarboxylase gene	Nicotine
A. rhizogenes	*Hyoscyamus muticus*	*A. belladonna* with 6-hydroxylase gene	Increased enzyme activity and a five-fold higher concentration of scopolamine

7.3.5.1.1 CROWN GALL DISEASE

Agrobacterium strain has the ability to transfer a part of its own DNA (T-DNA or transfer DNA) into plant cells. While understanding the oncogenesis in plant cells, most researchers were focusing on the bacterial origin of these neoplastic diseases. After the evident discovery of the causative agent (*A. tumefaciens*), interest in crown gall disease largely increased. *A. tumefaciens* infects the plant naturally at wound sites and the transferred DNA to produce crown gall disease. In addition, this strain also controls the plant machinery to produce unique sugars called opines that the bacterium uses as a nutrient supply. This bacterial strain contains a Ti (tumor-inducing) plasmid, which normally infects dicotyledonous plant cells. Replacement of tumor inducing gene with the gene of interest facilitates efficient transformation in plant cells. This tumor inducing DNA or T-DNA contains two types of genes. The first gene is called the oncogenic gene, which encodes for enzymes involved in the synthesis of auxins and cytokines and is responsible for tumor formation. The second gene encodes for the opine synthesis (condensation product between amino acids and sugars), produced and excreted by the tumor cells and consumed by bacteria as carbon and nitrogen sources. In addition to the T-DNA, there are some genes that are present for the opine catabolism, which assist in the T-DNA transfer from the bacteria to plant cell and bacterium/bacterium conjugation-mediated plasmid transfer. Recently a report on *A. tumefaciens*-mediated Bt corn transformation using a bacterial plasmid as a vector for the Bt gene brought a new genetic revolution in crop industry especially among dicotyledonous plants.

7.3.5.1.2 HAIRY ROOT SYNDROME

Hairy root syndrome is caused by the soil bacterium *A. rhizogenes*, resulting in the so-called hairy root disease (Figs 7.12 and 7.13). After infection with bacteria, hairy root accumulates the same component as accumulated by the roots of the intact plants and attains rapid growth in hormone-free medium. Infection caused by these bacteria lead to the transformation of plasmid, also called root-inducing (Ri) plasmid containing T-DNA, which is transferred into the plant cell and expressed therein. This Ri-plasmid is made up of T-DNA, located between TR and TL regions. Ri-plasmid once transferred integrates with the nuclear genome of the host plant. This infection furnishes a by-product near the site of infection called hairy root. As in the case of *A. tumefaciens*, transformation of plasmid of *A. rhizogenes* into the plant cell also leads to the production of opines, which serve as specific food for the bacteria [49]. Noncontiguous TL- and TR-DNA present at stretches of T-DNA are transferred separately into plant chromosomes. Integration of rol genes of TL-DNA into the plant genome is adequate to stimulate hairy root formation and ultimately produce hairy root syndrome [50–52]. On the other hand, *aux* genes of TR-DNA play a conditional but nonessential role in hairy root formation [52,53]. For successful establishment of hairy root culture several essential conditions should be taken into consideration such as *A. rhizogenes* strain, disease-free explant, suitable antibiotic to eliminate redundant bacteria after cocultivation, suitable culture medium, and screening after transformation [54]. The majority of plant materials can be used to induce hairy roots [55–58]. For inducing hairy roots, explants are initially wounded separately and then cocultivated or inoculated with *A. rhizogenes* (Fig. 7.12).

7.3.5.2 Electroporation

When cell suspension is mixed with DNA construct and exposed to pulses of high electrical voltage for shorter duration, permeability of the cell membrane is altered. This may increase the permeability of cell membrane and allows the foreign DNA to enter the cell. This foreign DNA successfully integrates with host genome and expresses the desired character. Direct transformation of DNA by electroporation into monocots was proved to be the successful method of DNA transformation (Fig. 7.12).

7.3.5.3 Microinjection

Microinjection is the conventional method of introducing DNA by microscopic examination of the targeted specimen, e.g., meristematic cells or any defined compartment of a cell. By microscopic visualization the targeted specimen cell is held in place with gentle suction followed by DNA insertion into the cytoplasm or nucleus with a fine pipette. This is preferred for plant protoplasts and tissues. This method often causes great damage to the tissue, thus it is not utilized for gene transfer (Fig. 7.12).

7.3.5.4 PEG-Mediated Gene Transfer

Lipid vesicles called liposomes, surrounded by a synthetic membrane of phospholipids having a hydrophobic shell and hydrophobic core, are used in this method for the drug delivery system. For gene transfer these vesicles are fused with protoplast in the presence of PEG. Protoplast allows these vesicles to enter the protoplasm by endocytosis.

7.3.5.5 Viral Transformation (Transduction)

In addition to bacteria, viruses also have the capability to move DNA (or RNA) into an organism and cause alteration in genetic organization in plant cells. Packaging of the desired genetic material (either DNA or RNA) into a capsid of suitable virus to allow stable infection of plant cells by a modified virus is a simple means of a virus-mediated gene transformation. Sometimes a chimeric gene is also packed inside the capsid to perform a variety of actions. Recombination with the chromosome in plant cells is possible when the transformable material is DNA. But if the transformable material is single-stranded RNA then replication occurs in the cytoplasm of the infected cell. This type of gene transfer is called transfection. Now it is well understood that it is not a transformation where foreign DNA enters the nucleus and integrates with the chromosomal material of plant cell. In this case, further generation of the infected plants is virus free and also free of the inserted gene.

7.3.5.6 Biolistics

Biolistics including particle bombardment is a commonly used method for genetic transformation of plants when either cells/tissues or intracellular organelles are impermeable to foreign DNA. The plant cell wall is usually impermeable to foreign DNA. Utilization of the gene gun method has shown better results against the various barriers that hinder the delivery of foreign DNA inside the organelle/cell/tissue. Gene transfer through a gene gun is part of the biolistic method. During this method DNA or RNA construct adheres to biological inert particles (such as gold or tungsten) to form a DNA/particle complex. The DNA/particle complex is bombarded on a targeted tissue in a vacuum. This bombardment is achieved by accelerating a powerful shot to the targeted tissue. The high density of the DNA/particle complex increases the bombardment speed toward the targeted tissue, which may result in effective transformation. Only inert metal particles can be bombarded through a solution containing DNA surrounding the cell. Such a complex once formed is directly transferred to the plant cell (Fig. 7.12).

7.3.6 Genetic Manipulation in Hairy Root Culture for Secondary Metabolite Production

A. tumefaciens and *A. rhizogenes* infected root furnish a promising platform for the genetic manipulation of plant cells. As discussed *A. rhizogenes*-mediated transformation of plants can be used in a similar manner to that used during *A. tumefaciens* transformation. Hairy root syndrome and production of transgenic hairy root cultures by genetic manipulation can be achieved by *A. rhizogenes*-mediated transformation. For the transformation border, sequences of T-DNA are required and the remaining T-DNA can be replaced with foreign DNA. After replacement whole plasmid is introduced into cells from which whole plants can be regenerated. Inheritance of these foreign DNA sequences follows the same pattern as inherited in Mendel's law of inheritance [59] *A. rhizogenes* has the potential to transfer foreign genes of interest present in binary vector to the transformed hairy root culture cells. In addition it is also possible to introduce gene encoding enzymes that catalyze certain hydroxylation, methylation, and glycosylation reactions selectively in some plant cells to produce large amounts of plant secondary metabolites. Various examples of transformation-influenced secondary metabolism in hairy root cultures are reported in Table 7.23.

Advantages of hairy root culture:

- Harvesting roots for extracting secondary metabolites can cause destruction to whole plants. Therefore, interest in producing secondary metabolites by developing hairy root culture has been raised.
- Hairy root culture potentially grows faster without needing an external supply of auxins. In certain cases, they do not need incubation under light.
- Due to their high genetic stability all hairy root cultures are stable in metabolite production.

TABLE 7.23   Recent Report on Valuable Metabolites Produced by Hairy Root Culture

Sr. no.	Plant species	Metabolite
1.	*Solidago altissima*	Polyacetylene
2.	*Saussurea medusa*	Jaceosidin
3.	*Rauvolfia micrantha*	Ajmalicine, ajmaline
4.	*Pueraria phaseoloides*	Puerarin
5.	*Plumbago zeylanica* L.	Plumbagin
6.	*P. rosea*	Plumbagin
7.	*P. somniferum*	Morphine, sanguinarine, codeine
8.	*Panax ginseng*	Ginsenoside
9.	*Linum flavum*	Coniferin
10.	*Gynostemma pentaphyllum*	Gypenoside
11.	*Gmelina arborea*	Verbascoside
12.	*C. acuminata*	Camptothecin
13.	*A. indica*	Azadirachtin

- Yield in hairy root cultures can be altered by optimizing various factors such as carbon source and its concentration, ionic concentration of the medium, pH of the medium, light, temperature, and inoculum [54].
- In addition utilization of techniques like precursor feeding, cell immobilization, elicitation, and biotranformation of hairy root culture can improve secondary metabolite production.

7.3.7 Scale-Up Technique

Various plants, especially higher plants, are rich sources of a wide range of biochemicals. Various active components that have different phytochemistry and are developed through the same or different metabolic pathways are grouped together under a broad heading of plant secondary metabolites. Extraction procedures followed for deriving these compounds may cause continued destruction of plants, which may lead to the extinction of plant species over the years. Alternative methods for the extraction of phytotherapeutic compounds are an issue of considerable socioeconomic importance. These factors have generated considerable interest in the use of plant cell culture technologies for the production of pharmaceuticals [60]. *In vitro* cultivation of plant cell or tissue has been considered as an alternative source of biochemicals over the last 40 years. Tobacco and various vegetables were first examined for the large-scale cultivation of plant cell culture techniques. Later on the first patent for the cultivation of plant tissue and its potential for the production of secondary metabolites was obtained by Routien in 1956 [61]. In addition, several Japanese companies started a number of joint venture programs for the commercial production of therapeutic compounds of plant origin (Table 7.24).

TABLE 7.24   Japanese Companies Involved in the Production of Secondary Metabolites at Larger Level [62]

Firm name	Product prepared
The Japan Tobacco Incorporation	Mass production of tobacco cells
Meiji Seika	Production of *P. ginseng* cells in large volumes
Nitto Denko Corporation	Cell mass of ginseng commercially
Ajinomoto and Nippon Shin-yaku	Accumulation of alkaloids, steroids, and other secondary products in cultured cells

Various bioreactors of different designs and capacities are used to produce secondary metabolites at a larger level. Bioreactor is defined as a vessel that carries out a biological reaction and is used to culture aerobic cells for conducting cellular or enzymatic immobilization. The bioreactor technique is also called the scale-up technique and was first applied to plant propagation in 1981 on *Begonia* using a bubble column bioreactor. This led to the development in bioreactor technology and aerobic bioreactor culture techniques for large-scale production of plant propagules [63].

Large-scale cultivation in bioreactors is promoted for following reasons [64,65]:

- This technique is advantageous for plants that are difficult to cultivate and has an extended cultivation period.
- The scale-up technique potentially produces therapeutic compounds that cannot be chemically synthesized at a larger scale.
- Bioreactors are suitable in those natural conditions where the cultivation process is either affected or limited due to change in environmental, ecological, or climatic conditions and/or insufficient agricultural lands.
- Secondary metabolites produced by this technique are independent of geographic and climatic conditions.

There are various advantages of bioreactors as a biological factory for the production of high-quality compounds [64,65]:

- Whole surface of culture always in contact with the medium, stimulated uptake of nutrients, and increased growth rate
- The opportunity to perform biosynthetic and/or biotransformation experiments related to metabolite production with enzyme availability
- Simpler and faster harvest of cells
- Reproducible yields of end product under controlled growth conditions
- Optimum aeration/agitation condition with respect to capacity of oxygen supply and intensity of hydrodynamic stress effects on the plant cells
- Maintenance of aseptic conditions for relatively longer cultivation period
- Large number of planlets produced in one batch in the bioreactor and scaling up of bioreactor
- Intensity of culture broth mixing and air-bubble dispersion
- Increased working volumes

- Homogeneous culture due to mechanical or pneumatic stirring mechanism
- Ease of handling of cultures such as inoculation or harvest, reducing the number of culture vessels, and the area of culture space resulting in the reduction of cost
- Forced aeration (oxygen supply) is performed, which improves the growth rate and final biomass
- Enhanced nutrient uptake stimulating multiplication rates and yielding a higher concentration of yield of bioactive compounds
- Easier separation of target compounds because of lower complexity of extract
- Controlled supply independent of plant availability
- Control of aggregate size (which may be important to enhance secondary metabolite production)
- Better control of cultural and physical environment, therefore easy optimization of growth parameters such as pH, nutrient media, temperature, etc. for achieving metabolite production
- Better control and ease of scale-up

7.3.7.1 Types of Bioreactors

Production of secondary metabolites and recombinant proteins in bioreactors minimized the variations in product yield and quality and as a result the product screening process is simplified. An optimum environment under controlled conditions can be achieved by using different bioreactor designs. This may enhance the cell growth and secondary metabolite production effectively. The bioreactors used for various plant cell cultures are classified as mechanically agitated, pneumatically driven, disposable, and nonagitated (Fig. 7.14). The stirred tank bioreactor is the most common bioreactor used in plant tissue culture. By employing a variety of impeller designs and seals numerous modifications have been made in the stirred tank bioreactor. These modifications are made to reduce the shear forces (Fig. 7.15, A1). There are various capacities of stirred tank bioreactors (1–2 L lab scale to 20,000 L industrial scale) reported in the literature. In spite of their various advantages, these bioreactors suffer from limitations, such as high power consumption, high shear, and problems with sealing and stability of shafts in tall bioreactors. Another type of mechanically agitated bioreactor is horizontal vessel or rotary drum reactors (Fig. 7.15, A2). These bioreactors have a considerably higher surface area to volume ratio than other reactor types. Therefore, mass transfer is achieved with comparably less power consumption. They are especially used for the cultivation of high-density plant suspensions and have advantages in terms of suspension homogeneity, low shear environment, and reduced wall growth, over either airlift or stirred tank reactors [65]. Rotary drum reactors have a disadvantage in their relatively high-energy consumption at large-scale operation.

A bubble column bioreactor (Fig. 7.15, B1) is a pneumatically driven type bioreactor, in the shape of a column. Reaction medium in this bioreactor is kept mixed and aerated by the introduction of air at the bottom [68]. Bubble column bioreactors have low capital costs, uncomplicated mechanical configurations, and not too high operational costs due to low energy requirements. In contrast they are not preferred for processes where highly viscous liquids exist. Another type of pneumatically driven reactor is the airlift bioreactor (Fig. 7.15, B1–5). It is defined as a reactor in which the reaction medium is continuously agitated and aerated by the introduction of air or another gas mixture and the circulation is enhanced by internal draught

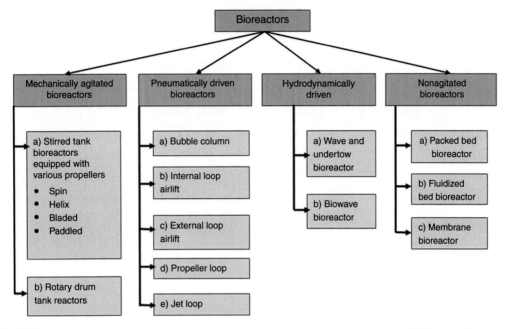

FIGURE 7.14 Depictions of bioreactor types for plant cell and tissue cultures [64–67]. Mechanically agitated bioreactors: (a) stirred tank reactor equipped with various propellers (spin, helix, bladed, and paddle), (b) rotary drum tank reactor. Pneumatically driven bioreactors: (a) bubble column, (b) internal loop airlift, (c) external loop airlift, (d) propeller loop, (e) jet loop. Hydrodynamically driven disposable bioreactors: (a) Wave and undertow bioreactor, (b) biowave reactor. Nonagitated bioreactors: (a) packed bed, (b) fluidized bed, (c) membrane reactor.

tubes or external loops. Thus, the reactor volume is separated into gassed and ungassed regions generating a vertically circulating flow [68]. Airlift bioreactors have the advantage of supplying low O_2 demands of plant cell cultures with low shear effects. In addition they have several benefits such as combining high loading of solid particles, providing good mass transfer, relatively low shear rate, low energy requirements, and simple design. The main limitation of this reactor is that it is not suitable for high-density plant cultures. In such cases stirred tank bioreactors are preferable for culturing plant cell suspensions at high densities [69].

Hydrodynamically driven bioreactors, also called disposable bioreactors, such as the wave and undertow bioreactors (Fig. 7.15, C1) and the biowave (Fig. 7.15, C2), are modern alternatives to traditional cultivation systems. These bioreactors contain a sterile plastic chamber, which is partially filled with media (10–50%). This plastic chamber is inoculated with cells and discarded after harvest. Utilization of these two novel, flexible, plastic-based disposable bioreactors has been explored recently. The wave and undertow reactor is based on the mechanism that provides continuous agitation while offering convenient mixing and aeration to the plant cell culture. The other bioreactor, also called a high aspect ratio bubble column bioreactor, is based on the mechanism of agitation and aeration. This can be achieved by intermittent generation of large diameter bubbles, "Taylor-like" or "slug bubbles." In these reactors, there is a possibility of raising the volume from a few liters up to several hundred liters with the use of multiple units. Disposable bioreactors have advantages over other bioreactors in

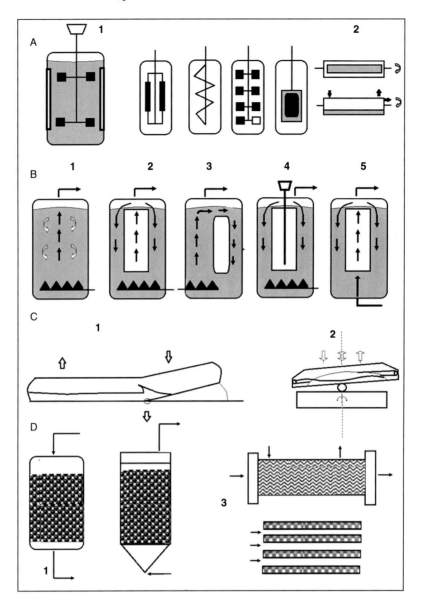

FIGURE 7.15   **Strategies for crop improvement.**

reducing or eliminating sterilization and maintenance operations [70]. In addition, packed bed (Fig 7.15, D1) and membrane reactors (Fig. 7.15, D3) are also advantageous in terms of immobilizing large amounts of cells per unit volume. In contrast diffusional limitations of mass transfer and difficulties in handling gaseous components can limit the use of both configurations [65]. Various reports of plant cell and tissue cultures with different types of reactors are listed in Table 7.25. Thus, it is clear from various reports that plant cell and tissue cultures

TABLE 7.25   Laboratory-Scale Plant Cell and Tissue Culture Studies Useful for Large-Scale Cultivation in Different Types of Bioreactors [64–67]

Bioreactor	Plant source	Volume	Type of culture	Product
Stirred tank	H. perforatum	2	Organ culture	Hypericin
	T. chinensis	2.5	Cell suspension	Taxoid
	D. carota	3	Cell suspension	Growth and differentiation
	A. indica	3	Cell suspension	Azadirachtin
	T. rugosum	5	High-density cell	Berberine
	P. ginseng	5	suspension	Biomass
	Picea mariana	7.5	Somatic embryogenesis	Cytoplasmic esterase
	M. sativa	14	Somatic embryogenesis	
Mist	Stizolobium hassjo	9	Hairy root	3,4-Dihydroxy phenylalanine
Immersion	C. arabica	1	Somatic embryogenesis	Germinated embryos
	C. arabica	1	Somatic embryogenesis	Germinated embryos
	Ananas comosus	10	Micropropagation	Shoot
	Potato atlantica	10	Micropropagation	Plantlets
Hanging stirrer bar	C. annuum	2	Somatic embryogenesis	Germinated embryos
Glass culture vessel	R. graveolens	5	Micropropagation	Shoots
Bubble column	Scopolia parviflora	0.6	Adventitious root	Scopolamine, hyoscyamine
	Lithospermum sp.	1.5	Hairy root	Shikonin
	Stevia rebaudiana	1.75	Shoot	Biomass
	Lavandula officinalis	5	Organ culture	Rosamarinic acid
Balloon type bubble	P. ginseng	5	Adventitious root	Ginsenoside
Airlift	F. alnus	0.25	Cell suspension	Anthraquinones

have been cultivated in reactors of various designs and configurations in scales ranging between 0.25 and 14 L.

7.3.8 Metabolic Engineering and Production of Secondary Metabolites

Plants synthesize their secondary metabolites by single or multiple biosynthetic pathways. Functioning of these pathways is dependent on the state of enzymes (activation or inactivation) and respective activator genes or transcription factors. These enzymes convert single precursor compounds or multiples to form several intermediates. Biotransformation of these intermediates is dependent on the key enzymes involved and their respective activator genes during the whole process. The targeted and purposeful alteration of metabolic pathways found in plant cells to achieve a better understanding and use of cellular pathways for chemical transformation, energy transduction, and supramolecular assembly is called plant cell metabolic engineering [71]. Plant cell metabolic engineering allows the manipulation of endogenous biochemical pathways, which results in development of transgenic crops. During this process the biosynthetic pathways of existing plants are manipulated in such a way as to provide beneficial commercial, agronomic, and/or postharvest processing characteristics. Metabolic engineering forms the foundation of an emerging branch called metabolomics, where secondary metabolites and their respective metabolic pathways are studied comprehensively.

In addition, metabolic engineering is an independent branch that investigates plant metabolic pathways and is a tool for triggering the production of commercial plant secondary metabolites. Metabolic engineering can provide various strategies to improve productivity where production of phytochemicals is too low for commercialization, e.g., shikonin, berberine, ginsenosides, and paclitaxel [29]. Metabolic engineering provides various strategies to improve productivity, such as: increasing the number of producing cells, increasing the carbon flux through a biosynthetic pathway by overexpression of genes codifying for rate-limiting enzymes or blocking the mechanism of feedback inhibition and competitive pathways; and decreasing catabolism. Genetic expression-mediated enzymatic activation always resulted in bioconversion of various compounds or intermediates to form secondary metabolites with improved quantity. Wide ranges of secondary metabolites of high therapeutic activity are being studied nowadays. Among various alkaloidal compounds tropane alkaloids are the well-known ones that are generated through this process. This class includes (–)-hyoscyamine, its racemate atropine, and scopolamine (hyoscine), which have an 8-azabicyclo[3.2.1]octane esterified nucleus.

Related to the tropane alkaloids, a new group of nortropane alkaloids, the calystegines, was discovered only 15 years ago. These tropane alkaloids are formed by various metabolic conversions of calystegines (water soluble compounds having three to five hydroxyl groups in various positions), yielding tropane alkaloids such as scopolamine, nicotine, and berberine. This process is dependent on the various enzymes and genes involved in the biosynthetic pathways. Expression of two branching point enzymes putrescine N-methyltransferase and (S)-scoulerine 9-O-methyltransferase was engineered. Putrescine N-methyltransferase was reported for its action in transgenic plants of *A. belladonna* and *Nicotiana sylvestris* whereas (S)-scoulerine 9-O-methyltransferase was reported in cultured cells of *C. japonica* and *E. californica*. Overexpression of putrescine N-methyltransferase increased the nicotine content in *N. sylvestris*, whereas suppression of endogenous putrescine n-methyltransferase activity decreased the nicotine content and induced abnormal morphologies. Similarly, ectopic expression of (S)-scoulerine 9-O-methyltransferase caused the accumulation of benzylisoquinoline alkaloids in *E. californica* [72].

7.3.9 Role of Endophytes in *In Vitro* Production of Secondary Metabolites

There is a great deal of speculation regarding endophytic fungi-mediated secondary metabolite production from plant cells [73]:

- It is thought that coinvolvement of both plant and endophytic microbe pathways produce these natural products.
- There is a suggestion that either plants or endophytic fungi produce these secondary metabolites and transfer them to the other symbiont.
- Based on biosynthetic pathway studies using radiolabeled precursor amino acids it is now revealed that plants and endophytic fungi have similar, but distinct, metabolic pathways for production of secondary metabolites.

Recently mutualistic association of both plants (*Taxus media*, yew species) and fungi (*Cladosporium cladosporioides*) in the independent production of Taxol was evidenced. In this report a gene 10-deacetylbaccatin-III-10-O-acetyltransferase was isolated from the endophytic fungus *C. cladosporioides*. This gene is involved in the biosynthetic pathway of Taxol and shares 99% identity with *T. media* (plant) and 97% identity with *T. wallichiana* var. *marirei* (plant). This report supported that plants and endophytic fungi produce secondary metabolites through mutualistic symbiosis. This mutualistic symbiosis-mediated secondary metabolite production was contraindicated after evidence that plants other than yew species also have endophytic fungi associated with them that make Taxol. So it has been concluded that plants and fungi are independently capable of producing these therapeutic secondary metabolites.

A combination of factors that promotes the plant/fungal association also promotes the accumulation of secondary metabolites in plants and fungi, respectively. Such an association can also produce various secondary metabolites that are essential for research [74].

7.3.10 Molecular Pharming in Crop Improvement

Molecular pharming furnishes a better way to produce biopharmaceuticals. It is a process that studies the strategies for the improvement of plants especially by transgenic means. Humans have consistently been trying to modify the various characteristics of plants for food and fiber for thousands of years. Various human efforts toward cultivation and harvesting have made certain pressure on some plant species in terms of their extinction from its natural resources. Over the last few years, molecular farming has emerged as an important field to enhance crop quality. Knowledge of these molecular processes gives an excellent idea about the production of recombinant proteins from the suitable host cell. These processes should be taken into consideration before conducting transgenesis. Trangenesis brings a major revolution in crop improvement. Genetically engineered plant and foods are synthesized in the laboratories to yield high-quality products. The monotypical nature of transgenic plants and their associated dangers to biodiversity has created various problems in the further development of these plants. Thus, an understanding of the complex molecular pathways helps to circumvent these problems. The usual strategy adopted in molecular pharming is illustrated in Fig. 7.16. Major breakthroughs in molecular pharming are highlighted in Fig. 7.17.

7.3.10.1 Strategies for Crop Improvement
- Plant host cell: By selecting suitable machinery for gene expression
- *Agrobacterium* – a natural DNA delivery system: *Agrobacterium* infects many plant species and delivers DNA that encodes for plant hormones.

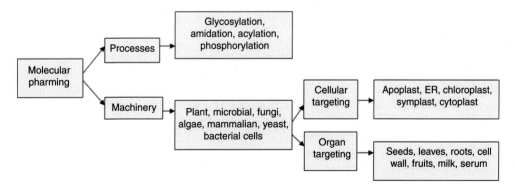

FIGURE 7.16   **Major breakthroughs in crop improvement.**

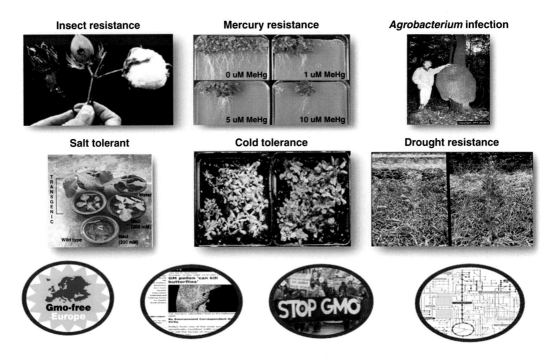

FIGURE 7.17　Major achievements and loopholes of plant tissue culture during crop improvement program.

- Vaccine production: But nature does not contain all the genetic variation that man desires. Human efforts toward development of medicines or vaccines in form of food or any plant part is now turns to reality with the achievement in production of edible vaccines in form of fruits.
- Golden rice (vitamin A): "Daffodil gene," which led to the high vitamin A content in the rice plant.
- Herbicide/drought/disease/pathogen resistant: "Roundup resistant plants."

7.4 PRODUCTION OF ANTITUMOR COMPOUNDS BY PLANT CELL CULTURE

For clinical medicines secondary metabolites in the form of therapeutic compounds having antitumor activity can be directly isolated from higher plants. Availability at lower concentrations and difficulty during its detection in plants limit its clinical availability as a potent medicine. In addition, slow growth rate of plants and geographical or environmental conditions-dependent accumulation of antitumor compounds hinder its clinical development in the world of medicine. Thus, large amounts and a stable supply of these compounds are required for further chemical or clinical studies. Plant tissue culture provides a clear solution to all of these problems. However, this method is still empirical and requires much trial and error to establish the stable cell lines. Moreover, optimal growth medium conditions of the chemicals are required to establish the stable cell lines to yield the maximum amount of antitumor compounds [75]. Various antitumor compounds are highlighted in Table 7.26.

TABLE 7.26   Antitumor Plants and Their Respective Components Explored in Plant Tissue Culture [75]

Product	Plant name	Plant dry weight (dry wt %)	Cultured cells (dry wt %)
Withanolide-A, Withaferin	*Withania somnifera*	–	–
Vinblastine, vincristine	*C. roseus*	5.0×10^{-3}	5.0×10^{-4}
Tripdiolide	*Tripterygium wilfordii*	1.0×10^{-3}	1.0×10^{-2}
Thalicarpine	*Thalictrum dasycarpum*	–	–
Taxol	*Taxus brevifolia*	5.0×10^{-1}	–
Podophyllotoxin	*P. hexandrum*	6.4×10^{-1}	7.1×10^{-1}
Maytansine	*Putterlickia verrucosa*	2.0×10^{-5}	5.0×10^{-7}
Indicine N-oxide	*Heliotropium indicum*	–	–
Homoharringtonine	*Cephalotaxus harringtonia*	1.8×10^{-5}	5.5×10^{-8}
Fagaronine	*Fagara zanthoxyloides*	–	–
Ellipticine	*Aspidosperma williansii, Ochrosia moorei*	3.2×10^{-5}	2.7×10^{-4}
Colchicine	*Colchicum autumnale*	–	–
Cesalin	*Caesalpinia gilliesii*	–	–
Camptothecin	*C. acuminata*	5×10^{-3}	2.5×10^{-4}
Bruceantin	*Brucea antidysenterica*	1.0×10^{-2}	5.8×10^{-5}
Baccharin	*Baccharis dracunculifolia*	2.0×10^{-2}	–

7.5 PRODUCTION OF FLAVORING COMPOUNDS THROUGH TISSUE CULTURE

Flavoring and aromatic compounds are an important part of the food, feed, cosmetic, and pharmaceutical industries. Globally they represent a value of almost US$7 billion per year. This figure is constantly increasing each year and forms 25% of the total food additives market [76,77]. Presently essential oils are one of the most important classes of natural compounds that are exploited commercially as perfumes, aroma products, flavoring agents in food and beverages, as cosmetic products, and as drugs. Flavors are the blend of volatile and nonvolatile components possessing diverse chemical and physicochemical properties. The nonvolatile compounds mainly contribute to taste whereas the volatile ones influence both taste and aroma. A variety of components are responsible for the aroma of food products, such as alcohols, aldehydes, esters, dicarbonyls, short- to medium-chain free fatty acids, methyl ketones, lactones, phenolic compounds, and sulfur compounds [78,79]. From earlier times various flavoring compounds (simple to complex) have been extracted from plant sources. Structural elucidation of these compounds offers foundation for the chemical synthesis of synthetic flavors. Flavoring compounds currently represent a quarter of the world market for food additives. Among these compounds most of the flavoring compounds are produced via chemical synthesis or by extraction from natural materials.

According to recent market investigations consumers prefer foodstuffs that are labeled as "natural." Synthetic flavors or flavors that are prepared by chemical transformation of natural substances cannot be legally labeled as natural. The main disadvantage of synthetic flavor is that chemical synthesis of the product may cause the formation of undesirable racemic mixtures, thus reducing process efficiency and increasing downstream costs. On the other hand, extraction of these compounds from natural resources, especially plants, causes various problems such as low yield, expensive extraction procedures, harvesting or availability of respective plants or their organs, lower production of these compounds under the influence of weather conditions, and disease state of the plants. Drawbacks of both methods directed many researchers toward the search for other strategies to produce natural flavors. These strategies involve microbial biosynthesis or bioconversion or plant cell culture-mediated production of flavoring compounds [80–83]. Microbial cultures or enzymatic preparations are known to be the most popular approach for production of these compounds. Microorganisms can synthesize flavors as secondary metabolites during fermentation on nutrients such as sugars and amino acids. Production of flavoring compounds by microbial means can be achieved by:

- Supplementation of precursors or intermediate compounds to the culture medium in order to promote the biosynthesis of specific flavors
- Microbial metabolism in food fermentation processes to develop suitable production systems for particular flavor additives
- The option of using various enzymes (i.e., lipases, proteases, glucosidases) for natural flavor biosynthesis by catalyzing them from precursor molecules. This enzyme technology is advantageous in providing higher stereoselectivity than chemical routes.

By using various nonclassical techniques plant cell cultures are also exploited nowadays for the higher production of flavoring compounds. Production of these flavoring compounds by means of plant cell cultures is often costly and most cultures are unable to produce an adequate yield of essential oils. A wide array of essential oils are isolated from cell cultures, e.g., paniculides instead of andrographolides. These essential oils are different from those occurring in the plant. In some cases these compounds are not even considered under the essential oils category. Most of the focus will be directed on monoterpenes (and to some extent also on sesqui-, di-, and triterpenes), phthalides, pyrethrins, valepotriates, cannabinoids, furanoterpenes, aromas, and derivatives of these compounds. These compounds are diversely present in dicotyledonae, monocotyledonae, coniferae, and bryophyta. *De novo* biosynthesis of complex molecules from simple molecules without being recycled after partial degradation was found to be unsuccessful in many cases. For improving this process various techniques such as biotransformation, precursor feeding, and metabolic engineering are extensively studied. Various examples of phytoflavors are highlighted in Fig. 7.18. Plant tissue culture is a potential method to produce a variety of flavoring and aromatic compounds (Tables 7.27 and 7.28). Synthesis and accumulation of these compounds is based on the unique biochemical and genetic capacity, and the totipotency of plant cells [84–86]. Each plant cell contains genes encoded with genetic information essential to produce numerous chemical components that constitute natural flavoring compounds. Feeding the precursor compounds and their intermediates assists in enhancing the production of flavor metabolites by precursor biotransformation. Advantages of plant cell culture technology over conventional agricultural production techniques [87,88] are:

- Costs can be decreased and productivity increased by automatization of cell growth control and regulation of metabolic processes.

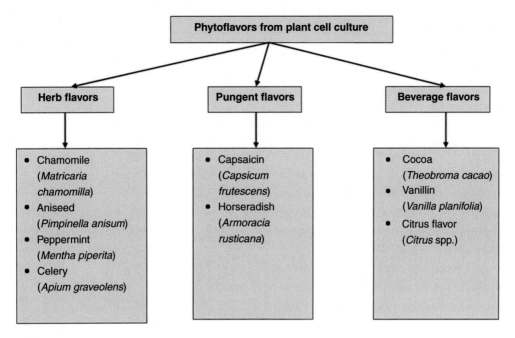

FIGURE 7.18 Various phytoflavours compounds through tissue culture technique.

TABLE 7.27 Examples of Various Flavoring Compounds Synthesized by Plant Tissue Culture Science [89]

Flavors from plant cell culture	
Vanillin	*V. planifolia*
Triterpenoid	*Glycyrrhiza glabra* *G. glandulifera*
Onion	*A. cepa*
Monoterpenes	*P. frutescens*
Garlic	*Allium sativum*
Flavanol	*Polygonum hydropiper*
Coriander	*Coriandrum sativum*
Cocoa flavor	*Theobroma cacao*
Citrus flavor	*Citrus* spp.
Cinnamic acid	*N. tabacum*
Caryophyllen	*Lindera strychnifolia*
Basmati flavor	*O. sativa*
Apple aroma	*Malus silvestris*
2,3 Butanedione	*Agastache rugosa*

TABLE 7.28   Various Types of Plant Cultures and Their Accumulated Flavoring Compounds [89]

Type of flavor and occurrence	Culture involved	Plant
Valepotriates – Dicotyledons	Cell suspensions	*V. wallichii*
Triterpenes – Dicotyledons	Suspension cultures	Rose
Sesquiterpenes – Dicotyledons	Callus cultures	*M. chamomilla*
Sesquiterpenes – Bryophyta	Suspension cultures	*Calypogeia granulatus*
Pyrethrins – Dicotyledons	Callus	*Chrysanthemum coccineum*
Phthalides – Dicotyledons	Callus and suspension cultures	*Apium graveolens*
Monoterpenes – Coniferae	Cell suspension cultures	*Thuja occidentalis*
Monoterpenes – Dicotyledons	Callus cultures	*Tanacetum vulgare* L.
Furano-terpenes – Dicotyledons	Callus cultures	*Ipomoea batatas*
Flavonoids – Dicotyledons	–	Citrus species and *Poncirus trifoliata*
Fatty acids – Monocotyledons	Callus cultures	*Iris sibirica*
Diterpenes – Dicotyledons	Callus and suspension cultures	*Andrographis paniculata*
Cannabinoids – Dicotyledons	Callus cultures	*C. sativa*
C_9-C_{11} compounds – Dicotyledons	Callus cultures	*R. graveolens*
Aromas – Monocotyledons	Callus cultures	*A. cepa*
Aromas – Dicotyledons	Cell suspension cultures	*T. cacao*

- Efficient downstream recovery and rapid production can be achieved.
- High productivity species can be selected.
- It also offers a defined production system, which ensures a continuous product supply, as well as uniform quality and yield.
- It is independent of geographical and seasonal variations, political interference, and other environmental factors.
- It is possible to produce novel compounds that are not normally found in parent plants, either directly or through stereo and regiospecific biotransformations of cheap precursors.

However, several factors should be taken into consideration while producing secondary metabolites from plant cell cultures, such as: sensitivity to shear stress, relatively long growth cycles, low yields, progressive loss of biosynthetic activity, development of large-scale suspension cultures, and rare product secretion. Moreover, utilization of certain strategies like optimization of culture conditions, selection of high producing strains, precursor feeding, elicitation, cell immobilization, hairy root transformation, and metabolic engineering helps in stimulating biosynthetic pathways. Accumulation of flavoring compounds can also be improved by regulation of plant secondary metabolism at the biochemical and genetic levels [88].

An initial effort in flavor production by plant cell culture was investigated by the synthesis of vanillin as a flavoring compound [90]. After the establishment of plant cell cultures of

V. planifolia various strategies such as elicitation and precursor feeding have been adopted [91] to induce vanillic acid synthesis [92]. Feeding of precursor such as ferulic acid resulted in an increase in synthesis of vanillin. Moreover, the use of charcoal in the production of vanillin from ferulic acid in vanilla aerial roots was also investigated. Bioconversion of vanillin from ferulic acid was also investigated in root cultures of *C. frutescens* [93]. Several research works related with production of monoterpenes (i.e., limonene, linalool, etc.) in callus tissues and cell suspensions of *P. frutescens* [94], and basmati rice volatile flavor components in callus cultures of *O. sativa* were studied. In certain cases it was observed that flavors obtained in plant cell cultures are different from those that are present in the parent plants, e.g., isolation of flavor-related alcohols (2-phenylethanol, a marked cucumber/wine-like aroma) in suspension cultures of *Agastache rugosa* Kuntze [95]. This type of modification can be achieved by the addition of precursors, as demonstrated in root cultures of *A. cepa* L. (onion) [96].

Approaches to improve the yield of essential oils produced by plant cell and tissue cultures are:

- Varying the physical conditions, such as light, temperature, and gaseous environment, under which the cultures are grown
- Induction of polyploidy cells
- Induction of morphological differentiation in tissue cultures
- Creating of artificial accumulation sites for these volatiles
- Altering the composition of the culture medium

7.6 ANTIMICROBIAL AGENTS FROM PLANT CELL CULTURE

Microorganisms infect plant tissue by activating its defense mechanisms. Activation of defense mechanisms results in production of secondary metabolites. But this process is not true for all microorganisms as some endophytic fungus symbiotically interact with plants to assist their secondary metabolite production. It was later found that these fungi are also capable of producing secondary metabolites independently. So interaction of plants with different microorganisms, including viruses, bacteria, and fungi, established the symbiotic relationships. This relationship stimulates the defense mechanism of plants, which may result in the strong adaptation of plant for its long survival in such microorganisms' prevailing environmental conditions. In addition to defense mechanism activation certain associations have benefited plants to improve their functions against harsh environmental conditions. A good example of such association is symbiotic association of certain bacteria such as rhizobia with leguminous plants, which results in the fixation of atmospheric nitrogen in root nodules. Other bacteria found close to the plant root (rhizobacteria) are able to control plant diseases caused by soil pathogens [97]. So now it is well understood that all microorganisms are not pathogenic for plants as some are essential to build the innate immunity of plants and others improve their functions for increasing their resistance against harsh conditions. Certain fungal strains (e.g., mycorrhizae) interactions can also be beneficial for the plant, stimulating its growth and development [98]. However, many plant-associated microbes are pathogens that affect plant development, reproduction, and ultimately yield. Control over these pathogens is a major challenge in agriculture industries. Plants prevent or resist infection and its spread among other plants by building an innate immunity that involves different layers of defense responses.

Some of these defenses are preformed and others are activated after recognition of pathogen elicitors [99], and include reinforcement of the cell wall, biosynthesis of lytic enzymes, production of secondary metabolites, and pathogenesis-related proteins [100].

7.6.1 Phytoanticipins versus Phytoalexins

A group of antimicrobial compounds produced to resist microbial attack and consequently control the defense mechanism of plants are called as phytoalexins. These compounds require *de novo* expression of the enzymes involved in their biosynthetic pathways after elicitation [98]. The exact molecular mechanism of phytoalexins production is not yet established; however, it has been reported that the production of phytoalexins requires transcriptional and/or translational activity in the plant once the pathogen has been detected. A pathogenic or microbial infection-induced response mechanism also involves the trafficking and secretion of antimicrobial compounds to the infection site [101]. Accumulation of these compounds at the specific site of infection indicates the role of these compounds in providing disease resistance against certain pathogens. However, this is not true for all as the function for plant defense is not always controlled by phytoalexins [102]. Another class of low molecular weight antimicrobial compounds that are present in plants before being challenged by microorganisms, or are produced after infection solely from preexisting constituents, is called phytoanticipin [103]. These are present at the plant surface. In addition, there are other compounds that are sequestered as preformed compounds in vacuoles or organelles and released through a hydrolyzing enzyme after pathogen challenge. Since the enzyme involved in the final release of the molecule is not formed *de novo*, these compounds are not called phytoalexins [104]. There is slight confusion related to definitions of phytoalexin and phytoanticipin as previous definitions are based on the dynamic of the synthesis of the antimicrobial molecule, since the same chemical can be a phytoalexin in one plant and a phytoanticipin in another. Moreover, the same molecule can be a phytoalexin or a phytoanticipin in different organs of the same plant [98]. Various examples of antimicrobial compounds synthesized from plant tissue culture are highlighted in Tables 7.29–7.31.

TABLE 7.29   Evidence of Production of Various Phytoalexins in Various Families of Plants [105]

Brassicaceae	Fabaceae	Vitaceae	Poaceae	Vitaceae
Camalexin	Medicarp	Resveratrol	Kauralexin A1	Resveratrol
Spirobrassinin	Wighteone	ε-Viniferin	Kauralexin B1	ε-Viniferin
Rutalexin	(+)-Pisatin		Zealexin A1	
Brassilexin	Arachidin 1		Zealexin B1	
	Arachidin 2		Avenanthramide A	
	Arachidin 3		Momilactone A	
	Resveratrol		Phytocassane A	
	Glyceollin I		Sakuranetin	
	Glyceollin II		Luteolin	

TABLE 7.30 Evidence of Production of Various Phytoalexins in Various Families of Plants

Plants	Phytoalexins	Pathogen infection
Brassicaceae: oilseed rape, canola, and mustard (*Brassica rapa* and *B. juncea*)		
B. rapa, *B. juncea*	Brassinin, spirobrassinin, cyclobrassinin, rutalexin, rapalexin A, and brassilexin	*Albugo candida* and *Alternaria brassicola*
Fabaceae (Leguminosae): alfalfa (*M. sativa*), barrel medic (*M. truncatula*), chickpea (*Cicer arietinum*), lupine (*Lupinus angustifolius*), pea (*Pisum sativum*), peanut (*Arachis hypogaea*), and soybean (*G. max*)		
M. sativa	Medicarpin and sativan	*Colletotrichum trifolii*
M. truncatula	Medicarpin and its isoflavone precursors	*Phoma medicaginis*
C. arietinum	Maackiain and medicarpin	
L. angustifolius	Luteone and wighteone	*C. lupini*
P. sativum	Pisatin	*Nectria haematococca*
A. hypogaea	Resveratrol, arachidin-1, arachidin-2, arachidin-3, isopentadienyl-4,30,50-trihydroxystilbene, SB-1, arahypin-1, arahypin-2, arahypin-3, arahypin-4, arahypin-5, arahypin-6, arahypin-7, aracarpene-1 and aracarpene-2	*Aspergillus* species: *A. caelatus, A. flavus, A. parasiticus,* and *A. niger*
G. max	Glyceollin	*Macrophomina phaseolina, Sclerotinia sclerotiorum,* and *Phytophthora sojae*
Solanaceae: pepper fruit (*Capsicum annuum*), tobacco (*N. tabacum*), and wild tobacco (*N. plumbaginifolia*)		
C. annuum	Capsidiol	
N. tabacum	Scopoletin and capsidiol	*Botrytis cinerea, Phytophthora nicotianae,* and *P. palmivora*
N. plumbaginifolia	Capsidiol	*Botrytis cinerea*
Vitaceae: grapevine (*V. vinifera*), *V. riparia*, *V. berlandieri*, and wild-growing grape (*Vitis amurensis*)		
V. vinifera	Resveratrol, viniferins, piceids, and pterostilbene	*Plasmopara viticola, Erysiphe necator,* and *Botrytis cinerea*
V. amurensis	Resveratrol	*A. rhizogenes*
Poaceae: maize (*Zea mays*), oat (*A. sativa*), rice (*O. sativa*) and sorghum (*Sorghum bicolor*)		
Z. mays	Kauralexins and zealexins	*Rhizopus microsporus, Colletotrichum graminicola, Fusarium graminearum, Cochliobolus heterostrophus,* and *Aspergillus flavus*
A. sativa	Avenanthramides	*Puccinia coronata*
O. sativa	Momilactone A, momilactone B, phytocassane A–phytocassane E, sakuranetin, and oryzalexin E	*Pyricularia oryzae, Magnaporthe grisea,* and *M. oryzae*
S. bicolor	Luteolin, apigenin, and 3-deoxyanthocyanidins	*Colletotrichum sublineolum* and *C. heterostrophus*

TABLE 7.31　Antimicrobial Plants Explored in Plant Tissue Culture

Components	Action	Plant
Tea tree oil	Antibacterial and antifungal agent	*Melaleuca alternifolia*
Shikonin	Antibacterial	*L. erythrorhizon*
Azadirachtin		
		Alfalfa (*M. sativa*)
	Antibacterial and antifungal agent	Ashwagandha (*Withania somniferum*)
Essential oils	*Salmonella*, bacteria	Basil (*Ocimum basilicum*)
Essential oils	Bacteria, fungi	
Essential oils	Antimicrobial	*Valeriana officinalis*
Essential oils	Antimicrobial	*Anthemis nobilis* L.
Essential oils	Antimicrobial	*Pelargonium fragrans*
Essential oils	Antimicrobial	Turmeric
Essential oils	Antimicrobial	*Vetiveria zizanioides*
Essential oils	Antimicrobial	*Thymus caespititius*
Essential oils	Antimicrobial	*Lavandula dentata*
Essential oils	Antimicrobial	*Telekia speciosa*
Essential oils	Antimicrobial	*Achillea millefolium*
Essential oils	Antimicrobial	*Aloysia citrodora*
Flavanoids	Antimicrobial	*Haloxylon salicornicum*
Flavanoids	Antimicrobial	*H. recurvum*
Flavanoids	Antimicrobial	*Salsola baryosma*
	Antimicrobial	*Ziziphus nummularia*
	Antibacterial	Castor (*R. communis*)
	Antimicrobial	*Alternanthera maritima*
	Bacteria, fungi	*Centella asiatica*
	Antimicrobial	Iranian *Arnebia euchroma*
	Antimicrobial	*Premna serratifolia*
Flavanoids	Antimicrobial	*Balanites aegyptiaca*
22β-Hydroxytingenone and tingenone	Antimicrobial	*Catha edulis*
	Antimicrobial	*M. sativa*
	Antimicrobial	*Ephedra strobilacea, E. procera, E. pachyclada*
Triterpene	Antimicrobial	*Tectona grandis*
	Antimicrobial	*Citrus hystrix*

TABLE 7.31 Antimicrobial Plants Explored in Plant Tissue Culture *(cont.)*

Components	Action	Plant
Trichosetin	Antimicrobial	Dual culture of *Trichoderma harzianum* and *C. roseus*
	Antimicrobial	*Alternanthera tenella*
	Antimicrobial	Petunia leaf
	Antimicrobial	*Mucuna pruriens* leaf
	Antimicrobial	*Thespesia populnea*
	Antimicrobial	*H. antidysenterica*
Flavanoids	Antimicrobial	*Gossypium* species

References

[1] Kaul B, Staba EJ. *Ammi visnaga* L. Lam. tissue cultures: multiliter suspension growth and examination for furanochromones. Planta Medica J Med Plant Res (Georg Thieme Verlag (Stuttgart)) 1967;15:145–56.

[2] Heble MR, Narayanaswamy S, Chadha MS. Diosgenin and sitosterol isolation from *Solanum xanthocarpum* tissue cultures. Science 1968;161:1145.

[3] Zenk MH, El-Shagi H, Arens H, Stockigt J, Weiler EW, Dens B. Formation of indole alkaloids serpentine and ajmalicine in cell suspension cultures of Catharabthus rosues. In: Barz W, Reinhard E, Zenk MH, editors. Plant tissue culture and its biotechnological applications. Berlin, Heidelberg, New York: Springer-Verlag; 1977. p. 27–43.

[4] Hannig E. Zur Physiologie pflanzlicher Embryonen. I. Über die Kultur von Cruciferen-embryonen ausserhalb des Embryosacks. Bot Ztg 1904;62:45–80.

[5] Simon S. Experimentelle Untersuchungen über die Entstehung von Gefäßverbindungen. Ber Dtsch Bot Ges 1908;26:364–96.

[6] Skoog F, Miller CO. Chemical regulation of growth and organ formation in plant tissue cultures *in vitro*. Symp Soc Exp Biol 1957;11:118–31.

[7] Gao SL, Zhu DN, Cai ZH, Jiang Y, Xu D. Organ culture of a precious Chinese medicinal plant *Fritillaria unibracteata*. Plant Cell Tiss Org Cult 2004;59:197–201.

[8] Vinterhalter B, Janković T, Šavikin K, Nikolić R, Vinterhalter D. Propagation and xanthone content of *Gentianella austriaca* shoot cultures. Plant Cell Tiss Org Cult 2008;97:329–35.

[9] Do CB, Cormier F. Accumulation of anthocyanins enhanced by a high osmotic potential in grape (*Vitis vinifera* L.) cell suspensions. Plant Cell Rep 1990;9:143–6.

[10] Sasse F, Knobloch K, Berlin J. Induction of secondary metabolism in cell suspension cultures of Catharanthus roseus, Nicotiana tabacum and Peganum harmala. In: Fujiwara A, editor. Proceedings of the 5th International Congress of Plant Tissue and Cell Culture. Tokyo: Abe Photo Printing, 1982; p. 343–344.

[11] Ikeda T, Matsumoto T, Noguchi M. Effects of inorganic nitrogen source and physical factors on the formation of ubiquinone by tobacco plant cells in suspension culture. Agric Biol Chem 1977;41:1197–201.

[12] Courtois D, Guren J. Temperature response of Catharanthus roseus cells cultivated in liquid medium. Plant Sci Lett 1980;17:473–82.

[13] Seitz HU, Hinderer W. Anthocyanins. In: Constabel F, Vasil I, editors. Cell culture and somatic cell genetics of plants, 5. San Diego: Academic Press; 1988. p. 49–76.

[14] Kreis W, Reinhard E. The production of secondary metabolites by plant cells cultivated in bioreactors. Planta Med 1989;55:409–16.

[15] Ambid C, Fallot J. Role of the gaseous environment on volatile compound production by fruit cell suspension cultured *in vitro*. In: Schreier P, editor. Flavour '81. Berlin: de Gruyter; 1981. p. 529–38.

[16] Kobayashi Y, Fukui H, Tabata M. Effect of carbon dioxide and ethylene on berberine production and cell browning in Thalictrum minus cell cultures. Plant Cell Rep 1991;9:496–9.

[17] Toivonen L, Laakso S, Rosenqvist H. The effect of temperature on hairy root cultures of Catharanthus roseus: growth, indole alkaloid accumulation and membrane lipid composition. Plant Cell Rep 1992;11:395–9.

[18] Namdeo AG. Plant cell elicitation for production of secondary metabolites: a review. Pharmacog Rev 2007;1(1):69–79.

[19] DiCosmo F, Misawa M. Eliciting secondary metabolism in plant cell cultures. Trends Biotechnol 1985;3(12):322–91.

[20] Patel H, Krishnamurthy R. Elicitors in plant tissue culture. J Pharmacog Phytochem 2013;2(2):60–5.

[21] Vasconsuelo A, Boland R. Molecular aspects of the early stages of elicitation of secondary metabolites in plants. Plant Sci 2007;172:861–75.

[22] Angelova Z, Georgiev S, Roos W. Elicitation of plants. Biotechnol Biotechnol Eq 2006;20(2).

[23] Aijaz A, Jain S, Hariharan AG. Effect of elicitation on the production of phytoconstituents through plant tissue culture technique – a review. Int J Drug Discov Herb Res 2011;1(2):84–90.

[24] Namdeo AG, Jadhav TS, Rai PK, Gavali S, Mahadik KR. Precursor feeding for enhanced production of secondary metabolites. Pharmacog Rev 2007;1(2):227–31.

[25] Giri A, Dhingra V, Giri CC, Singh A, Ward OP, Narasu ML. Biotransformations using plant cells, organ cultures and enzyme systems: current trends and future prospects. Biotechnol Adv 2001;19(3):175–99.

[26] Pras N, Woerdenbag HJ. Production of secondary metabolites by bioconversion. In: Ramawat KG, Merillon JM, Editors. Biotechnology: secondary metabolites, Science Publisher, Inc.: USA; 1999.

[27] Johnson TS, Ravishankar GA, Venkataraman LV. Biotransformation of ferulic acid and vanyllylamine to capsicin and vanillin in immobilized cell cultures of Capsicum frutescens. Plant Cell Tiss Org Cult 1996;44:117–21.

[28] Rao SR, Ravishankar GA. Biotransformation of protocatechuic aldehyde and caffeic acid to vanillin and capsaicin in freely suspended and immobilized cell cultures of Capsicum frutescens. J Biotechnol 2000;76:137–46.

[29] Rao SR, Ravishankar GA. Plant cell cultures: chemical factories of secondary metabolites. Biotechnol Adv 2002;20:101–53.

[30] Williams PD, Mavituna F. Immobilized plant cells. In Plant biotechnology: comprehensive biotechnology, Second Supplement, Fowler M.W., Warren G.S., Moo-Young M. Pergamon Press, Oxford, 1992.

[31] Tyler RT, Kurz WGW, Paiva NL, Chavadej S. Bioreactors for surface immobilized cells. Plant Cell Tiss Org Cult 1995;42:81–90.

[32] Brodelius P, Deus B, Mosbach K, Zenk MH. Immobilized plant cells for the production and transformation of natural products. FEBS Lett 1979;103:93–7.

[33] Brodelius P, Nilsson K. Entrapment of plant cells in different matrices. FEBS Lett 1980;122:312–6.

[34] Lindsey K, Yeoman MM, Black GM, Mavituna F. A novel method for the immobilization and culture of plant cells. FEBS Lett 1983;155:143.

[35] Hu ZD, Yuan YJ. Fuzzy growth kinetics of immobilized C. roseus cells in polyurethane foams. Chem Eng Sci 1995;50:3297–301.

[36] Kobayashi Y, Fukui H, Tabata M. An immobilized cell culture system for berberine production by Thalictrum minus cells. Plant Cell Rep 1987;6:185–6.

[37] Wilkinson A, Williams P, Mavituna F. The effect of oxygen stress on secondary metabolites production by immobilized plant cells in bioreactors. In Plant cell biotechnology, Ed. Pais M., Mavituna F., Novais J. Springer, Berlin 1988.

[38] Kim DJ, Chang HN. Enhance shikonin production from Lithospermum erythrorhizon by in situ extraction and calcium alginate immobilization. Biotechnol Bioeng 1990;36:460–6.

[39] Facchini PJ., DiCosmo F. Plant cell bioreactor for the production of protoberberine alkaloids from immobilized Thalictrum rugosum cultures. Biotechnol Bioeng 1991;37:397–403.

[40] Ryu OH, Ju JY, Shin CS. Continuous L-cysteine production using immobilized cells reactors and product extractors. Process Biochem 1996;32:201–9.

[41] Archambault J, Volesky B, Kurz WGW. Surface immobilization of plant cells. Biotechnol Bioeng 1989;33:293–9.

[42] Facchini PJ, DiCosmo F. Plant cell bioreactor for the production of protoberberine alkaloids from immobilized Thalictrum rugosum cultures. Biotechnol Bioeng 1991;37:397–403.

[43] Kurata H, Furusaki S. Immobilized Coffea arabica cell cultures using a bubble column reactor with controlled light intensity. Biotechnol Bioeng 1993;42:414–502.

[44] Kurata H, Seki M, Furusaki S. Light effect to promote secondary metabolite production of plant cell culture in advances in plant biotechnology, Ryu D.D.Y., Furusaki S. Elsevier, Amsterdam 1994.

[45] Lambie AJ. Commercial aspects of the production of secondary compounds by immobilized plant cells in secondary product from plant tissue culture, Charlwood B.V., Rhodes M.J.C. (Eds). Clarendon Press, Oxford 1990.

[46] Downs CG, Christey MC, Davies KM, King GA, Seelye JF, Sinclair BK, et al. Hairy roots of Brassica napus: II. Glutamine synthetase overexpression alters ammonia assimilation and the response to phosphinothricin. Plant Cell Rep 1994;14:41–6.

[47] Berlin J, Rügenhagen C, Dietze P, Fecker LF, Goddijn OJM, Hoge JHC. Increased production of serotonin by suspension and root cultures of Peganum harmala transformed with a tryptophan decarboxylase cDNA clone of *Catharanthus roseus*. Transgenic Res 1993;2:336–44.

[48] Hashimoto T, Yun DJ, Yamada Y. Production of tropane alkaloids in genetically engineered root cultures. Phytochemistry 1993;32:713–8.

[49] Chilton MD, Tepfer DA, Petit A, David C, Casse-Delbart F, Tempe J. *Agrobacterium rhizogenes* inserts T-DNA into the genomes of the host plant root cells. Nature (Lond) 1982;295:432.

[50] Nilsson O, Olsson O. Getting to the root: the role of the *Agrobacterium rhizogenes* rol genes in the formation of hairy roots. Physiol Plant 1997;100:463–73.

[51] Spena A, Schmulling T, Koncz C, Schell JS. Independent and synergistic activity of rol A, B and C loci in stimulating abnormal growth in plants. EMBO J 1987;6:3891–9.

[52] White FF, Taylor BH, Huffman GA, Gordon MP, Nester EW. Molecular genetic analysis of the transferred DNA regions of the root inducing plasmid of *Agrobacterium rhizogenes*. J Bacteriol 1985;164:33–44.

[53] Cardarelli M, Mariotti D, Pomponi M, Spano L, Capone I, Costanino P. *Agrobacterium rhizogenes* T-DNA genes capable of inducing hairy root phenotypes. Mol Gen Genet 1987;209:475–80.

[54] Hu Z, Du M. Hairy root and its application in plant genetic engineering. J Integr Plant Biol 2006;48(2):121–7.

[55] Mugnier J. Establishment of new axenic hairy root lines by inoculation with *Agrobacterium rhizogenes*. Plant Cell Rep 1988;7:9–12.

[56] Han KH, Keathley DE, Davis JM, Gordon MP. Regeneration of transgenic woody legume (*Robinia pseudoacacia* L. Black locust) and morphological alterations induced by *Agrobacterium rhizogenes* transformation. Plant Sci 1993;88:149–57.

[57] Drewes FE, Staden JV. Initiation of and solasodine production in hairy root culture of *Solanum mauritianum* Scop. Plant Growth Regul 1995;17:27–31.

[58] Giri A, Rafindra ST, Dhingra V, Narasu ML. Influence of different strains of *Agrobacterium rhizogenes* on induction of hairy roots and artemisinin production in *Artemisia annua*. Curr Sci 2001;81:378–82.

[59] Zambryski P. Agrobacterium-plant cell DNA transfer. In: Mobile DNA. Berg D.E., Howe M.M., eds., American Society for Microbiology, Washington D.C., pp. 309-333:1989.

[60] DiCosmo F, Facchini PJ, Kraml MM. Cultured plant cells: the chemical factory within. Chem Brit 1989;25:1001–4.

[61] Routien JR., Nickel LG. Cultivation of plant tissue, US Patent No. 2,747,334, 1956.

[62] Misawa M. Plant tissue culture: an alternative for production of useful metabolite. FAO Agricultural Services Bulletin 1994;108.

[63] Takayama S, Akita M. The types of bioreactor used for shoots and embryos. Plant Cell Tiss Org Cult 1994;39:147–56.

[64] Chattopadhyay S, Farkya S, Srivastava AK, Bisaria VS. Bioprocess considerations for production of secondary metabolites by plant cell suspension cultures. Biotechnol Bioprocess Eng 2002;7:138–49.

[65] Sajc L, Grubisic D, Vunjak-Novakovic G. Bioreactors for plant engineering: an outlook for further research. Biochem Eng J 2000;4:89–99.

[66] Sharma S, Shahzad A. Bioreactors: a rapid approach for secondary metabolite production. Recent Trends Biotechnol Therapeut Appl Med Plants 2013;25–49.

[67] Yesil-Celiktas O, Gurel A, Vardar-Sukan F. Large Scale Cultivation of Plant Cell and Tissue Culture in Bioreactors 2010:1-54.

[68] International Union of Pure and Applied Chemistry (IUPAC). Compendium of chemical terminology (2nd ed.). Oxford: Blackwell Scientific, 1997.

[69] Tanaka H. Technological problems in cultivation of plant cells at high density. Biotechnol Bioeng 2000;67(6):775–90.

[70] Terrier B, Courtois D, Henault N, Cuvier A, Bastin M, Aknin A, et al. Two new disposable bioreactors for plant cell culture: the wave and undertow bioreactor and the slug bubble bioreactor. Biotechnol Bioeng 2007;96(5):914–23.

[71] Lessard P. Metabolic engineering, the concept coalesces. Nat Biotechnol 1996;14:1654–5.

[72] Sato F, Hashimoto T, Hachiya A, Tamura KI, Choi KB, Morishige T, et al. Metabolic engineering of plant alkaloid biosynthesis. Proc Natl Acad Sci USA 2001;2:367–72.

[73] Wink M, Alfermann AW, Franke R, Wetterauer B, Distl M, Windhovel J, et al. Sustainable bioproduction of phytochemicals by plant in vitro cultures: anticancer agents. Plant Genetic Resour 2005;3:90–100.

[74] Engels B, Dahm P, Jennewein S. Metabolic engineering of taxadiene biosynthesis in yeast as a first step towards Taxol (Paclitaxel) production. Metab Eng 2008;10:201–6.

[75] Nakanishi TM. Antitumor Compounds: production by plant cell cultures. M. Misawa, Medicinal and Aromatic Plants I. Biotechnology in Agriculture and Forestry 1988;4:191–208.

[76] Berger RG., Drawert F, Hadrich S. Microbial sources of flavour compounds. In Bioflavour '87. AnaIysis-BiochemistryBiotechnology, ed. Schreier P, Gruyter WD. Berlin, pp. 1988:415-434.

[77] Armstrong DW., Gillies B, Yemazaki H. Natural flavors produced by biotechnological processing. In Flavor chemistry: trends and developments. ed. Teranishi R, Buttery RG., Shahldi F. Chemical Society, Washington, DC, 1989:105-120.

[78] Urbach G. The flavor of milk and dairy products: II. cheese: contribution of volatile compounds. Int J Dairy Technol 1997;50:79–89.

[79] Gatfield IL. Production of flavor and aroma compounds by biotechnology. Food Technol 1988;10:110–22.

[80] Janssens L, de Pooter HL, Vandamme EJ, Schamp NM. Production of flavors by microorganisms. Process Biochem 1992;27:195–215.

[81] Krings U, Berger RG. Biotechnological production of flavors and fragrances. Appl Microbiol Biotechnol 1998;49:1–8.

[82] Vandamme EJ, Soetaert W. Bioflavours and fragrances via fermentation and biocatalysis. J Chem Technol Biotechnol 2002;77:1323–32.

[83] Aguedo M, Ly MH, Belo I, Teixeira JA, Belin JM, Waché Y. The use of enzymes and microorganisms for the production of aroma compounds from lipids. Food Technol Biotechnol 2004;42:327–36.

[84] Harlander S. Biotechnology for the production of flavoring materials. In: Source book of flavours, Reineccius, G. (Ed.). Chapman and Hall, New York, USA 1994:151–175.

[85] Sahai OM. Plant tissue culture. In: Gabelman A, editor. Bioprocess production of flavor, fragrances, color ingredients. New York, USA: Wiley; 1994. p. 239–75.

[86] Scragg AH. The production of aromas by plant cell cultures. In: Advances in biochemical engineering biotechnology, Vol. 55, P. Scheper (Ed.). Springer, Berlin, Germany, 1997, 239–263.

[87] Rao SR, Ravishankar GA. Plant cell cultures: chemical factories of secondary metabolites. Biotechnol Adv 2002;20:101–53.

[88] Mulabagal V, Tsay HS. Plant cell cultures – an alternative and efficient source for the production of biologically important secondary metabolites. Int J Appl Sci Eng 2004;2:29–48.

[89] Longo MA, Sanromán MA. Production of food aroma compounds. Food Technol Biotechnol 2006;44(3):335–53.

[90] Rao SR, Ravishankar GA. Vanilla flavor: production by conventional and biotechnological routes. J Sci Food Agric 2000;80:289–304.

[91] Davidonis G, Knorr D. Callus formation and shoot regeneration in *Vanilla planifolia*. Food Biotechnol 1991;5:59–66.

[92] Funk C, Brodelius P. Phenylpropanoid metabolism in suspension cultures of *Vanilla planifolia* Andr. IV. Induction of vanillic acid formation. Plant Physiol 1992;99:256–62.

[93] Escamilla-Hurtado ML, Valdes-Martinez S, Soriano-Santos J, Tomasini-Campocosio A. Effect of some nutritional and environmental parameters on the production of diacetyl and on starch consumption by *Pediococcus pentosaceus* and *Lactobacillus acidophilusin* submerged cultures. J Appl Microbiol 2000;88:142–53.

[94] Nabeta K, Ohnishi Y, Hirose T, Sugisawa H. Monoterpene biosynthesis by callus tissues and suspension cells from Perilla species. Phytochemistry 1983;22:423–5.

[95] Kim TH, Shin JH, Baek HH, Lee HJ. Volatile flavor compounds in suspension culture of *Agastache rugosa* Kuntze (Korean mint). J Sci Food Agric 2001;81:569–75.

[96] Prince CL, Shuler ML, Yamada Y. Altering flavor profiles in onion (*Allium cepa* L.) root cultures through directed biosynthesis. Biotechnol Progr 1997;13:506–10.

[97] Bais HP, Weir TL, Perry LG, Gilroy S, Vivanco JM. The role of root exudates in rhizosphere interactions with plants and other organisms. Annu Rev Plant Biol 2006;57:233–66.

[98] Grayer RJ, Kokubun T. Plant-fungal interactions: the search for phytoalexins and other antifungal compounds from higher plants. Phytochemistry 2001;56:253–63.

[99] Jones JD, Dangl JL. The plant immune system. Nature 2006;444:323–9.

[100] Lindsay WP, Lamb CJ, Dixon RA. Microbial recognition and activation of plant defense systems. Trends Microbiol 1993;1:181–7.

[101] Bednarek P, Osbourn A. Plant-microbe interactions: chemical diversity in plant defense. Science 2009;324:746–8.

[102] Müller KO, Börger H. Experimentelle Untersuchungen über die Phytophtora-Resistenz, Kartoffel [In German]. Arb Biol Reichsanstalt Landw Forstw Berlin 1940;23:189–231.

[103] VanEtten HD, Mansfield JW, Bailey JA, Farmer EE. Two classes of plant antibiotics: phytoalexins versus phyto-anticipins. Plant Cell 1994;6:1191–2.

[104] Osbourn AE. Preformed antimicrobial compounds and plant defense against fungal attack. Plant Cell 1996;8:1821–31.

[105] González-Lamothe R, Mitchell G, Gattuso M, Diarra MS, Malouin F, Bouarab K. Plant antimicrobial agents and their effects on plant and human pathogens. Int J Mol Sci Aug 2009;10(8):3400–19.

Plant-Based Biotechnological Products With Their Production Host, Modes of Delivery Systems, and Stability Testing

Saurabh Bhatia, Randhir Dahiya

Modern Applications of Plant Biotechnology in Pharmaceutical Sciences. http://dx.doi.org/10.1016/B978-0-12-802221-4.00008-X

8.1 INTRODUCTION

The uses of herbal drugs and their secondary metabolites for the treatment of various human ailments predate the earliest stages of recorded civilization, dating back at least to the Neanderthal period. By the end of sixteenth century, botanical gardens provided a wealth of *Materia Medica* for teaching therapeutic use. Herbal medicine flourished until the seventeenth century when more scientific "pharmacological" remedies were discovered. Subsequently, the pharmacologically active principles in herbal drugs were identified and purified for their therapeutic use. Even today, about one-fourth of current prescription drugs have a botanical origin. Modern biotechnology has led to a resurgence of interest in obtaining new medicinal agents from botanical sources.

Through genetic engineering (GE), plants can now be used to produce a variety of proteins, including mammalian antibodies, blood substitutes, vaccines, and other therapeutic entities. Recently, the production of foreign proteins in GE plants has become a viable alternative to conventional production systems such as microbial fermentation or mammalian cell culture. GE plants, acting as bioreactors/biofactories, can efficiently produce recombinant proteins in larger quantities than those produced using mammalian cell systems. Plant-derived proteins are particularly attractive, since they are free of human diseases and mammalian viral vectors. Large quantities of biomass can be easily grown in the field, and may permit storage of material prior to processing. Thus, plants offer the potential for efficient, large-scale production of recombinant proteins with increased freedom from contaminating human pathogens [1].

Biopharmaceuticals represent the fastest growing segment in the pharmaceutical industry, accounting for approximately 10% of the pharmaceutical market in 2007, 20% of newly approved drugs in recent years, and 40% of new entities in the pipeline. In 2006, it was estimated that approximately 2500 biotechnology drugs were in the discovery phase, 900 in preclinical, and over 1600 in clinical trials. Sales of many top-selling biopharmaceuticals are increasing, with US sales of the monoclonal antibody Herceptin used for the treatment of breast cancer growing by 82% from 2005 to 2006 alone. In 2007, the three top-selling pharmaceutical products sold by the Swiss drugmaker Roche were therapeutic monoclonal antibodies (Rituxan/Mabthera, Herceptin, and Avastin), contributing to sales of €9311 million [2]. Various applications of biotechnology to improve yield and quality of crops and various well-known biopharmaceuticals with their respective functions are listed in Tables 8.1 and 8.2.

8.2 PLANT-BASED BIOTECHNOLOGICAL PRODUCTS WITH THEIR RESPECTIVE PRODUCTION HOST

Most of the biopharmaceuticals, especially peptides and proteins, are produced by recombinant DNA technology using various expression systems. Expression systems used for this purpose are *Escherichia coli*, *Bacillus*, yeast (*Saccharomyces cerevisiae*), fungi (*Aspergillus*), animal cells, plant cells, and insect cells. Among them *E. coli* and mammalian cells are the most widely used expression systems. The most common biopharmaceuticals produced by recombinant DNA technology are cytokines and other proteins of therapeutic interest. Each expression system displays its own unique set of advantages and disadvantages. Various factors such as expression level (soluble form), glycosylation, easy purification, cultivation process, cell density, cost effectiveness, and feasibility play an important role in designing suitable expression systems for the production of specific biopharmaceuticals. Additionally production systems for therapeutic proteins should be efficient in multiplication so that hosts could be cultured in large quantities, inexpensively, and in a short time by standard cultivation methods [3]. Various applications of host as a suitable expression system are highlighted in Fig. 8.1.

8.2.1 Plant Cell

Proteins can be used as diagnostic as well as therapeutic agents and this creates a strong demand for the production of recombinant proteins on an industrial scale. Commercial protein production has traditionally relied on microbial fermentation and mammalian cell lines, but these systems have disadvantages in terms of cost, stability, and safety, which prompted research into alternatives. Despite industry apathy and conservatism, plants have emerged as one of the most promising sources for the production of biological active components. Plants allow the cost-effective production of recombinant proteins on an agricultural scale, while eliminating risks of product contamination with endotoxins or human pathogens [4].

Another advantage of the use of plants in recombinant protein production is that vaccine candidates can be expressed in edible plant organs, allowing them to be administered as unprocessed or partially processed material. Current limitations of plant bioreactor technology include low yield, difficulties with downstream processing (leading to inconsistent product quality), and the presence of nonauthentic glycan structures on recombinant human proteins. These limitations raise regulatory issues and have prevented the routine approval of plant-derived biopharmaceuticals for use in clinical trials [5].

8.2.1.1 Emerging Production Platforms for Biopharmaceuticals
8.2.1.1.1 SELECTION OF HOST SPECIES

Many of the early, plant-derived recombinant proteins were produced in transgenic tobacco plants and were extracted directly from harvested leaves. The continuing

TABLE 8.1   List of Various Well-Known Biopharmaceuticals With Their Respective Functions

Biopharmaceutical	Products	Function
Clotting factors	Factor VIIa	Factor VII, proconvertin, causes blood coagulation in the coagulation cascade
	Factor IX	Hemophilia B is the second most common type of hemophilia. It can also be known as factor IX deficiency, or Christmas disease. It was originally named "Christmas disease"
	Antihemophilic factor (factor VIII (FVIII))	Factor VIII (FVIII) is an essential blood clotting protein, also known as antihemophilic factor (AHF). In humans, factor VIII is encoded by the *F8* gene. Defects in this gene result in hemophilia A, a recessive X-linked coagulation disorder
Colony stimulating factors (CSF)	Macrophage CSF	Cells to proliferate and differentiate into a specific kind of blood cell in bone marrow stimulation
Dismutases	Superoxide dismutase	These are enzymes that catalyze the dismutation of superoxide into oxygen and hydrogen peroxide. Thus, they are an important antioxidant defense in nearly all cells exposed to oxygen
Erythropoietins	Epoetin	Glycoprotein hormone that controls erythropoiesis, or red blood cell production in anemia
Growth factors	Epidermal growth factor (EGF)	Epidermal growth factor or EGF is a growth factor that stimulates cell growth, proliferation, and differentiation by binding to its receptor
	Fibroblast growth factor	Fibroblast growth factors, or FGFs, are a family of growth factors involved in angiogenesis, wound healing, and embryonic development
	Insulin-like growth factor	The insulin-like growth factors (IGFs) are proteins with high sequence similarity to insulin. They consist of two cell-surface receptors (IGF1R and IGF2R) and two ligands (IGF-1 and IGF-2)
	Platelet-derived growth factor	Platelet-derived growth factor (PDGF) is one of the numerous growth factors or proteins that regulate cell growth and division. In particular, it plays a significant role in blood vessel formation (angiogenesis), the growth of blood vessels from already-existing blood vessel tissue. All these factors play a major role in wound healing
Growth hormone	Somatotropin	Growth hormone (GH) is a peptide hormone that stimulates growth, cell reproduction and regeneration in humans and other animals and is clinically used for short stature and multiple sclerosis. Somatotropin (STH) refers to the growth hormone 1 produced naturally in animals, whereas the term somatotropin refers to growth hormone produced by recombinant DNA technology, and is abbreviated "HGH" in humans
Somatostatin	Somnidren GH	(Also known as growth hormone-inhibiting hormone (GHIH) or somatotropin release-inhibiting factor (SRIF).) Somatotropin release-inhibiting hormone is a peptide hormone that regulates the endocrine system and affects neurotransmission and cell proliferation via interaction with G-protein-coupled somatostatin receptors and inhibition of the release of numerous secondary hormones. Plays a major role in glucose regulation

(Continued)

TABLE 8.1 List of Various Well-Known Biopharmaceuticals With Their Respective Functions *(cont.)*

Biopharmaceutical	Products	Function
Insulin	Humulin	Insulin is a hormone, produced by the pancreas, which is central to regulating carbohydrate and fat metabolism in the body. Insulin causes cells in the liver, muscle, and fat tissue to take up glucose from the blood, storing it as glycogen inside these tissues
Proinsulin		Glucose regulation
Triproamylin		Glucose regulation
Interferons	Interferon-β α-Interferon γ-Interferon	Multiple sclerosis Viral diseases/hairy cell leukemia Carcinoma
Interleukins	PEG interleukin-2 Interleukin-1α Interleukin-1β Interleukin-3, -4, -6	The majority of interleukins are synthesized by helper CD4⁺ T lymphocytes, as well as through monocytes, macrophages, and endothelial cells. They promote the development and differentiation of T, B, and hematopoietic cells. Interleukin receptors on astrocytes in the hippocampus are also known to be involved in the development of spatial memories in mice
Monoclonal antibodies (MoAb)	Anti-EGF receptor MoAb Anti-EGF Anti-IL-2 receptor Anti-LPS MoAb Antipseudomonas MoAb	Monoclonal antibodies (mAb or MoAb) are monospecific antibodies that are the same because they are made by identical immune cells that are all clones of a unique parent cell. Monoclonal antibodies have monovalent affinity, in that they bind to the same epitope; used in cancer treatment and autoimmune disease
	Antitumor necrosis factor	The epidermal growth factor receptor (EGFR; ErbB-1; HER1 in humans) is the cell-surface receptor for members of the epidermal growth factor family (EGF-family) of extracellular protein ligands. The epidermal growth factor receptor is a member of the ErbB family of receptors, a subfamily of four closely related receptor tyrosine kinases: EGFR (ErbB-1), HER2/c-neu (ErbB-2), Her 3 (ErbB-3), and Her 4 (ErbB-4). Mutations affecting EGFR expression or activity could result in cancer
	Chimeric anti-CD4 MoAb Chimeric anti-TNF MoAb, HA-IA MoAb, E5 MoAb Antifibrin MoAb HER-2 MoAb Human MoAb to cytomegalovirus Technetium 99m-FAB fragments	Chimera is an organism from different zygotes and in opposite mosaic are two organisms from same origin. Technetium-99m is a medical isotope, which can be easily detected in the body for diagnosis purposes. HER-2 Amplification or overexpression of this gene has been shown to play an important role in the pathogenesis and progression of certain aggressive types of breast cancer and in recent years it has evolved to become an important biomarker and target of therapy for the disease
Recombinant soluble CD4s	CD4-IgG rsCD4	CD4 (cluster of differentiation 4) is a glycoprotein found on the surface of immune cells such as T helper cells, monocytes, macrophages, and dendritic cells. It is a coreceptor that assists the T cell receptor (TCR) with an antigen-presenting cell

(Continued)

TABLE 8.1　List of Various Well-Known Biopharmaceuticals With Their Respective Functions *(cont.)*

Biopharmaceutical	Products	Function
Tissue plasminogen activators	Tissue plasminogen activator (fibrinolytic)	Tissue plasminogen activator (abbreviated TPA or PLAT) is a protein involved in the breakdown of blood clots. It is a serine protease found on endothelial cells, the cells that line the blood vessels. As an enzyme, it catalyzes the conversion of plasminogen to plasmin, the major enzyme responsible for clot breakdown. tPA is used in clinical medicine to treat embolic or thrombotic stroke. Use is contraindicated in hemorrhagic stroke and head trauma
Streptokinase		Fibrinolytic enzyme
Hirudin	Desirudin, a recombinant form of hirudin	Fibrinolytic (hirudin) is a naturally occurring peptide in the salivary glands of medicinal leeches (such as *Hirudo medicinalis*) that has a blood anticoagulant property
Tumor necrosis factors	TNF	Tumor necrosis factors (or the TNF-family) refer to a group of cytokines whose family can cause cell death (apoptosis). The first two members of the family to be identified were TNF and lymphotoxin-alpha
Vaccines	AIDS vaccine Herpes vaccine Malaria vaccine Melanoma vaccine	A vaccine is a biological preparation that improves immunity to a particular disease
Murine MoAb to human B-cell lymphomas	Mifarmonab Anti-B4-blocked ricin Celogovab Orthoclone OKT4A Muromonab CD5-RTA, Pancarcinoma Re-186 MoAb, Anti-CD5 MoAb-ricin Xomazyme[R]-791, CD7 plus, mel	These are the antibodies that fight against cancer. These antibodies come from a variety of sources, but mouse (or Chinese hamster) antibodies are a common source. Moabs called "murine" are made entirely from mouse antibodies. In chimeric antibody a portion of a mouse antibody has been replaced with a human part so that the body will not reject it as quickly. Humanized antibodies are entirely human
Others Interleukin-1 receptor antagonist Atrial natriuretic peptide Monophosphoryl lipid A Retroviral vector with TNF gene		Interleukin-1 receptor antagonist modulates a variety of interleukin-1 related immune and inflammatory responses. A polymorphism of this gene is reported to be associated with increased risk of osteoporotic fractures and gastric cancer. Atrial natriuretic peptide (ANP) is a powerful vasodilator, and a protein (polypeptide) hormone secreted by heart muscle cells. ANP acts to reduce the water, sodium, and adipose loads on the circulatory system, thereby reducing blood pressure. Monophosphoryl lipid A is a derivative of the lipid A molecule found in the membrane of Gram-negative bacteria. A drug delivery virion, which contains an expression system for the desired protein active ingredient packaged in an envelope derived from a retrovirus, is especially useful in administering materials that need to cross cell membranes in order to serve their function
α-1 Antitrypsin (aat)		Alpha-1 antitrypsin (AAT) deficiency is a condition in which the body cells are unable to make enough protein that protects the lungs and liver from damage

TABLE 8.2 Applications of Biotechnology to Improve Yield and Quality of Major Field Crops

Crops	Areas of improvement
Rice	Drought and salinity tolerance Resistance to stem borers, brown hoppers, gall midge, and leaf sheath blight Nutritional and table quality of grains
Wheat	Yield, quality, and adaptation Resistance to rusts
Maize	Yield and quality Resistance to lodging and stem borers
Sorghum	Yield, quality, and adaptation to drought Resistance to shoot fly, stem borer, midge, head bugs, and grain molds
Pearl millet	Yield, and adaptation to drought Resistance to downy mildew, stem borers, and head mine
Pigeonpea	Yield, and adaptation to drought Resistance to Helicoverpa and Fusarium wilt
Chickpea	Adaptation to drought and chilling tolerance Resistance to wilt, Ascochyta blight, and Helicoverpa
Mustard	Yield, and adaptation to drought, oil content, and quality Resistance to aphids
Groundnut	Yield, oil content, and adaptation to drought Resistance to foliar diseases, aflatoxins, and leaf miner
Cotton	Yield, fiber quality, and oil content Resistance to jassids and bollworms
Sugarcane	Resistance to stem borers Yield and induction of early maturity
Tobacco	Yield and quality Resistance to aphids, tobacco caterpillar, and viruses

popularity of tobacco reflects its status as a well-established expression host for which robust transformation procedures and well-characterized regulatory elements for the control of transgene expression are available. Furthermore, its high biomass yields and rapid scalability make tobacco very suitable for commercial molecular farming. It is also a nonfood, nonfeed crop, and so carries a reduced risk of transgenic material or recombinant proteins contaminating feed and human food chains. Tobacco has been adopted as a platform system by several biotechnological companies, including Planet Biotechnology Inc. (http://www.planetbiotechnology.com/) and Meristem Therapeutics (http://www.meristem-therapeutics.com/), the only two companies to have plant-derived pharmaceuticals undergoing Phase II clinical trials. One disadvantage of tobacco is its high content of nicotine and other toxic alkaloids, which must be removed completely during downstream processing steps. Although low-alkaloid tobacco cultivars are available, attention has turned to other leafy crops for pharmaceutical production [6]. These crops include lettuce, which has been used for clinical trials with a hepatitis B virus subunit vaccine, and alfalfa, which is being promoted as a platform

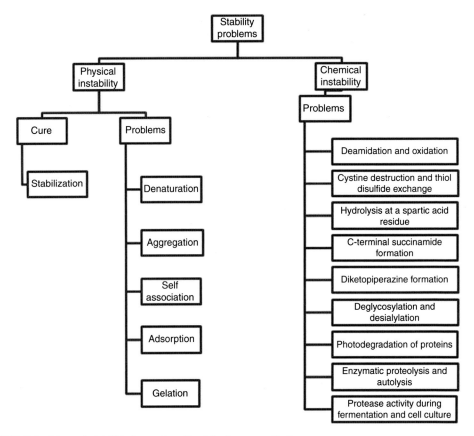

FIGURE 8.1   General stability issues faced by biopharmaceuticals.

system by Medicago Inc. This Canadian biotech company has isolated novel promoters that allow high-level protein expression in alfalfa leaves, and has focused on the early part of the production pipeline by developing alfalfa cell culture and transient-expression technology [7]. Advantages of alfalfa include its high biomass yield and the fact that it is a perennial plant that fixes its own nitrogen. A strong advantage of alfalfa for pharmaceutical production is that fact that glycoproteins synthesized in alfalfa leaves tend to have homogeneous glycan structures, which is important for batch-to-batch consistency. However, alfalfa is a feed crop and its leaves contain large amounts of oxalic acid, which might interfere with processing.

   Although leafy crops are advantageous in terms of biomass yield, proteins that are expressed in leaves tend to be unstable, which means the harvested material has a limited shelf-life and must be processed immediately after harvest. By contrast, proteins that are expressed in cereal seeds are protected from degradation by proteolytic enzymes; they can remain stable for longer periods at room temperature (unpublished data) and refrigerator temperatures without significantly affecting biological activity [8]. Several different cereals, including rice, wheat, barley, and maize, have been investigated as potential hosts for recombinant protein production. Maize has been chosen by Prodigene Inc., an industry leader in cereal-based commercial protein production because it has a high biomass yield, it is easily transformed and manipulated *in vitro*, and the production of transgenic maize can be scaled up conveniently. Maize has been used for the commercial production of the technical proteins avidin and β-glucuronidase (GUS) [9]. In addition, Prodigene is exploring its use for the production of subunit vaccines, recombinant antibodies, and further technical enzymes, such as aprotinin and laccase.

Although it is beneficial to focus on a small number of platform technologies for the bulk production of biopharmaceuticals, the delivery of recombinant vaccines in edible plant organs is exceptional because it would be advantageous to use locally grown plants for vaccination campaigns. Therefore, a variety of different expression hosts have been evaluated. Potato was the first major system to be used for vaccine production, and transgenic potato tubers have been administered to humans in at least three clinical trials to date. Over the past few years, potatoes have been evaluated for the production of human serum albumin, novel vaccines, tumor necrosis factor-α (TNF-α), and antibodies. Other production hosts that have been used to express vaccines include tomatoes, bananas, carrots, lettuce, maize, alfalfa, white clover, and *Arabidopsis*. Oil crops are useful hosts for protein production because the oil bodies can be exploited to simplify protein isolation. An example is the oleosin-fusion platform developed by SemBioSys Genetics Inc., in which the target recombinant protein is expressed in oilseed rape or safflower as a fusion with oleosin. The Finnish biotech company UniCrop is also developing an oilseed technology platform, although in this case, the idea is to isolate recombinant proteins from the rapidly developing sprouts cultivated in bioreactors.

Finally, there have been significant recent developments in the use of more diverse plant species, which can easily be contained, propagated, and transformed to produce recombinant proteins. Mayfield et al. have described a protein expression system that is based on the unicellular green alga *Chlamydomonas reinhardtii*. In this system, chloroplast-targeted transgenes were used to express an antibody that recognized herpes simplex virus glycoprotein D [10]. Other simple plants that have been adopted as bioreactors include *Lemna* (duckweed), which is being developed as a platform technology by Biolex Inc., and the moss *Physcomitrella patens*, which is being developed by Greenovation Inc., Freiburg, Germany. The advantages and disadvantages of different expression hosts are summarized in Table 8.3.

8.2.1.1.2 ALTERNATIVE PLANT-BASED EXPRESSION SYSTEMS

The majority of plant-based recombinant pharmaceutical proteins have been produced by nuclear transformation and the regeneration of transgenic plant cell lines, followed by the extraction and purification of proteins from the transgenic tissues (Table 8.4). Although nuclear gene transfer is now routine in many species, it has disadvantages in terms of production time scales, which are being addressed or circumvented by the development of alternative plant-based production technologies (Table 8.5). Transient expression is generally used to verify transformation construct activity and to validate small amounts of recombinant protein (Table 8.4). It can be achieved by the vacuum infiltration of leaves with recombinant *Agrobacterium tumefaciens*, resulting in the transient transformation of many cells. High levels of protein expression are achieved for a short time, but generally the technique is insufficient for commercial-scale production. Recently, however, several reports have described how this

TABLE 8.3 Proteins/Peptides Obtained From Plant Sources

Anticoagulants			
Protein C pathway	Tobacco	Human protein C (serum protease)	AMT
Indirect thrombin inhibitors	Ethiopian mustard	Human hirudin variant 2	AMT
Recombinant hormones/proteins			
Neutropenia	Tobacco	Human granulocyte-macrophage colony-stimulating factor	AMT
Anemia	Tobacco	Human erythropoietin	AMT
Antihyperanalgesic by opiate activity	Tobacco	Human erythropoietin	AMT
Wound repair/control of cell proliferation	Thale cress, oilseed	Human enkephalins	AMT
Hepatitis B and C treatment	Rice, turnip	Human interferon-α	AMT
Liver cirrhosis	Potato, tobacco	Human serum albumin	AMT
Blood substitute	Tobacco	Human hemoglobin	AMT
Collagen	Tobacco	Human homotrimeric collagen	AMT
Protein/peptide inhibitors			
Cystic fibrosis, liver disease and hemorrhage	Rice	Human α-1-antitrypsin	PB
Trypsin inhibitor for transplantation surgery	Maize	Human aprotinin	PB
Hypertension	Tobacco/tomato	Angiotensin-1-converting enzyme	AMT
HIV therapies	N. benthamiana	α-Trichosanthin from TMV-U1 subgenomic coat protein	AMT
Recombinant enzymes			
Gaucher's disease	Tobacco	Glucocerebrosidase	AMT

AMT, Agrobacterium-mediated transformation; PB, particle bombardment.

agro-infiltration process could be scaled up more efficiently [11]. Baulcombe and colleagues have shown that the loss of protein expression seen after a few days is predominantly caused by gene silencing. They managed to increase the expression levels of several proteins at least 50-fold by coexpressing the p19 protein from tomato [12]. Furthermore, researchers at Medicago Inc. have described how the agro-infiltration of alfalfa leaves can be scaled up to 7500 leaves per week, producing micrograms of recombinant protein per week. Similarly, we have shown that up to 100 kg of wild-type tobacco leaves could be processed by agro-infiltration, resulting in the production of several hundred milligrams of protein.

Another emerging tobacco transient-expression technology is based on the use of plant viruses as expression vectors. Virus-infected plants have been used to produce several pharmaceutical proteins, including vaccine candidates and antibodies, one of which is now

TABLE 8.4 Stable Transformation Versus Transient Expression

	Nuclear transformation	Chloroplast transformation	Transient expression
Transgene silencing	Yes	Not known	No
Scale-up potential	Large	Large	Moderate due to labor-intensive inoculation
Protein processing	Eukaryotic	Prokaryotic	
Possibility for simultaneous expression of multiple transgenes	Possible via crossing of different transgenic lines	Possible by the use of polycistronic messages	Low because of gene size limitation
Inheritance of trait	Mendelian	Maternal (except few species)	No
Expression levels	Low/moderate	High	High
Exclusive expression in certain parts of the plant (fruits, grains, etc.)	Achievable by the use of specific promoters	Unlikely, maybe some fruits such as tomatoes	No
Environmental concerns	Medium	Low	High
Development time	High	Very high	Low
Applicability	Most species	Very limited	Most species

undergoing Phase I clinical trials. The advantages of virus-based production include the rapid onset of expression, the systemic spread of the virus so that recombinant protein is produced in every cell, and the fact that more than one vector can be used in the same plant, allowing multimeric proteins to be assembled. The tobacco chloroplast transgenic system is another promising variant, which was boosted this year by the launch of a new company, Chlorogen, to capitalize on its pharmaceutical potential. Transplastomic plants are generated by introducing DNA into the chloroplast genome, usually by particle bombardment. The advantages of chloroplast transformation are many: the transgene copy number is high because of the many chloroplasts in a typical photosynthetic cell, there is no gene silencing, multiple genes can be expressed in operons, the recombinant proteins accumulate within the chloroplast, thus limiting toxicity to the host plant, and the absence of functional chloroplast DNA in the pollen of most crops provides natural transgene containment [13].

The chloroplast transgenic system has achieved remarkably high expression levels, recently exceeding 25% total soluble protein (TSP) for a tetanus toxin fragment, 11% TSP for human serum albumen, and 6% TSP for a thermostable xylanase. At present, chloroplast transformation is routine only in tobacco and *C. reinhardtii*. However, plastid transformation has been achieved in a growing number of plant species, including carrot and tomato. The ability to transform the chromoplasts of fruit and vegetable crops has obvious advantages for the expression of subunit vaccines. Plant cell cultures can be used for the production of small molecule drugs, but they are also advantageous for molecular farming because of the high level of containment that they offer and the possibility of producing proteins under current good manufacturing practice (cGMP) conditions. Tobacco suspension cells are the most popular

TABLE 8.5   Features of Different Plant Host Systems

Plant	Advantages	Disadvantages
Tobacco	Facile, efficient transformation system Abundant material for protein characterization	Toxic alkaloids incompatible w/oral delivery Potential for outcrossing in field
Potato	Facile, efficient transformation system Tuber is edible raw Tuber-specific promoters available Microtuber production for quick assay Clonally propagated, low potential for outcrossing in field Industrial tuber processing well established	Relatively low tuber protein content Unpalatable in raw form; cooking may cause denaturation and poor immunogenicity of vaccine
Tomato	Relatively efficient transformation system Fruit is edible raw Fruit-specific promoters available Crossing possible to stack antigen genes Industrial greenhouse culture well established Industrial fruit processing well established	Relatively low fruit protein content Acidic fruit may be incompatible with some antigens or for delivery to infants No *in vitro* system to test fruit expression
Alfalfa	Relatively efficient transformation system High protein content in leaves Leaves edible uncooked Ideal system for animal vaccines	Potential for outcrossing in field Deep root system problematic for cleaning field
Legumes or cereals	Production technology widely established High protein content in seeds Stable protein in stored seeds Well suited for animal vaccines Industrial seed processing well established	Inefficient transformation systems Heating or cooking for human use may cause denaturation and poor immunogenicity of vaccine (corn meal is exception) Potential for outcrossing in field for some species
Banana	Cultivated widely in developing countries where vaccines are needed Eaten raw by infants and adults Clonally propagated, low potential for outcrossing in field Once established, abundant and inexpensive fruit is available on a 10–12-month cycle	Inefficient transformation system Little data available on gene expression, especially for fruit-specific promoters High cultivation space requirement; very expensive in greenhouse
Simple plants *P. patens,* *C. reinhardtii,* *Lemna*	Containment, clonal propagation, secretion into medium, regulatory compliance, homologous recombination in *Physcomitrella*	Scalability

system at present, although pharmaceutical proteins have also been produced in soybean, tomato, and rice cells, and in tobacco hairy roots. More than 20 pharmaceutical proteins have been produced in plant cell-suspension cultures, including antibodies, interleukins, erythropoietin, human granulocyte-macrophage colony stimulating factor (hGM-CSF), and hepatitis B antigen. Unfortunately, few of these proteins have been expressed at yields sufficient for commercial production. As discussed below, the problem of poor yields could be addressed in part by the use of optimized regulatory elements. For example, the expression of hGM-CSF in rice suspensions using an inducible promoter produced far greater yields than was possible using tobacco cells and a constitutive promoter [14].

8.2.1.1.3 STRATEGIES TO IMPROVE PROTEIN YIELDS

The factors that affect recombinant protein yields in transgenic plants and other plant systems have recently been reviewed in detail. The general approach is to maximize both the efficiency of all stages of gene expression and protein stability by appropriate subcellular targeting. Transgene expression in plants used for molecular farming is often driven by the strongest available constitutive promoters. However, regulated promoters are increasingly used, particularly those that allow external regulation by physical or chemical stimuli. Several novel inducible promoters that may be useful in molecular farming applications have been described recently. For example, a peroxidase gene promoter isolated from sweet potato (*Ipomoea batatas*) was used to drive the *gus A* reporter gene in transgenic tobacco. This promoter produced 30 times more GUS activity than did the cauliflower mosaic virus (CaMV) 35S promoter following exposure to hydrogen peroxide, wounding, or ultraviolet light. The wounding response is interesting as it would allow postharvest induction of gene expression in the same manner as the Crop Tech mechanical gene activation (MeGA) system, which is based on a tomato hydroxy-3-methylglutaryl CoA reductase 2 (HMGR2) promoter. A novel seed-specific promoter from the common bean (*Phaseolus vulgaris*) has been used to express a single chain antibody in *Arabidopsis thaliana*. In contrast to the CaMV 35S promoter, which resulted in antibody accumulation to 1% TSP, the beanarc 5-Ipromoter resulted in antibody levels in excess of 36% TSP in homozygous seeds, and the antibody retained its antigen binding activity and affinity. A trichome-specific promoter that might be useful for the secretion of recombinant proteins into the leaf guttation fluid has also been described in tobacco. Another secretion system, which is being commercialized by Phytomedics Inc., involves the secretion of recombinant proteins into tobacco root exudates and the leaf guttation fluid. This was developed for the production of human secreted alkaline phosphatase and has recently been used for the secretion of recombinant antibodies.

Subcellular targeting plays an important role in determining the yield of recombinant proteins because the compartment in which a recombinant protein accumulates strongly influences the interrelated processes of folding, assembly, and posttranslational modification. Comparative targeting experiments with full-size immunoglobulins and single-chain fragment variable (scFv) fragments have shown that the secretory pathway is more suitable for folding and assembly than the cytosol, and is therefore an advantageous site for high-level protein accumulation. Antibodies that are targeted to the secretory pathway using either plant or animal amino-terminal signal peptides usually accumulate to levels that are several orders of magnitude greater than those of antibodies expressed in the cytosol. Occasional exceptions to this general observation suggest that the intrinsic features of each antibody might also contribute to overall stability. The endoplasmic reticulum (ER) provides an oxidizing environment and an abundance of molecular chaperones but few proteases. These features are likely to be the most important factors affecting protein folding and assembly. It has been shown recently that antibodies that are targeted to the secretory pathway in transgenic plants interact specifically with the molecular chaperone BiP. In the absence of further targeting information, proteins that accumulate in the secretory system are secreted to the apoplast. Depending on its size, the protein can be retained in the apoplast or might leach from the cell, with important implications for production systems that are based on cell-suspension cultures. The stability of antibodies in the apoplast is lower than that in the lumen of the ER. Therefore, antibody expression levels can be increased even further if the protein is retrieved to the ER lumen using an H/KDEL carboxy-terminal tetrapeptide tag. Accumulation levels of proteins tagged in this way are generally 2- to 10-fold greater than those of identical proteins that lack the KDEL signal. Targeting is especially important if the recombinant protein is toxic to the production host. For example, the accumulation of avidin in the cytosol of transgenic tobacco plants is toxic, but plants can be regenerated successfully when this molecule is targeted to the vacuole [15].

8.2.1.1.4 DOWNSTREAM PROCESSING

Although high-level expression is necessary to provide good yields in plant-based production systems, the efficient recovery of recombinant proteins must also be optimized. Secretion systems are advantageous because no disruption of plant cells is necessary during protein recovery; hence, the release of phenolic compounds is avoided. Nevertheless, the recombinant proteins may be unstable in the culture medium. The use of affinity tags to facilitate the recovery of proteins is a useful strategy as long as the tag can be removed after purification to restore the native structure of the protein. In the oleosin fusion system mentioned earlier, the fusion protein can be recovered from oil bodies using a simple extraction procedure and the recombinant protein separated from its fusion partner by endoprotease digestion. Recent strategies that have been described include the expression of His-tagged GUS-fusion proteins in tobacco chloroplasts, the extraction of His-tagged proteins by foam fractionation, and the release of recombinant proteins using a modified expression system.

Therapeutic proteins have been produced in plants since 1986 when human growth hormone was expressed in engineered tobacco and sunflower callus cultures. The first description of a plant-made vaccine antigen appeared in a patent application filed in 1990 by inventors Curtiss and Cardineau who expressed *Streptococcus mutans* surface protein A in transgenic tobacco plants. Two years later the expression of hepatitis B surface antigen, also in tobacco, was published in what was to be the first report of a plant-made antigen in a peer-reviewed journal. Fourteen years later, the first plant-made vaccine received regulatory approval. Chickmate Newcastle disease virus vaccine for chickens was approved by the US Department of Agriculture Center for Veterinary Biologics in 2006. The vaccine was produced in a contained, tobacco, plant cell production system, the cells lysed and delivered by subcutaneous injection to chickens. Although this landmark example demonstrated the feasibility of licensing plant-made biopharmaceuticals within the current regulatory framework, it remains the only licensed plant-made vaccine. One of the greatest hurdles in plant protein expression has been achieving sufficient yields of the protein of interest to warrant further development. While the challenge to improve yields has been addressed for many proteins with recombinant protein yields of up to 80% of total soluble protein (TSP) reported using transient viral-based systems, 51% of TSP reported for stable chloroplast transformation and up to 37% of TSP in seed derived from stable nuclear transformation, protein-specific solutions may be required in some cases. Recombinant protein yields need to be assessed on a case-by-case basis; a strategy that may work for the production on one protein may not be applicable to another. Efforts devoted to improving recombinant protein yields in plants have led to the development of novel and varied strategies, including stable or transient, nuclear or plastid production systems, subcellular organelle targeting, codon optimization, or choice of promoter, plant tissue, or species. If sufficient yields can be obtained the next challenge facing development of plant-made vaccines and therapeutics is an understanding of the optimal routes of delivery, which can deliver therapeutics in bioactive forms that are safe, consistent, and efficacious [16].

8.2.1.1.5 ANTIBODIES

Monoclonal antibodies (mAbs) have been critical both for the development of biotechnology itself and as products for both therapeutic and diagnostic importance. Traditional therapeutic monoclonal antibodies have been derived from mice. These proteins were readily identified by the human immune system as foreign, limiting the utility of these antibodies for therapeutic use, especially with repeated dosing. Even in the absence of anaphylaxis or serum sickness, the occurrence of neutralizing antibodies, which inactivate the drug, often precluded further therapeutic use. However, recombinant technologies have allowed murine antibodies to be replaced with partially humanized or chimeric antibodies, and now allow the production of fully human antibodies. The latter may be derived from mice carrying the human immunoglobulin genes or produced using yeast or other gene expression array technologies. Recombinant technology can also be used to selectively "evolve" an antibody gene to produce higher affinity binding (affinity maturation). Thus, compared with earlier monoclonal antibodies, current recombinant antibodies exhibit reduced immunogenicity and increased biological activity.

Recently, the first fully human therapeutic monoclonal antibody has been commercialized (Humira, Adalimumab, Abbott Laboratories), and one would anticipate a low rate of neutralizing antibody development. Currently, there are over a dozen FDA-approved mAbs, and as many as 700 therapeutic Abs may be under development. Plants now have potential as a virtually unlimited source of mAbs, referred to by some as "plantibodies." Tobacco plants have been used extensively for antibody expression systems [17]. However, several other plants have been used including potatoes, soybeans, alfalfa, rice, and corn. Antibody formats can be full-size, Fab fragments, single-chain antibody fragments, bispecific scFv fragments, membrane anchored scFv, or chimeric antibodies. Plant cells, unlike mammalian cell expression systems, can express recombinant secretory IgA (sIgA). sIgA is a complex multisubunit antibody that may be useful in topical immunotherapy, and has been successfully expressed in the tobacco plant. Transgenic soybeans are capable of producing humanized antibodies against herpes simplex virus-2. GE corn reportedly is capable of producing human antibodies at yields of up to 1 kg per acre, and has been demonstrated to preserve antibody function through 5 years of storage under ordinary conditions.

Antibodies derived from plants have a multitude of applications, including binding to pathogenic organisms, binding to serum or body fluid effector proteins (e.g., interleukins), binding to tumor antigens to deliver imaging or antitumor agents, or binding to a cellular receptor site to up- or down-regulate receptor function. However, plant glycosylation patterns differ from those in mammalian systems, and glycosylation is essential for antibody-mediated activation of complement or the initiation of cellular immune responses. Plantibodies may carry plant glycoproteins or may be nonglycosylated as a result of genetically deleting glycosylation sites, but are incapable of inducing the latter phenomenon in either case. This does not appear to be a major limitation, however, since therapeutic applications of monoclonal antibodies are often mediated by binding and inactivation of proteins or receptor molecules and do not require complement or cell-mediated immunity. While glycosylation sequences are poorly immunogenic and hence unlikely to precipitate immunological adverse reactions, the presence of mammalian glycosylation sequences not required for therapeutic function may only serve to produce undesired complement- or cell-mediated side effects.

As of 2001, four antibodies expressed in plants had shown potential to be useful as therapeutics. A chimeric secretory IgG/IgA antibody effective against a surface antigen of *S. mutans* has been expressed in tobacco, and has been demonstrated to be effective against dental caries. Soybeans can express a humanized antiherpes simplex virus (HSV), which has been effective in preventing the transmission of vaginal HSV-2 in animals. Rice and wheat expression systems can produce antibodies against carcinoembryonic antigen, which may be useful for *in vivo* tumor imaging. Finally, a plant viral vector has been used to produce a transiently expressed tumor-specific vaccine in tobacco for the treatment of lymphoma. Currently, seven plant-derived antibodies have reached the advanced stages of clinical product development. These include products directed at the treatment and/or diagnosis of cancer, dental caries, herpes simplex virus, and respiratory syncytial virus. No plantibodies have currently reached the commercialized stage, although at least one product has been tested clinically, and several have been examined *in vitro* and in animal systems and appear to be equivalent to mammalian-cell-derived analogs. Given the high levels of production, purification cost, apparent efficacy, and low immunogenicity of recombinant human antibodies derived from plants, plants appear to hold great potential for future production of monoclonal antibodies [18].

8.2.1.1.6 VACCINES

There has been considerable interest in developing low-cost, edible (i.e., oral) vaccines. Traditional edible vaccines, as for polio, use whole, attenuated organisms or semipurified materials to induce both systemic (Ig-G-mediated) and local membrane (Ig-A-mediated) immunity. Plant-based vaccines cover various proteins in form of antigens obtained from DNA encoded with antigenic sequences from pathogenic viruses, bacteria, and parasites. Key immunogenic proteins or antigenic sequences can be synthesized in plant tissues and subsequently ingested as edible subunit vaccines. The mucosal immune system can induce protective immune responses against pathogens or toxins, and may also be useful to induce tolerance to ingested or inhaled antigens. The production of secretory Ig-A (sIg-A) and provocation of specific immune lymphocytes can occur in mucosal regions, and these regions take on special importance in the development of edible vaccines. Aside from intrinsic low production cost, plant-based vaccines offer a number of unique advantages, including increased safety, stability, versatility, and efficacy. Plant produced vaccines can be grown locally where needed, avoiding storage and transportation costs. Relevant antigens are naturally stored in plant tissue, and oral vaccines can be effectively administered directly in the food product in which they are grown, eliminating purification costs.

In many instances, it appears that refrigeration will not be needed to preserve vaccine efficacy, removing a major impediment to international vaccination efforts of the past. Plants engineered to express only select antigenic portions of the relevant pathogen may reduce immunotoxicity and other adverse effects, and plant-derived vaccines are free of contamination with mammalian viruses. Finally, the development of multicomponent vaccines is possible by insertion of multiple genetic elements or through cross-breeding of transgenic lines

TABLE 8.6   Recombinant Vaccines Expressed in Plants

Year	Vaccine antigen	Species
1992	Hepatitis virus B surface antigen	Tobacco
1995	Malaria parasite antigen	Virus particle
1995	Rabies virus glycoprotein	Tomato
1995	E. coli heat-labile	Tobacco, enterotoxin, potato
1996	Human rhinovirus 14 (HRV-14) and human immunodeficiency virus type (HIV-1) epitopes	Virus particle
1996	Norwalk virus capsid protein	Tobacco, potato
1997	Diabetes-associated autoantigen	Tobacco, potato
1997	Hepatitis B surface proteins	Potato
1997	Mink enteritis virus epitope	Virus particle
1997	Rabies and HIV epitopes	Virus particle
1998	Foot and mouth disease virus VP1 structural protein	Arabidopsis
1998	E. coli heat-labile enterotoxin	Potato
1998	E. coli heat-labile enterotoxin	Potato
1998	Rabies virus	Virus particle
1998	Cholera toxin B subunit	Potato
1998	Human insulin-cholera toxin B subunit fusion protein	Potato
1999	Foot and mouth disease virus VP1 structural protein	Alfalfa
1999	Hepatitis B virus surface antigen	Yellow lupin, lettuce
1999	Human cytomegalovirus glycoprotein B	Tobacco
1999	Dental caries (S. mutans)	Tobacco
1999	Diabetes-associated autoantigen	Tobacco, carrot
2002	Respiratory syncytial virus	Tomato

expressing antigens from various pathogenic organisms. There are, however, some limitations associated with the use of transgenic plants for vaccine production. A major limitation of the expression of recombinant antigens in transgenic plants is obtaining a protein concentration adequate to confer total immunity, given varying protein expression among and within the various plant species. Tight control of expression yields will likely be necessary to reduce variability and assure consistent, effective immunization.

During the last decade, nearly a dozen vaccine antigens have been expressed in plants (Table 8.6). Transgenic potatoes can produce antigens of enterotoxigenic E. coli heat labile enterotoxin B subunit, and is effective in immunizing against viruses and bacteria that cause diarrhea. Still other "edible vaccines" are under development for rabies, foot and mouth disease (veterinary), cholera, and autoimmune diabetes. Transgenic lupin and lettuce plants can express hepatitis B surface antigen. Efforts are under way to develop an "edible vaccine" against the measles virus using the tobacco plant. A plant-based oral subunit vaccine for the respiratory syncytial virus (RSV) using either the apple or the tomato is under development. The plant species to be used for the production and delivery of an oral vaccine can be specifically selected to achieve desired goals. A large number of food plants (e.g., alfalfa, apple, asparagus, banana, barley, cabbage, canola, cantaloupe, carrots, cauliflower, cranberry, cucumber, eggplant, flax, grape, kiwi, lettuce, lupin, maize, melon, papaya, pea, peanut, pepper, plum, potato, raspberry, rice, service berry, soybean, squash, strawberry, sugar beet, sugarcane, sunflower, sweet potato, tomato, walnut, and wheat) have been transformed. Many of the high volume, high acreage plants such as corn, soybean, rice, and wheat may offer advantages. Corn, since it is a major component in the diet of the domestic animal, is a good candidate for vaccine production. In humans, particularly infants, the plant of choice to produce the vaccine might be the banana. Bananas are a common component of many infant diets and can be consumed uncooked, thus eliminating the possibility of protein denaturation due to high temperatures. Unfortunately, it is relatively difficult to create transgenic bananas and the production time is longer than for certain other food crops. Cereals and other edible plants are advantageous for vaccine production over plant species such as tobacco because of the lower levels of toxic metabolites. It is evident that there are numerous opportunities to identify and develop low-cost plant-derived vaccine materials, including edible plant-based vaccines [19].

8.2.1.1.7 OTHER THERAPEUTIC AGENTS

A wide variety of other therapeutic agents have been derived from plants (Tables 8.7 and 8.8), including hormones (somatotropin), enzymes, interleukins, interferons (IFN), and human serum albumin (HSA). Similar biotherapeutic agents have also been expressed from mammalian and bacterial cell systems. There is a worldwide demand for HSA, and plant production would offer the advantage of freedom from contamination with human pathogenic viruses. Modified rice plants are capable of producing human α-1-antitrypsin, a protein that may realize therapeutic potential in emphysema and hepatic diseases. Hirudin, originally isolated from leeches, is a blood anticoagulant that can now be expressed from oilseed rape, tobacco, and mustard. Transgenic potato plants can encode for at least two subtypes of human TNF, some of which may moderate certain cancers and diseases caused by viral agents. Erythropoietin (EPO) can also be expressed in transgenic tobacco plants. Erythropoietin, a

TABLE 8.7 List of Transformed Products

Year	Format	Antibody/antigen	Plant organ	Cellular location	Transformed species
1989	IgG1	Phosphonate ester	Leaf	ER	Tobacco
1990	IgM	NP hapten	Leaf	ER chloroplast	Tobacco
1991	VH domain	Substance P (neuropeptide)	Leaf	Intra- and extracellular	N. benthamiana
1992	scFv	Phytochrome	Leaf	Cytosol	Tobacco
1993	IgG1	Fab human creatine kinase	Leaf	Nucleolus	Tobacco
1993	scFv	Phytochrome	Leaf	Apoplast	Tobacco

TABLE 8.7   List of Transformed Products *(cont.)*

Year	Format	Antibody/antigen	Plant organ	Cellular location	Transformed species
1993	scFv	AMCV	Leaf	Cytosol	*N. benthamiana*
1994	IgG	Fungal cutinase	Root	Apoplast	Tobacco
1994	IgG1	*S. mutans* adhesin	Leaf	Apoplast	Tobacco
1995	IgA/G	*S. mutans* adhesin	Leaf	Apoplast	Tobacco
1995	IgG	TMV	Leaf	Apoplast	Tobacco
1996	scFv	Cutinase	Leaf	ER	Tobacco
1996	IgM	RKN secretion	Leaf root	Apoplast	Tobacco
1996	scFv	BNYVV	Leaf	Apoplast	*N. benthamiana*
1996	scFv	Human creatine kinase	Leaf	Cytoplasm ER	Tobacco
1996	IgG1Fab	Human creatine kinase	Leaf	Apoplast	*A. thaliana*
1997	scFv	β-1,4-Endoglucanase	Root	Cytosol	*Symphytum tuberosum*
1997	scFv	Oxazolone	Leaf	ER	Tobacco
1997	scFv	Abscisic acid	Leaf	ER	Tobacco
1997	scFv	Abscisic acid	Seed	ER	Tobacco
1997	scFv-IT	CD-40	Plant	Apoplast	Tobacco tissue culture
1998	scFv	Oxazolone	Tuber	ER	Potato
1998	Humanized IgG	HSV-2	Plant	Secretory pathway	Soybean
1998	scFv	Dihydro-flavonol 4-reductase	Leaf	Sytosol	*Petunia hybrida*
1999	IgG	Human IgG	Plant	Apoplast	Alfalfa
1999	scFv	CEA	Leaf	Transient expression	Tobacco
1999	scFv	Topoviruses	Plant	ER, apoplast	*N. benthamiana*
1999	bi-scFv	TMV	Leaf	ER, apoplast	Tobacco cell suspension
1999	scFv	TMV	Plant	Cytosol	Tobacco
1999	scFv	CEA	Cell	ER, apoplast	Rice suspension cells
1999	scFv	38C13 mouse B-cell lymphoma A	Leaf	Apoplast	*N. benthamiana*
2000	scFv	CEA	Plant ER	Apoplast	Rice, wheat
2000	scFv	TMV	Leaf	Apoplast, membrin	Tobacco

CEA, carcinoembryonic antigen; ER, endoplasmic reticulum; AMCV, artichoke mottle crinkle virus; TMV, tobacco mosaic virus; RKN, root knot nematode; BNYVV, beet necrotic yellow vein virus; HSV-2, herpes simplex virus-2; scFv-IT, scFv-bryodin-immunotoxin. *N. benthamiana*, tobacco (*Nicotiana*)-related species; *A. thaliana*, *Arabidopsis*, an experimental species.
Table modified from Fischer and Emansv [20].

TABLE 8.8   Comparison of Recombinant Protein Production in Plants, Yeast, and Mammalian Systems

	Transgenic plants	Plant viruses	Yeast	Bacteria	Mammalian cell cultures	Transgenic animals
Cost/storage	Cheap/RT	Cheap/20°C	Cheap/20°C	Cheap/20°C	Expensive	Expensive
Distribution	Easy	Easy	Feasible	Feasible	Difficult	Difficult
Gene size	Not limited	Limited	Unknown	Unknown	Limited	Limited
Glycosylation	Correct?	Correct?	Incorrect	Absent	Correct	Correct
Multimeric protein assembly (SigA)	Yes	No	No	No	No	Yes
Production cost	Low	Low	Medium	Medium	High	High
Production scale	Worldwide	Worldwide	Limited	Limited	Limited	Limited
Production vehicle	Yes	Yes	Yes	Yes	Yes	Yes
Propagation	Easy	Feasible	Easy	Easy	Hard	Feasible
Protein folding accuracy	High?	High?	Medium	Low	High	High
Protein homogeneity	High?	Medium	Medium	Low	Medium	High
Protein yield	High	Very high	High	Medium	Medium–High	High
Public perception of risk	High	High	Medium	Low	Medium	High
Safety	High	High	Unknown	Low	Medium	High
Scale-up costs	Low	Low	High**	High**	High**	High
Therapeutic risk*	Unknown	Unknown	Unknown	Yes	Yes	Yes
Time required	Medium	Low	Medium	Low	High	High

Residual viral sequences, oncogenes, endotoxins.
Large, expensive fermenters. Table modified from Fischer and Emans [20].

glycoprotein used to treat anemia, was commercialized from mammalian systems nearly 20 years ago. Blood substitutes such as human hemoglobin have long been pursued, and human hemoglobin derived from transgenic tobacco is being tested to ensure the molecules' function and oxygen carrying capacity. In general, the levels of pharmaceutical proteins produced by transgenic plants have been low, often <1% of total soluble protein. While this is quite sufficient to allow for economical production of highly active pharmaceutical molecules, improved technologies for high-level expression of protein will be probably needed to allow practical production of high volume human replacement proteins such as HSA, hemoglobin, or blood coagulation factors [21].

8.2.1.1.8 ADVANTAGES OF TRANSGENIC PLANTS AS HOST

- Potentially attractive recombinant protein producer
- Low cost of plant cultivation
- Harvest equipment/methodologies are inexpensive and well established
- Ease of scale-up
- Proteins expressed in seeds are generally stable
- Plant-based systems are free of human pathogens (e.g., HIV) [22]

8.2.1.1.9 DISADVANTAGES OF TRANSGENIC PLANTS AS HOST

- Variable/low expression levels of proteins
- Potential occurrence of posttranslational gene silencing
- Different glycosylation pattern from that in humans
- Seasonal/geographical nature of plant growth

The most likely focus of future transgenic plants is the production of oral vaccines in edible plants or fruit, such as tomatoes and bananas. Ingestion of transgenic plant tissue expressing recombinant subunit vaccines induces the production of antigen-specific antibody responses. Direct consumption of this type of plant material provides a cheap, efficient, and technically straightforward mode of large-scale vaccine delivery. On the contrary, edible vaccines have some serious concerns, as immunogenicity of orally administered vaccines varies widely, stability of antigens in the digestive tract varies widely, and genetics of many potential systems remain poorly characterized (inefficient transformation systems and low expression levels) [22].

8.2.2 Bacteria

Production in *E. coli* lacks the machinery to perform posttranslational modifications (such as N- and O-glycosylation, fatty acid acylation, phosphorylation, and disulfide bond formation), which are often required for proper assembly and functionality of a protein. Simple proteins that are not glycosylated (such as insulin and human growth hormone) or that, while glycosylated in their native form, do not require glycosylation for pharmacological activity [such as α-, β-, and γ-interferon (IF), interleukin-2 (IL-2), or TNF-α] are mainly produced in *E. coli* [23].

The most common microbial species to produce heterologous proteins (proteins that do not occur in host cells) of therapeutic interest is *E. coli*. The first therapeutic protein produced by *E. coli* was human insulin (Humulin) in 1982 and tPA (tissue plasminogen activator) in 1996.

8.2.2.1 *Major Advantages of* E. coli

- Because of its well-characterized molecular biology, it serves as the model system for prokaryotic genetics.
- It has high-level expression of heterologous proteins [high expression promoters (~30% of total cellular protein)].
- Easy and simple process ensures rapid growth, simple and inexpensive media, appropriate fermentation technology, large-scale cultivation.

8.2.2.2 *Major Disadvantages of* E. coli

- Intracellular accumulation of proteins in the cytoplasm.
  - Complicated downstream processing compared to extracellular production
  - Additional primary processing steps: cellular homogenization, subsequent removal of cell debris by filtration or centrifugation
  - Extensive purification steps to separate the protein of interest
- Inclusion body.
  - Insoluble aggregates of partially folded protein
  - Formation via intermolecular hydrophobic interactions and high-level expression of heterologous proteins overload the normal cellular protein-folding mechanisms: hydrophobic patch is exposed, promoting aggregate formation via intermolecular hydrophobic interactions
- Inability to undertake posttranslational modification, especially glycosylation: limitation to the production of glycoproteins
- The presence of lipopolysaccharide (LPS) on its surface induces a pyrogenic nature, which leads to a more complicated purification procedure

8.2.3 Mammalian Cell Culture

There are currently many established mammalian cell lines for the production of proteins, especially those needed for therapeutic applications. The cell lines are often considered ideal since they are, in many cases, capable of producing proteins with all of the posttranslational modifications required for clinical efficacy. Chinese hamster ovary cells, or CHO cells, are the most well known and commonly used in industry today, with some companies claiming that more protein species are being produced in CHO cells than *E. coli* or yeast. Other mammalian cell lines used for production include Syrian hamster kidney or baby hamster kidney (BHK) cells, and hybridoma cells. In addition to production of recombinant proteins such as human factor VII, BHK cells are also known for their susceptibility to viruses and therefore have been used extensively for virus growth and vaccine production. Other cell lines available are Madine Darby canine kidney (MDCK), Vero cells (derived from the kidney of a normal, adult, African green monkey), and Per.C6 cells (human fetal retinoblast cells immortalized by transfection with the E1 mini gene of adenovirus); all of which have proven useful for the production of influenza vaccine. It should be noted, however, that mammalian cells do have variations in glycosylation depending on the animal species from which the cells were derived. Other disadvantages are that the development of large-scale expression techniques is time consuming and requires high initial financial investment [24]. Furthermore, mammalian cells require a nutrient media that is more complex than that of bacteria, fungi, or plants, and susceptible to carry human pathogens.

Ultimately, when all these variables are taken into consideration the cost of the resulting product is quite substantial. For the production of more complex proteins requiring posttranslational modifications, the CHO cell is mainly used. Blockbuster therapeutic mAbs such as trastuzumab (Herceptin), bevacizumab (Avastin), and rituximab (Rituxan/Mabthera) are produced in CHO cells. Further, mammalian cell types used for the commercial production of approved protein drugs are BHK cells, mouse myeloma cell lines (used for the production of palivizumab/Synagis) such as NS0, J558L, or Sp2/0, as well as hybridoma cell lines (for the production of antibodies such as muromonab-CD3/Orthoclone OKT3 or basiliximab/Simulect). While mammalian cells provide the full posttranslational machinery, their handling, media, and fermentation requirements are far from trivial, and low titers of the transgenic proteins produced are a problem despite recent developments [25].

8.2.3.1 *Major Advantage*

- CHO and BHK cells are most common cell lines used for this purpose and the typical proteins produced in animal cells are EPO, tPA, interferons, immunoglobulin antibodies, blood factors, etc. Animal cells are suitable for production of glycoprotein, especially glycosylation.

8.2.3.2 *Major Disadvantages*
- Very complex nutritional requirements: growth factors are expensive and complicate the purification procedure.
- Slow growth rate, that is, long cultivation time and more susceptible to physical damage.
- Higher production cost.

8.2.4 Yeast

S. cerevisiae is also an established fungus for the production of biopharmaceuticals such as human insulin, glucagon, and hirudin, in cases where the yeast-specific glycosylation is not an issue. It grows rapidly and to high cell densities, is neither pyrogenic nor pathogenic, and has a GRAS (generally recognized as safe) status indicating that it is considered as a safe production host [26].

8.2.4.1 *Major Advantages*
- The molecular biology of yeast is well characterized to facilitate genetic manipulation.
- Yeast is considered as GRAS-listed organism with a long history of industrial applications (e.g., brewing and baking).
- Fast growth in relatively inexpensive media and suitable industrial-scale fermentation equipment/technology are already available.
- Posttranslational modifications of proteins, especially glycosylation, occur in yeast (host) that offers the better yield of biopaharmaceuticals.

8.2.5 Fungi

Fungi have shown great promise in the production of foreign proteins and several species are most commonly exploited. *Saccharomyces*, *Pichia*, and *Hansenula* have been used for their efficient protein expression, capacity for posttranslational protein modification, and relatively high fermentation rates. One of the most well-known examples is the utilization of *S. cerevisiae* for the production of a hepatitis B surface antigen-based vaccine (Engerix-B made by GlaxoSmithKline and Recombivax HB made by Merck). Similarly, molds such as *Trichoderma* and *Aspergilli* have been used for their high protein expression levels. Though these lower eukaryotes show great promise, they have a number of technical issues that need to be resolved. Two of the most prevalent issues are the loss of plasmid and dramatic decrease in protein yield during large-scale production. It also has been shown that both N- and O-linked oligosaccharide structures in these systems are much different than their mammalian counterparts. Hypermannosylation is a common occurrence in yeast leading to compromised protein structure and therefore loss of the desired activity. *Aspergillus niger* is mainly used for production of industrial enzymes such as α-amylase, glucoamylase, cellulase, lipase, protease, etc. [27].

8.2.5.1 *Advantages*
- High-level expression of heterologous proteins (~30 g/L)
- Secretion of proteins into extracellular media (easy and simple separation procedure)
- Posttranslational modifications: glycosylation and different glycosylation pattern compared to that in humans

8.2.5.2 *Disadvantage*

- Produces significant quantities of extracellular proteases (degradation of heterologous proteins and use of mutant strain with reduced level of proteases).

8.2.6 Insect Cells

In this system, laboratory-scale production of proteins is done by infection of cultured insect cells with an engineered baculovirus (a viral family that naturally infects insects) carrying the gene coding for a target protein. The most commonly used systems are silkworm virus *Bombyx mori* nuclear polyhedrovirus (BmNPV) in conjunction with cultured silkworm cells and the virus *Autographa californica* nuclear polyhedrovirus (AcNPV) in conjunction with cultured armyworm cells [28].

In 1983, a cell line derived from *Spodoptera frugiperda*, infected with an expression vector based on the Baculoviridae virus *A. californica*, was used to produce human β-interferon. Since then, this approach has been increasingly used for the production of foreign proteins. Insect cells have posttranslational protein modification machinery suitable for making complex mammalian proteins. In addition, baculoviruses are not infectious to vertebrates and their promoters are inactive in mammalian cells, giving them an advantage over other systems for the expression of a broad range of targets, including oncogenes [29]. In 2007, the first insect cell-derived vaccine, a vaccine against human papilloma virus with relevance to the control of human cancer, was licensed by GlaxoSmithKline. Though this system has a number of advantages, several disadvantages exist. It has been shown that internal cleavage at arginine- or lysine-rich sequences is extremely inefficient and leads to improperly processed proteins. Furthermore, glycosylation capability is limited only to the high mannose type and not processed to complex oligosaccharides containing fucose, galactose, and sialic acid [30].

8.2.6.1 Advantages
- High-level intracellular protein expression
- Use of strong promoter derived from the viral polyhedrin: ~30–50% of total intracellular protein, cultivation at high growth rate, and less expensive media than animal cell lines
- No infection of human pathogens, for example, HIV

8.2.6.2 Disadvantages
- Low level of extracellular secreted target protein
- Glycosylation patterns: incomplete and different
- No therapeutic protein approved for human use

8.2.7 Transgenic Animals

Transgenic technology has allowed for recombinant protein production in living animals such as rabbits, goats, pigs, and cows. For example, the production of human hemoglobin A in pig's blood. However, due to the inherent chemical complexity of blood, target protein purification requires the use of high-cost and complicated procedures. Also, blood cannot be used as a site of accumulation for biologically active proteins such as cytokines and hormones without creating serious health problems for the transgenic animal, as seen in transgenic pigs producing high levels of human growth hormone. This does not rule out the production of normal constituents of blood such as hemoglobin, antibodies, and α-1-antitrypsin. Recombinant proteins are expressed in mammary glands of animals including mice, rabbits, goats, sheep, and cows. The natural secretory properties of this gland are expected to decrease the risk to transgenic animals, potentially allowing for the production of highly bioactive proteins. One of the most encouraging examples of protein production in transgenic animals was the expression of human α-1-antitrypsin where 50% of the total milk protein was the protein of interest. Though recent data for these systems are encouraging, the technology is still young and has many obstacles to overcome. The process of producing transgenic animals is costly, tedious, time consuming, and technically challenging, and like mammalian cell lines, animals are susceptible to human pathogens [31–33].

Goats and sheep are the most attractive host system and they have following advantages:

- High milk production capacities: 700–800 L/year in the case of goat
- Ease of handling and breeding and ease of harvesting of crude product, that is, simply requires the animal to be milked
- Preavailability of commercial milking systems with maximum process hygiene
- Low capital investment: relatively low-cost animals replace high-cost traditional cultivation equipment, and low running costs
- High expression levels of proteins are potentially attained: >1 g protein/L milk

8.3 DIFFERENT MODES OF DELIVERY SYSTEMS USED FOR PLANT-BASED BIOPHARMACEUTICALS

8.3.1 Parenteral Delivery

The parenteral route remains the most effective route of vaccine administration. There are some perceived disadvantages of parenteral delivery including the need to purify vaccines to a standard compliant with cGMP, which often results in a soluble product that requires cold chain logistics to maintain product integrity during transportation and storage. Not only does this increase the financial burden of therapy but can be logistically problematic given that regions of the world that are in greatest need experience a warm–hot climate and/or may be inaccessible by vehicle. Injected therapeutics requires administration by health care professionals and imposes risks of needle-stick injury and contamination by infectious agents if appropriate practices are not adhered to. There is also reduced patient compliance due to the physical discomfort and even fear involved with needle delivery.

Parenteral delivery refers to a route of administration that usually involves one or more injections to penetrate the skin or mucosal membrane, bypassing the gastrointestinal tract. This includes subcutaneous, intramuscular, intradermal, intraperitoneal, intralymphatic, and intravenous injection. In human drug delivery, intramuscular and intravenous are the predominant delivery routes due to their convenience of administration and in the case of intravenous, speed of circulation. The epidermal and dermal layers of the skin comprise an important network of frontline immunity including antigen-presenting cells (APCs) such as dendritic cells (DCs) (Langerhans cells), keratinocytes, and lymphocytes. Also between these two layers is a dense network of lymphatic vessels draining into lymph nodes. Immunogens injected into the skin are delivered from the peripheral tissue at the site of injection to the lymph nodes in a size-dependent manner by either direct drainage or cellular transport. DCs residing at both the periphery and lymph nodes are key players in trafficking the antigen and directing protective immune responses. Traffic of larger molecules or particles (500–2000 nm) is mediated by Langerhans cells. Once activated the Langerhans cells mature, take up, process, and transport the immunogen to lymph nodes. In contrast, smaller molecules or particles (20–200 nm), including free antigens and virus-like particles (VLPs), drain freely to the lymph nodes where they are taken up by the residing DCs. The route of parenteral administration may dictate the type and quality of immune response elicited based on the type of APCs encountered. Intraperitoneal immunization is often associated with uptake by macrophages, while intradermal immunization is associated with uptake by DCs.

Comparison of subcutaneous, intradermal, intramuscular, and intralymphatic administration of ovalbumin (two doses of 20 μg) suggests that while all routes efficiently deliver antigen to lymphoid organs to evoke antigen-specific T-helper (Th) 2-type immune responses, Th1 responses were more sensitive to the route of administration with only weak responses observed for subcutaneous, intradermal, and intramuscular routes. The inclusion of adjuvants improved the strength of the elicited immune responses across all administration routes. Earlier studies indicate that the Th response is dose sensitive with low doses preferentially stimulating Th2 responses while Th1 responses require higher doses. These observations suggest that while adjuvants may generally improve immune responses, improved Th1 responses may benefit from increased doses when administering antigens via subcutaneous, intradermal, or intramuscular routes.

The first parenterally (subcutaneous) delivered plant-made vaccine to undergo human Phase I clinical trial was an idiotype vaccine for treatment of non-Hodgkin's lymphoma. Patient-specific tumor-derived single chain variable fragments were transiently expressed in *Nicotiana benthamiana* leaves using a plant virus-based vector. Production and purification to cGMP standards occurred within 12–16 weeks of receiving patient biopsy samples, comparing favorably with animal cell approaches [34]. A rapid production system means that vaccines could be administered to newly diagnosed patients before exposure to immunosuppressive treatments such as chemotherapy. This unique feature suggests a niche application for plant-made, patient-specific, recombinant, idiotype vaccines for the treatment of tumors. Subcutaneous administration of the plant-made, patient-specific, non-Hodgkin's lymphoma vaccines was found to be safe, well tolerated, and in most cases vaccine-specific humoral responses and/or cell responses were reported [35].

8.3.1.1 *Processing and Purification*

All plant biomass for use as a therapeutic or vaccine, particularly if delivered parenterally, will require some form of processing in order to obtain a homogeneous batch with a uniform distribution of the antigen or therapeutic to ensure accurate dosage. Plant biomass will also require a level of processing compliant with cGMP of relevant regulatory agencies such as the US Food and Drug Administration (FDA), European Medicines Agency (EMA), or the World Health Organization (WHO), to yield a safe and well-defined product. The feasibility for purification of commercial quantities of recombinant plant-made proteins of pharmaceutical value has been demonstrated previously for avidin, aprotinin, monoclonal antibodies, bovine trypsin, human insulin, and apolipoprotein AI.

The way forward in the development of plant-made vaccines and therapeutics is to improve bioavailability of the delivered material. This can be achieved through rational and innovative design strategies for better protection and targeting of relevant cellular pathways and immune responsive sites. Also, less invasive alternatives to traditional injections in the form of microneedles should be explored as a means of parenteral delivery with improved patient compliance.

8.3.1.2 *Adjuvants and Biodegradable Carrier Vehicles*

Adjuvants are defined as molecules that modulate the immune response when coadministered with an antigen, but are themselves not immunogenic. They are often used to improve upon weak immunogenic responses associated with subunit vaccines and can direct the immune system to favor Th1 or Th2 responses. Although their mode of action is often unclear, adjuvants can improve immune responses by acting as a depot to guide antigens to relevant sites, protect them from degradation, control release, and activate APCs. They can be naturally occurring in plants, such as lectins and saponins, or can be produced in plants as recombinant proteins. A benefit of using plants as a production platform is that they are capable of expressing, processing, and assembling complex, recombinant immunogenic complexes. These self-adjuvanting complexes may comprise ligands for pattern recognition receptors, antigen and self-specific antibodies, or cytokines. Adjuvants can be codelivered with an antigen at the time of administration or incorporated with the antigen into particulate delivery systems. Biodegradable particle carriers or delivery vehicles are composed of various materials such as lipids, proteins, starch, polysaccharides, or polyesters, and like adjuvants are immunogenically inert.

Incorporation of antigens and adjuvant into the delivery vehicle ensures that both reach the same population of APCs. The therapeutic cargo can be either encapsulated by the particle by entrapment, or linked to the surface by chemical conjugation or physical adsorption. The method chosen to associate antigen and particle should be that which affords minimal risk of damage to the antigen. Encapsulated antigens are afforded protection from extracellular proteases during trafficking to the target immune responsive sites. Ideally the carrier particle will erode at a rate sufficient to sustain prolonged exposure to APCs including DCs, macrophages, and monocytes. Consequently, the choice of material used to form the particle is critical to maximize bioavailability of its cargo. A fine balancing act is required to avoid overprotection of the encapsulated antigen, inhibiting release of the therapeutic or premature release if protection is inadequate. In either case the reduced bioavailability of the therapeutic would result in weakened host immune responses. If controlled and sustained release can be achieved it may permit single dose immunization schedules. Particulate carriers may offer better targeting for parenteral delivery. In this respect, size is important. Nanoparticles ($\leq$100 nm) are able to move through biological barriers such as membranes and along blood and lymph vessels after injection more efficiently than larger particles. Alternatively, incorporation of ligands for pattern recognition receptors, such as toll-like receptors, into the design of the particle carrier can facilitate delivery to specific immune responsive sites or cells [36].

Structures such as liposomes, VLPs, virosomes, and immunostimulatory complexes (ISCOMs) combine the advantages of both particulate carrier and adjuvant. Moreover, they are particularly well recognized by APCs because they have characteristics, including size, shape, and surface properties that are similar to viral and bacterial pathogens that the immune system has evolved to attack. VLPs, for example, comprise viral envelope proteins that enable them to self-assemble to closely resemble viruses, but lack the genetic material rendering them noninvasive but readily identifiable by the host immune system. VLP-based vaccines have the added benefit of having been successfully produced in plants. ISCOMs are comprised of antigen, cholesterol, phospholipid, and an adjuvant of Quil A saponin from the bark of *Quillaja saponaria*. They are within the size range of viruses (~40 nm) and are readily taken up by DCs, macrophages, and monocytes [37]. Furthermore, they are stable for up to 3 months at 37°C, 2 years at 2–8°C, can sustain multiple freeze–thaw cycles, and are manufactured at pH 6.2 in phosphate buffered saline. Clinical studies have shown that ISCOM adjuvanted viral vaccines are well tolerated both orally and parenterally in humans and stimulate both cellular and humoral immune responses against antigens for human immunodeficiency virus, herpes simplex virus, human papilloma virus, hepatitis C virus, influenza, as well as cancer. These attributes may make ISCOMs an ideal formulation partner for purified plant-made vaccines, providing a means not only to enhance immunogenicity but also to confer the stability required to avoid the cold chain when distributing to warmer climates [38].

8.3.1.3 *Nonbiodegradable Particles*

An alternative to biodegradable, particulate carriers is solid nanoparticle carriers. It has been hypothesized that if gold, silver, latex, silica, or polystyrene particles remain in tissues for extended periods of time, antigen presentation will also be prolonged resulting in strengthened immune responses. The potential for solid nanoparticles as carriers for parenteral delivery of therapeutics and vaccines has been demonstrated in mice. Metal nanoparticles can be engineered in plants in diverse species including alfalfa, cucumber, red clover, ryegrass, sunflower, and oregano, or from plant extracts. The system is flexible, allowing size and geometry of metal particles to be manipulated by simply altering plant growth conditions. Antigens or peptides can be coupled to the metal particle but unfortunately few conjugation sites are available, often resulting in inadequate epitope presentation. Additionally, the coupling processes are inconsistent and can result in aggregates and precipitates [39].

8.3.1.4 Microneedles

A promising alternative to injections are dissolving microneedle patches developed by Sullivan et al. in 2010. The microneedles are 650 μm in length and made from a biocompatible water-soluble polymer (polyvinylpyrrolidone). The microneedles deliver the encapsulated vaccine through the epidermis to a depth that optimizes exposure to APCs in the skin. Upon application, the microneedles become inserted into the skin and dissolve to within 89% of its mass in 5 min. As the needles dissolve the vaccine load is released and deposited within the epidermis. Studies in mice showed that delivery of a lyophilized inactivated influenza virus vaccine using the microneedle patch produced antibody and cellular immune responses equivalent to a single intramuscular injection. In challenge studies, the microneedle patch outperformed intramuscular injection. Although both routes of administration were protective 30 days after vaccination, at 90 days mice immunized by a microneedle patch showed a 1000-fold better clearance of the virus, had better cellular immune responses and more antibody-secreting cells in the spleen and lungs than those immunized intramuscularly. Microneedle technology overcomes many of the problems associated with injections. The patches are stable at ambient temperature, by dissolving upon application they eliminate the risk of needle-stick injury and biohazard waste disposal, and they can be self-administered, overcoming needle phobia and improving patient compliance. The technology should be applicable to any plant-made antigens or therapeutic that will withstand lyophilization and encapsulation during polymerization. However, no matter the method, the antigen to be entrapped or carried requires purification. This purification and association with the delivery vehicle add extra time and cost to the processing of the vaccine and therefore would most likely prohibit use in the developing world and some veterinary industries such as poultry.

8.3.2 Mucosal Delivery of Therapeutics and Vaccines

The mucosal surfaces are a popular site for delivering therapeutic small molecules due to the ease of administration and speed of uptake across the large surface areas. However, development of orally delivered peptide and protein therapeutics has been hampered by the inherent proteolytic and hydrolytic environment of the mucosal surfaces. The physical encapsulation within plant cells has been suggested as a means by which protein therapeutics may be protected during transit in the gastrointestinal tract, and several studies have indicated that plants are also successful at delivering recombinant proteins and therapeutics orally. However, in addition to transit across the epithelium, a strong tolerating response to therapeutic proteins including proinsulin and clotting factor IX has been observed. In a conundrum, the principal mucosal immunoglobulin (Ig) IgA, involved in protective mucosal immune responses (in its secretary form), also appears to be extensively implicated in tolerating responses to mucosally delivered antigens when not secreted. The mechanism that determines whether a tolerating or immunogenic response is made is unknown and poses the conundrum: how can therapeutics be delivered orally without inducing an undesirable immune response?

One of the oldest aims of plant-produced therapeutics is to activate the mucosal immune response to enable immunization against infectious disease. While parenteral delivery of vaccine antigens is capable of generating protective systemic immune responses, the administration of vaccines at mucosal surfaces is often immunologically superior at protecting mucosal sites than needle-based delivery. However, due to the inherent problems determining the dose, release kinetics, and host variability, there have been limited oral vaccines reaching the market. Recent advances in understanding the complex environment of the mucosal immune response system are driving improvement of the efficacy, consistency, and versatility of mucosa vaccination [39].

8.3.2.1 Plants as Delivery Vehicles for Mucosal Vaccines

There have been many preclinical trials with minimally processed plant cells, but only a few trials in which unpurified plant materials have been orally administered to humans. These include two trials using the B subunit of heat-labile enterotoxin from enterotoxigenic *E. coli* delivered in potato tubers and maize seed, the viral capsid protein of Norwalk virus delivered in potato tubers, hepatitis B surface antigen from transgenic lettuce leaves and potato tubers, and lettuce leaves expressing a genetic fusion of peptides from the rabies virus glycoprotein and nucleoprotein with the viral coat protein of alfalfa mosaic virus. In all trials, serum and mucosal immune responses were variable; however, no toxic safety concerns were observed. Protection during digestion of antigens may be facilitated by plant cells themselves, and modern plant expression techniques can extend this encapsulation either via the aggregation of proteins into chloroplasts, protein bodies, nonlytic vacuoles, or within the endomembrane system of the plant cell [40].

8.3.2.2 Receptor-Targeting Ligands

There has been significant investigation into identifying receptor-mediated pathways for targeting epithelial cells, rather than simply flooding the luminal space with formulated antigen and relying on standard antigen uptake processes. While not highly immunogenic itself, the plant lectin UAE-1 from *Ulex europaeus*-I has been extensively characterized for binding the apical surfaces of epithelial and endothelial cells and is one of the classical markers of epithelial cells, leading to the suggestion for a role as a localizing molecule for vaccine development. When used as an epithelial localizing agent in the formulation of poly(DL-lactide-*co*-glycolide) microparticles containing human immunodeficiency virus peptides, UAE-1-coated particles generated a more rapid response than uncoated particles when administered via the oral route, and an increased rate and intensity of response to human immunodeficiency virus peptides were observed when delivered via the intranasal route. UAE-1 and other plant lectins have also been shown to be effective targeting molecules for many types of delivery vehicle. An advantage of plant biotechnology is that recombinant lectin can be expressed in plants as a genetic fusion with an antigen of interest [41]. The potential for such a strategy was successfully demonstrated by Medina-Bolivar et al. who expressed ricin B in tobacco as a fusion with GFP. In this study, ricin B retained its specificity to bind galactose/galactosamine cell surface receptors and deliver its fusion partner to the mucosal surface to elicit systemic and mucosal immune responses. Other receptor-targeting ligands include invasin from *Yersinia* sp. and the RGD motif of fibronectin. Both have been shown to increase the binding of latex nanoparticles to human immune follicle-associated epithelium and induce an improved immune response to poly(DL-lactide-*co*-glycolide) particles containing ovalbium [42].

8.3.2.3 *The AB5 Toxins as Adjuvants*

Cholera toxin was first suggested as an oral adjuvant after it was found to prevent oral tolerance to another otherwise tolerogenic protein, keyhole limpet hemocyanin, when coadministered orally to mice. Mutants that fully or partially abrogate the catalytic function of the A or B ganglioside-binding subunits have also been extensively investigated as both adjuvants and carrier proteins. Moreover, the B subunit of heat-labile enterotoxin from enterotoxigenic *E. coli* was one of the first vaccine antigens or adjuvants expressed in plant cells. Paradoxically, when chemically conjugated to other antigens the cholera toxin subunit B can in some cases induce oral tolerance. The relationship between tolerance or immune induction and dose, schedule, conjugation method, antigen, and species has not yet been elucidated, and there is growing evidence that suggests that the B subunits may directly stimulate the innate immune system in the absence of the A subunit, steering a Th2 and Th17 response instead of the canonical whole toxin Th1 response. The interaction between these two subunits has been explored using chimeric proteins with only the holotoxin-interacting domain of the A subunit fused to streptococcal adhesion antigen, and in similar fusions including tuberculosis antigens early secretory antigenic target 6 and antigen 85b in plants (Claire Penney, unpublished data); no tolerogenic effects have been observed following oral immunization in mice [43].

8.3.2.4 *Saponins*

Saponins are a diverse group of metabolic glycosides present in many higher plants. Of importance to therapeutic and vaccine delivery is the ability of many saponins to potentiate systemic and oral delivery of antigens. Crudely processed saponin extracts may be too toxic for parenteral delivery in humans, yet crudely prepared saponins from the *Q. saponaria* Molina have been used extensively in injected veterinary vaccines since the 1950s, and have been investigated for their adjuvant function during oral delivery. Early animal studies indicated that many viral proteins formulated with Quil A containing ISCOMs became highly potent at inducing IgA, IgG2a, and cytotoxic T-lymphocyte responses upon oral delivery. Investigation of saponins as adjuvants during oral delivery suggests that saponin and ISCOMs are more rapidly transcytosed by APCs including DCs and macrophages compared to antigen alone, and are more rapidly transported to the draining lymph nodes than soluble protein [44]. Despite being already produced in plants and well tolerated orally, saponins and ISCOMs have been infrequently investigated in plant-vaccine trials, with only four trials using saponins delivered orally. When orally coadministered with a crudely purified plant-made measles virus H protein vaccine, food-grade *Quillaja* bark extract was a more efficient adjuvant than the nontoxic enterotoxigenic *E. coli* heat labile toxin mutant, LTR192G, cholera toxin/cholera toxin B subunit. This response may be due to a possible adjuvant role for saponins in increasing the permeability of the intestinal epithelium to facilitate transit of high molecular compounds across the mucosa. For low-cost oral vaccine purposes, it would be ideal to express an antigen complex in a host plant capable of direct or indirect modulation [45]. The principal saponin in unripe coperscium fruit and leaves is the glycoside alpha-tomatine, which exhibits diverse bioactivity similar to *Quillaja*-derived saponins, making it a potential candidate for oral vaccine formulation. Alpha-tomatine has been shown to act as a potent adjuvant to steer oral and subcutaneous delivery of the Norwalk virus capsid protein expressed in tomato and delivered as a crude, dried preparation toward a Th1, IgG2a dominant response in rats (Robert Shepherd, unpublished data). The large hollow tubular structures of 100–160 nm width and up to 3000 nm length formed by alpha-tomatine have been suggested to act not only as an antigen "depot" slowing release of antigen into the major histocompatibility complex (MHC) class II pathway following phagocytosis by APCs, but also to directly stimulate loading of antigen onto MHC class I molecules, and the potent cholesterol-binding ability of alpha-tomatine may be trafficked via lipid rafts on epithelial cells [46].

8.3.2.5 *Genetic-Encoded Particles*

In addition to receptor-mediated and encapsulated strategies for transporting antigens across epithelial membranes, nonreplicating VLPs may also be a key tool in generating immunity instead of tolerance at the mucosal surface. By their inherent adaptation to environmental stresses, many nonenveloped mammalian mucosal viruses are also stable at low pH and are resistant to proteolytic degradation. When expressed in plant cells, many recombinant VLPs have been shown to correctly assemble into tertiary structures indistinguishable from their native conformation. Of those mammalian VLPs produced in plant systems, many have been shown to be orally immunogenic in rodents, including the hepatitis B surface antigen VLPs, Norwalk VLPs, and human papilloma VLPs. Of these, Norwalk and hepatitis B surface antigen are also orally immunogenic in humans [47].

8.4 STABILITY OF PROTEINS AND PEPTIDES

Proteins are biochemical compounds consisting of one or more polypeptides typically folded into a globular or fibrous form, facilitating a biological function. Peptide chains in peptides and proteins are seldom linear and adapt a variety of specific folded three-dimensional patterns and conformations. Conformation in a peptide chain is determined by the covalently bonded amino acids sequence, by disulfide bridges between cysteine residues, and by total conformational energy [48]. Various stability issues faced by biopharmaceuticals are highlighted in Fig. 8.2.

8.4.1 Properties Affected by Instability

- Physical properties include solubility and spectral properties such as circular dichorism.
- Chemical properties include alteration of stabilized reactive group or group sterically shielded from the reagents.
- Biological properties include 3D structures that place catalytic groups into proper orientation for enzymatic activity or place backbone and side-chain groups into proper orientation for hormone receptor interaction.
- Stability to enzymatic cleavage is affected since some of the amide groups susceptible to proteolysis are deterred due to sterical peptide chain orientation.

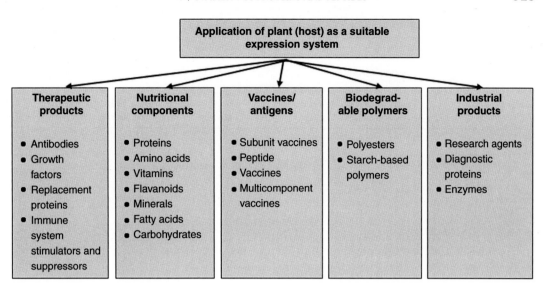

FIGURE 8.2   Applications of host as a suitable expression system.

8.4.1.1 Physical Stability

- Physical instability involves transformations in the secondary, tertiary, or quaternary structure of the molecule.

8.4.1.1.1 DENATURATION

- Any nonproteolytic modification of the unique structure of a native protein affects definite changes in physical, chemical, and biological properties.
- Peptides and proteins are comprised of both polar amino residues and nonpolar amino acid residues.

Factors that favor denaturation

- Change of solvent from an aqueous to organic solvents or to a mixed solvent.
- Breakup of hydrophobic and hydrogen bonds.
- pH changes – alters the ionization of the carboxylic acid and amino acids and therefore the charges carried by the molecules.
- Alteration in the ionic strength and rise in temperature.
- Denaturation may be reversible or irreversible.

Denaturation may lead to decrease in solubility, alteration in surface tension, loss of crystallizing ability, changes in constituent group reactivity and molecular profile, vulnerability to enzymatic degradation, loss or alteration of antigenicity, and loss of specific biological activity [49]. Several denaturing agents and their respective mechanism of actions are described in Table 8.9.

TABLE 8.9   Denaturing Agents

Category	Mechanism	Examples
Polar and protic chemicals	Disrupt H-bonds	Urea, guanidine HCl, alcohol, acetic acid
Surfactants	Hydrophobic disruption and charge group separation	Sodium dodecyl sulfate, polyethylene glycol, dodecyl ammonium chloride

Methods to prevent denaturation

- Denaturated protein is restored on removal of denaturants.
- pH, ionic strength, and temperature are maintained.

8.4.1.1.2 ADSORPTION

Peptides and proteins are amphiphilic in nature, hence they tend to adsorb at interfaces such as air/water and air/solid (polar, hydrophilic; nonpolar, hydrophobic). After adsorption, they form some short-range bonds (van der Waals, hydrophobic, electrostatic, hydrogen, ion-pair bonds) with the surface resulting in further denaturation of polypeptide moieties. Adsorption of peptides and proteins at the interfaces is rapid, but the rates of conformational changes are relatively slower. Conformational rearrangement leading to denaturation can be induced by their interfacial adsorption. On adsorption there may be a loss or change in biological activity as the molecular structure is rearranged. If peptide and protein drug entities are adsorbed at interfaces there may be a reduction in the concentration of drug available to elicit its function. Such loss of proteinaceous drug(s) may occur during purification, formulation, storage, and/or delivery [50].

Methods to prevent adsorption

- Insulin adsorption may be minimized by the addition of 0.1–1% albumin.
- Excess agitation should be prevented during production.
- The headspace within the confines of the container should be small.
- Surfactants are used to reduce adsorption with smooth glass walls.

Aggregation and Precipitation

- The denatured, unfolded protein may rearrange in such a manner that hydrophobic amino acid residue of various molecules associate together to form the aggregates.
- If the aggregation is on a macroscopic scale, precipitation occurs.
- Interfacial adsorption may be followed by aggregation and precipitation.
- The extent to which aggregation and precipitation occurs is defined by the relative hydrophilicity of the surfaces in contact with the polypeptide/protein solution.

Causes of aggregation and precipitation

- The presence of a large air/water interface generally accelerates this process.
- Presence of large headspace within the confines of the container also accelerates the course of precipitation.
- Insulin forms finely divided precipitates on the walls of the containers, referred to as frosting. The presence of a large air/water interface generally accelerates this process.

- Thermal motion of the molecules increases due to agitation.
- Solvent composition, solvent dielectric profile, ionic strength, and pH should be carefully controlled at every step in production.

Methods to prevent aggregation and precipitation

- Organic solvent such as 10–15% propylene glycol can suppress the formation of peptide liquid crystals.
- Excess agitation should be prevented during production.
- The headspace within the confines of the container should be small.
- The ionic strength, solvent composition, solvent dielectric profile, and pH should be carefully controlled at every step in production.
- Surfactants should be used to reduce aggregation.

8.4.2 Chemical Instability

This involves alteration in the molecular structure producing a new chemical entity, by bond formation or cleavage. The stability of peptide and proteins against a chemical reagent is decided by temperature, length of exposure, and the amino acid composition, sequence, and conformation of the peptide/protein [51].

8.4.2.1 Deamidation

This reaction involves the hydrolysis of the side chain amide linkage of an amino acid residue leading to the formation of a free carboxylic acid, which then leads to conversion of a neutral residue to a negatively charged residue and primary sequence isomerization. *In vivo* deamidation is observed with human growth hormone, bovine growth hormone, prolactin, adrenocorticotropic hormone, insulin, lysozyme, and secretin.

8.4.2.1.1 FACTORS THAT FAVOR THE RATE OF DEAMIDATION

- pH, temperature, ionic strength.
- The deamidation of Asn residues is accelerated at neutral and alkaline pH.
- The tertiary structure of the protein also affects its stability, as observed with trypsin in which the tertiary structure prevents deamidation.

8.4.2.1.2 METHODS TO PREVENT DEAMIDATION

- The use of genetic engineering and recombinant DNA technology.
- The asparagine residues can be selectively eliminated and replaced by other residues, provided conformations and bioactivity of protein can be maintained.

8.4.3 Oxidation and Reduction

- Major degradation pathways.
- Oxidation commonly occurs during isolation, synthesis, and storage of proteins

8.4.3.1 Factors that Favor Oxidation and Reduction

The oxidative degradation reactions can even occur in atmospheric oxygen under mild conditions (autoxidation). Temperature, pH, trace amounts of metal ions, and buffers influence these reactions. Oxidation may take place involving side chains of histidine (His), lysine (Lys), tryptophan (Trp), and thyronine (Tye) residues in proteins. The thioether group of methionine (Met) is particularly susceptible to oxidation. Under acidic conditions Met residues can be oxidized by atmospheric oxygen. Oxidizing agents like hydrogen peroxide, dimethylsulfoxide, and iodine can oxidize Met-to-Met sulfoxides. The thiol group of cysteine can be oxidized to sulfonic acid; oxidation by iodine and hydrogen peroxide is catalyzed by metal ions and may occur spontaneously by atmospheric oxygen. Usually the oxidation of amino acid residues is followed by a significant loss of biological activity as observed after oxidation of Met residues in calcitonin, corticotrophin, and gastrin. Glucagon is an exception as it retains biological activity even after oxidation.

8.4.3.2 Methods to Prevent Oxidation and Reduction

- Oxidation scavengers may block these acid or base catalyzed oxidations. Example phenolic compounds, propyl gallate.
- Reducing agents – methionine, ascorbic acid, sodium sulfate, thioglycerol, and thioglycolic acid.
- Chelating agents – EDTA and citric acid.
- Nitrogen flush, refrigeration, protection from light, and adjustment of pH.
- Avoiding vigorous stirring and exclusion of air by degassing solvents can prevent air-initiated oxidation.

8.4.4 Proteolysis

The hydrolysis of peptide bonds within the polypeptide or protein destroys or at least reduces its activity. The vulnerability of peptide bonds to cleavage is dependent on the other residues involved. In comparison to other residues, Asn residues are unstable and in particular the Asn–proline bond.

8.4.4.1 Factors that Favor Proteolysis and Prevention

- Proteolysis may occur on exposing the proteins to harsh conditions, such as prolonged exposure to extremes of pH or high temperature or proteolytic enzymes.
- Bacterial contamination is the most common source of proteases. This can be avoided by storing the protein in the cold under sterile conditions.
- Proteases may also gain access during the isolation, purification, and recovery of recombinant proteins from cell extracts or culture fluid.
- This problem can be minimized by manipulation of the solution conditions during the stage of purification and/or by addition of protease inhibitors.
- Some proteins even have autoproteolytic activity. This property aids in controlling the level or function of protein *in vivo*.

8.4.5 Disulfide Exchange

Thiol–disulfide exchange results into formation of an intermediate in which the charge is shared among the three sulfur atoms. The thiolate group attacks a sulfur atom of the disulfide bond, displacing the other sulfur atom, and forming a new disulfide bond. Disulfide bonds may break and reform with incorrect pairings. This results in an alteration in the three-dimensional structure followed by a resultant change in biological activity. A peptide chain with more than one disulfide can enter into disulfide exchange reactions, leading to scrambling of disulfide bridges and thereby a change in conformation. By analogous reactions, trimers and dimers can be formed. The reaction is concentration dependent, particularly for oligomer formation. These oligomers appear at low R_f value on TLC and are readily removed by gel filtration.

8.4.5.1 Methods to Prevent Disulfide Exchange

- Disulfide exchange can be prevented by thiol scavengers such as *p*-mercuribenzoate, *n*-ethylmaleimide, and copper ions.

8.4.6 Racemization

Racemization is the alteration of L-amino acids to D, L-mixtures. With the exception of Gly, all the mammalian amino acids are chiral at the carbon bearing chain and are susceptible to base-catalyzed racemization. Racemization may form peptide bonds that are sensitive to proteolytic enzymes. This reaction can be catalyzed in neutral and alkaline media by thiols, which may arise as a result of hydrolytic cleavage of disulfides.

8.4.6.1 Methods to Prevent Racemization

- The thiolated ions carry out nucleophilic attack on a sulfur atom of the disulfide.
- Addition of thiol scavengers such as *p*-mercuribenzoate, *N*-ethylmaleimide, and copper ions may prevent susceptible sulfur and disulfide.

8.4.6.2 Beta-Elimination

- The mechanism involved in beta-elimination is similar to racemization, that is, it proceeds through a carbanion intermediate. Higher elimination rate prevails under alkaline conditions, which ultimately lead to loss of biological activity. Protein residues susceptible to beta-elimination under alkaline conditions include Cys, Lys, Phe, and Ser. Proteins should be stabilized against thiol–disulfide exchange by chemically blocking the thiol group(s) involved in the process. For example, S-alkylating the Cys-34 of albumin stabilizes the protein not only during high temperature and high humidity storage, but also when loaded within a polymeric matrix.

References

[1] Gerlach JQ, Kilcoyne M, McKeown P, Spillane C, Joshi L. Plant-produced biopharmaceuticals. In: Kole C, editor. Transgenic crop plants. Heidelberg, Germany: Springer-Verlag; 2010. p. 269–99.
[2] Roche. Annual Finance Report; 2007.
[3] Doran PM. Foreign protein production in plant tissue cultures. Curr Opin Biotechnol 2000;11:199–204.
[4] Desai PN, Shrivastava N, Padh H. Production of heterologous proteins in plants: strategies for optimal expression. Biotechnol Adv 2010;28:427–35.
[5] Sparrow PAC, Irwin JA, Dale PJ, Twyman RM, Ma JKC. Pharma-planta: road testing the developing regulatory guidelines for plant-made pharmaceuticals. Transgen Res 2007;16:147–61.
[6] Staub JM, Garcia B, Graves J, Hajdukiewicz PT, Hunter P, Nehra N, et al. High-yield production of a human therapeutic protein in tobacco chloroplasts. Nat Biotechnol 2000;18:333–8.

[7] Kapusta J, Modelska A, Figlerowicz M, Pniewski T, Letellier M, Lisowa O, et al. A plant-derived edible vaccine against hepatitis B virus. FASEB J 1999;13:1796–9.

[8] D'Aoust MA, Lerouge P, Busse U, Bilodeau P, Trépanier S, Gomord V, et al. Efficient and reliable production of pharmaceuticals in alfalfa. In: Fischer R, Schillberg S, editors. Molecular farming: plant-made pharmaceuticals and technical proteins. New York: John Wiley & Sons; 2000.

[9] Hood EE, Witcher DR, Maddock S, Meyer T, Baszczynski C, Bailey M, et al. Commercial production of avidin from transgenic maize: characterization of transformant, production, processing, extraction and purification. Mol Breed 1997;3:291–306.

[10] Mayfield SP, Franklin SE. Expression of human antibodies in eukaryotic microalgae. Vaccine 2005;23:1828–32.

[11] Merle C, Perret S, Lacour T, Jonval V, Hudaverdian S, Garrone R, et al. Hydroxylated human homotrimeric collagen I in *Agrobacterium tumefaciens*-mediated transient expression and in transgenic tobacco plants. FEBS Lett 2002;515:114–8.

[12] Voinnet O, Rivas S, Mestre P, Baulcombe D. An enhanced transient expression system in plants based on suppression of gene silencing by the p19 protein of tomato bushy stunt virus. Plant J 2003;33:949–56.

[13] Leelavathi S, Reddy VS. Chloroplast expression of His-tagged GUS fusions: a general strategy to overproduce and purify foreign proteins using transplastomic plants as bioreactors. Mol Breed 2003;11:49–58.

[14] Molina A, Hervás-Stubbs S, Daniell H, Mingo-Castel AM, Veramendi J. High yield expression of a viral peptide animal vaccine in transgenic tobacco chloroplasts. Plant Biotechnol J 2004;2:141–53.

[15] Schouten A, Roosien J, van Engelen FA, de Jong GAM, Borst-Vrenssen AWM, Zilverentant JF, et al. The C-terminal KDEL sequence increases the expression level of a single chain antibody designed to be targeted to both the cytosol and the secretory pathway in transgenic tobacco. Plant Mol Biol 1996;30:781–93.

[16] Daniell H, Streatfield SJ, Wycoff K. Medical molecular farming: production of antibodies, biopharmaceuticals and edible vaccines in plants. Trends Plant Sci 2001;6:219–26.

[17] Drake PMW, Chargeleuge DM, Vine ND, van Dolleweerd CJ, Obregon P, Ma JKC. Rhizosecretion of a monoclonal antibody protein complex from transgenic tobacco roots. Plant Mol Biol 2003;52:233–41.

[18] Ko K, Brodzik R, Steplewski Z. Production of antibodies in plants: approaches and perspectives. Curr Top Microbiol Immunol 2009;332:55–78.

[19] Kathuria S, Sriraman R, Nath R, Sack M, Pal R, Artsaenko O, et al. Efficacy of plant-produced recombinant antibodies against HCG. Hum Reprod 2002;17:2054–61.

[20] Fischer R, Emans N. Molecular farming of pharmaceutical proteins. Transgenic Res 2000;9:279–99.

[21] Shadwick FS, Doran PM. Foreign protein expression using plant cell suspension and hairy root cultures. In Molecular Farming: Plant-made Pharmaceuticals and Technical Proteins. Edited by Fischer R, Schillberg S. New York: John Wiley & Sons; In Press.

[22] Ma JKC, Drake PMW, Christou P. The production of recombinant pharmaceutical proteins in plants. Nature Rev Genet 2003;4:794–805.

[23] Demain AL, Vaishnav P. Production of recombinant proteins by microbes and higher organisms. Biotechnol Adv 2009;27:297–306.

[24] Dietmair S, Nielsen LK, Timmins NE. Mammalian cells as biopharmaceutical production hosts in the age of omics. Biotechnol J 2012;7:75–89.

[25] Zhu J. Mammalian cell protein expression for biopharmaceutical production. Biotechnol Adv 2012;30:1158–70.

[26] Harashima S. Heterologous protein production by yeast-host vector systems. Bioprocess Technol 1994;19:137–58.

[27] Gerngross TU. Advances in the production of human therapeutic proteins in yeast and filamentous fungi. Nat Biotechnol 2004;22:1409–14.

[28] Ikonomou L, Schneider Y-J, Agathos SN. Insect cell culture for industrial production of recombinant proteins. Appl Microbiol Biotechnol 2003;62:1–20.

[29] Summers MD. Milestones leading to the genetic engineering of baculoviruses as expression vector systems and viral pesticides. Adv Virus Res 2006;68:3–73.

[30] Drugmand J-C, Schneider Y-J, Agathos SN. Insect cells as factories for biomanufacturing. Biotechnol Adv 2012;30:1140–57.

[31] Houdebine LM. Transgenic animal bioreactors. Transgenic Res 2000;9:305–12.

[32] Houdebine LM. Antibody manufacture in transgenic animals and comparisons with other systems. Curr Opin Biotechnol 2002;13:625–9.

[33] Houdebine LM. Use of transgenic animals to improve human health and animal production. Reprod Domest Anim 2005;40:269–81.

[34] D'Aoust MA, Lavoie PO, Couture MM, Trépanier S, Guay JM, Dargis M. Influenza virus-like particles produced by transient expression in *Nicotiana benthamiana* induce a protective immune response against a lethal viral challenge in mice. Plant Biotechnol J 2008;6:930–40.

[35] McCormick AA, Reddy S, Reinl SJ, Cameron TI, Czerwinkski DK, Vojdani F. Plant-produced idiotype vaccines for the treatment of non-Hodgkin's lymphoma: safety and immunogenicity in a phase I clinical study. Proc Natl Acad Sci USA 2008;105:10131–6.

[36] Hans ML, Lowman AM. Biodegradable nanoparticles for drug delivery and targeting. Curr Opin Solid State Mater Sci 2002;6:319–27.

[37] Kensil CR, Patel U, Lennick M, Marciani D. Separation and characterization of saponins with adjuvant activity from *Quillaja-saponaria molina* cortex. J Immunol 1991;146:431–7.

[38] Barr IG, Sjolander A, Cox JC. ISCOMs and other saponin based adjuvants (review). Adv Drug Deliv Rev 1998;32:247–71.

[39] Jha AK, Prasad K, Prasad K, Kulkarni AR. Plant system: nature's nanofactory. Colloid Surf B Biointerfaces 2009;73:219–23.

[40] Gardea-Torresedey JL, Armendariz V, Herreira I, Parsons JG, Peralta-Videa JR, Teimann KJ, et al. Binding of silver ions by alfalfa biomass (*Medicago sativa*): batch pH, time, temperature, and ionic strength studies. J Hazardous Subs Res 2003;4:1–15.

[41] Lambkin I, Pinilla C, Hamashin C, Spindler L, Russell S, Schink A. Toward targeted oral vaccine delivery systems: selection of lectin mimetics from combinatorial libraries. Pharm Res 2003;20:1258–66.

[42] Medina-Bolivar F, Wright R, Funk V, Sentz D, Barroso L, Wilkins TD, et al. A non-toxic lectin for antigen delivery of plant-based mucosal vaccines. Vaccine 2003;21:997–1005.

[43] Norton EB, Lawson LB, Mahdi Z, Freytag LC, Clements JD. The A subunit of *Escherichia coli* heat-labile enterotoxin functions as a mucosal adjuvant and promotes IgG2a, IgA, and Th17 responses to vaccine antigens. Infect Immun 2012;80:2426–35.

[44] Morelli AB, Becher D, Koernig S, Silva A, Drane D, Maraskovsky E. ISCOMATRIX: a novel adjuvant for use in prophylactic and therapeutic vaccines against infectious diseases. J Med Microbiol 2012;61:935–43.

[45] Kamstrup S, San Martin R, Doberti A, Grande H, Dalsgaard K. Preparation and characterisation of Quillaja saponin with less heterogeneity than Quil-A. Vaccine 2000;18:2244–9.

[46] Friedman M. Anticarcinogenic, cardioprotective, and other health benefits of tomato compounds lycopene, α-tomatine, and tomatidine in pure form and in fresh and processed tomatoes. J Agric Food Chem 2013;61:9534–50.

[47] Al-Barwani F, Donaldson B, Pelham SJ, Young SL, Ward VK. Antigen delivery by virus-like particles for immunotherapeutic vaccination. Ther Deliv 2014;5:1223–40.

[48] Teekamp N, Duque LF, Frijlink HW, Hinrichs WL, Olinga P. Production methods and stabilization strategies for polymer-based nanoparticles and microparticles for parenteral delivery of peptides and proteins. Expert Opin Drug Deliv 2015;19:1–21.

[49] Delgado Y, Morales-Cruz M, Hernández-Román J, Martínez Y, Griebenow K. Chemical glycosylation of cytochrome c improves physical and chemical protein stability. BMC Biochem 2014;15:16.

[50] Radhakrishna M, Grimaldi J, Belfort G, Kumar SK. Stability of proteins inside a hydrophobic cavity. Langmuir 2013;29:8922–8.

[51] Goldstein DA, Thomas JA. Biopharmaceuticals derived from genetically modified plants. Q J Med 2004;97:705–16.

Edible Vaccines

Saurabh Bhatia, Randhir Dahiya

9.1 INTRODUCTION

Vaccines are considered primary tools for health intervention in both humans and animals. Vaccines can be used more widely, especially in developing countries, if their cost of production can be reduced and they can be preserved without refrigeration. In developing countries certain limitations, like vaccine affordability, the need for "cold chains" from the producer to the site of use of the vaccine, and the dependence on injection, are barriers to health care services. Plant-derived vaccines do not face such limitations. Research under way is dedicated to solving these limitations by finding ways to produce oral (edible) vaccines from transgenic plants. Plant-derived vaccines offer increased safety, envisage low-cost programs for mass vaccination, and propose a wider use of vaccination for veterinary use [1].

Modern Applications of Plant Biotechnology in Pharmaceutical Sciences. http://dx.doi.org/10.1016/B978-0-12-802221-4.00009-1

With the advent of modern molecular biology techniques in the 1980s, new strategies were developed for the production of vaccines. These vaccines are comprised of proteins derived from pathogenic viruses, bacteria, or parasites (generally proteins are produced not by the pathogens themselves, but by expression of the gene encoding the protein in a "surrogate organism") [2]. In the last decade, it was found that green plants can also be used as the "surrogate production organism" to produce antigens of human pathogens (including HB-sAg). These proteins can elicit priming and also can boost the immune response in humans when administered orally. In addition, unlike almost all other cell lines used for production of vaccines, components of plant cells have always been an important part of the normal human diet. Plants, therefore, offer significant new opportunities for making safe and effective oral vaccines [3].

9.2 PRODUCTION OF EDIBLE VACCINES

9.2.1 Selection of the Desired Gene and Plant

The introduction of selected desired genes into plants and then inducing these altered plants to produce the encoded proteins is the primary condition for the development of edible vaccines. This process is known as transformation and altered plants are called transgenic plants. Selection of important epitope region(s) from the pathogen of interest is the one of the key factors that determines the success of potential edible vaccines. Edible vaccine development has been challenged by low expression levels of foreign proteins in transgenic plants. Reported expression rates range from 0.01% to 2% total soluble protein (TSP), which can render edible vaccine proteins less immunogenic. Selection of strong plant-specific super promoters to improve expression levels is another key factor that can determine the success of edible vaccines [4].

9.2.2 Plant Transformation

9.2.2.1 Antigenic Gene Transformation through a Suitable Vector

After transformation of tobacco, great efforts have been made to develop efficient methods for genetic transformation and optimizing expression of foreign genes in plants. The techniques used to introduce foreign genes into plants have been extended to major crops, vegetables, and ornamental and medicinal plants. Various foreign proteins including serum albumin, human α-interferon, human erythroprotein, and murine IgG and IgA immunoglobulins have been successfully expressed in plants. In recent years, several attempts have been made to produce various antigens and antibodies in plants. Antigens or antibodies expressed in plants can be administered orally as any edible part of the plant, or by the parenteral route (such as intramuscular or intravenous injection) after isolation and purification from the plant tissue. The edible part of the plant to be used as a vaccine is fed raw to experimental animals or humans to prevent possible denaturation during cooking, and avoid cumbersome purification protocols [5].

While *Agrobacterium*-mediated transformation still remains the method of choice for dicots, a general method, the biolistics method, of transformation of plants, including

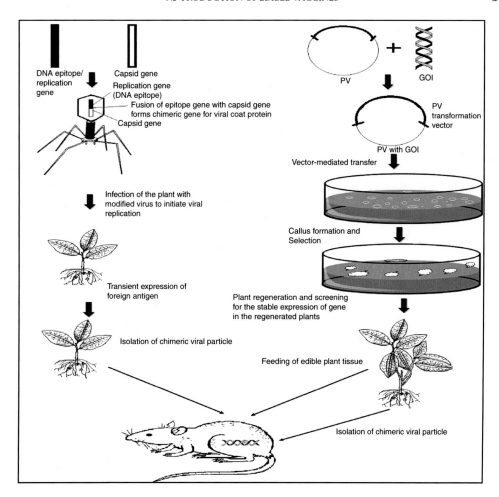

FIGURE 9.1 Strategies for the production of edible vaccine. PV (plasmid vector); GOI (gene of interest).

monocots, has come into existence. Other strategies for expression of foreign genes in plants include use of strong and organ-specific plant promoters, targeting of the protein into endoplasmic reticulum (ER) by incorporating ER-targeting and ER-retention signals, creation of an optimized translation start site context, as well as alteration of codons to suit the expression of prokaryotic genes in a plant. For the production of edible vaccines or antibodies, it is desirable to select a plant whose products can be consumed raw to avoid degradation during cooking. Thus, plants like tomato, banana, and cucumber are generally the plants of choice. While expression of a gene into the genome allows maintenance of the material in the form of seeds, some virus-based vectors can also be used to express the gene transiently to develop the products in a short period (Fig. 9.1). This may have the additional advantage of allowing expression of the product at a very high level; not always attainable in transgenic systems [6].

9.2.2.2 *Transformation of Chimeric Gene through Viral Infection*

Plus-sense, single-stranded plant RNA viruses have been proposed as an effective alternative to produce vaccine antigens in plants. In this technique, the epitope of interest is engineered into a plant virus, usually within the coat protein gene. Infection of a susceptible non-GM-plant results in intracellular production and accumulation of the epitope. The epitope sequence, as well as the viral genome, never become integrated into the plant genome and hence are only expressed by the generation of infected cells. A recombinant cowpea mosaic virus has shown to elicit protective immunity in mink when engineered to express the antigenic epitope against mink enteritis virus. Recombinant alfalfa mosaic virus (AlMV) has enabled expression of significant quantities of rabies virus and HIV epitopes upon integration of their respective coding sequence into the AlMV coat protein. The extra sequences were found to protrude from the virion surface without interfering with virus assembly. Recombinant AlMV coat protein molecules have also demonstrated the ability to assemble into particles containing three different epitopes from HIV and rabies. This demonstrates the ability of plant viruses to produce multicomponent vaccines [7]. Claimed advantages of transient viral expression of transgenes over transgenic plants are: lesser time for cloning of the foreign gene in the viral genome as compared to time required for transformation of plants; the ease at which antigen production can be scaled up; and the wide host range of plant viruses, which allows use of multiple plant species as biofactories.

9.2.3 Evaluation of the Protein in Animal Models

Each single antigen expressed in plants must be verified by animal studies and Western blots, and quantified by enzyme-linked immunosorbent assay (ELISA).

9.3 MECHANISM OF ACTION

Most pathogens enter at mucosal surfaces lining the digestive, respiratory, and urino-productive tracts, which are collectively the largest immunologically active tissue in the body. The mucosal immune system is the first line of defense and the most effective site for vaccination against pathogens. Nasal and oral vaccines are most effective for mucosal infections. The goal of oral vaccine is to stimulate both mucosal and humoral immunity against pathogens. Edible vaccines when taken orally undergo mastication, and degradation of plant cells occurs in the intestine due to the action of digestive enzymes. Peyer's patches are an enriched source of IgA producing plasma cells and have the potential to populate mucosal tissue and serve as mucosal immune effector site. The breakdown of edible vaccine occurs near Peyer's patches, which consist of 30–40 lymphoid nodules on the outer surface of the intestine and also contain follicles from which the germinal center develops after antigenic stimulation. These follicles act as a site for the penetration of antigens in intestinal epithelium. The antigen then comes in contact with M-cells. M-cells express class-2 major histocompatibility complex molecules, and antigens transported across the mucous membranes by M-cells can activate B-cells within these lymphoid follicles. The activated B-cells leave the lymphoid follicles and migrate to diffuse mucosal associated lymphoid tissue where they differentiate into plasma cells that secrete the IgA class of antibodies. These IgA antibodies are transported across the

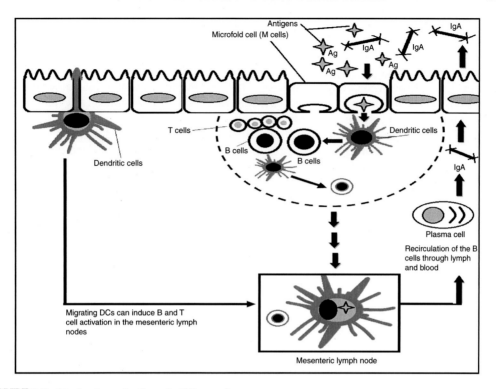

FIGURE 9.2   Mechanism of action of edible vaccines.

epithelial cells into secretions of the lumen where they can interact with antigens present in the lumen (Figure 9.2).

9.4 ADVANTAGES AND DISADVANTAGES OF EDIBLE VACCINES

9.4.1 Advantages of Edible Vaccine

- Edible vaccines are effective as a delivery vehicle for immunization because adjuvants that enhance the immune response are not required.
- Edible vaccine can elicit mucosal immunity, which is not observed in traditional vaccines.
- Edible vaccines are also cost effective in availability, storage, preparation, production, and transportation. Vaccines produced by biotechnological methods are stable at room temperature, unlike traditional vaccine, which needs cold chain storage, which multiplies the yearly cost to preserve vaccines. Moreover, the seeds of transgenic plants could be dried as there is less moisture content in seeds and the plants with oil or their aqueous extracts possess more storage opportunities. Manufacturing cost is low as there is no need for special premises to manufacture them. Edible vaccine can be easily produced at mass level in comparison to an animal system.

- Edible vaccines are well tolerated, as they do not require administration by injection unlike traditional vaccines. Thus, there is also a reduced need for medical personnel and risk of contamination is low. The feasibility of oral administration compared to injection is also an advantage.
- Plant-derived vaccines could be the source for new vaccines combining numerous antigens. These multicomponent vaccines are called second generation vaccines as they allow for several antigens to approach M-cells simultaneously.
- Edible vaccines are subunit preparations, do not involve attenuated pathogens, and improve the safety of individuals as compared to traditional vaccine since there is no possibility of proteins reforming into infectious organisms.
- The separation and purification of vaccines from plant materials is very easy and pathogenic contamination from animal cells can be effectively prevented.

9.4.2 Disadvantages of Edible Vaccines

- There is the possibility of development of immunotolerance to the vaccine protein or peptide.
- Consistency of dosage form differs from plant to plant and generation to generation.
- Protein content varies from plant to plant and generation to generation.
- Ripeness also affects the proteins that are present in form of antigens in the fruits.
- Limitations of methods for standardization of plant material/product.
- Stability of vaccine differs from plant to plant.
- Some food cannot be eaten raw (e.g., potato) and needs to be cooked, which will denature or weaken the protein present in it.
- Variable conditions for edible vaccine are also a major problem. Potatoes containing vaccine can be stored at 4°C for longer time, while tomato does not last long at this temperature. Thus, these vaccines need to be properly stored to avoid infection through microbial spoilage.
- Another concern regarding edible vaccine is the need for proper distinguishing characters to identify between "vaccine fruit" and "normal fruit" to avoid maladministration of vaccine, which could lead to tolerance.
- The glycosylation pattern of plants and humans is different, which could affect the functions of vaccines.

9.5 MOST POPULAR EDIBLE VACCINES PRODUCED BY PLANTS [8,9]

9.5.1 Tobacco

The first report of the production of edible vaccine (a surface protein from *Streptococcus*) in tobacco, at 0.02% of total leaf protein level, appeared in 1990 in the form of a patent application published under the International Patent Cooperation Treaty. Subsequently, a number of attempts were made to express various antigens in plants (Table 9.1). Since acute watery diarrhea is caused by enterotoxigenic *Escherichia coli* and *Vibrio cholerae* that colonize the small intestine and produce one or more enterotoxin, an attempt was made to produce edible vaccine by expressing heat-labile enterotoxin (LT-B) in tobacco.

TABLE 9.1 Benefits Envisaged in Plant-Derived Edible Vaccines

Benefit	Characteristics
Oral delivery	The plant cell wall, consisting essentially of cellulose and sugars, provides protection in the stomach and gradual release of the antigen in the gut
Use as raw food or dry powder	The vaccinogenic plant tissue may be used as raw food or, alternatively, proteins may be partially or fully purified and administered in capsules as dry powder
No need for "cold chain"	The vaccinogenic plant parts or plant extracts can be stored and shipped at room temperature
Mucosal and serum immune response	Plant-derived vaccines are primarily designed to trigger the mucosal immune system (IgA)
Cost efficiency	Production cost will be reduced 100–1000 times as compared with that of traditional vaccines
Optimized expression system	Plants may be engineered to accumulate the antigen in convenient intracellular compartments (endoplasmic reticulum, chloroplast)
Ease of genetic manipulation	Procedures essentially rely on established molecular and genetic manipulation protocols; these are already available
Ease of production and scale-up	GM plants can be stored as seeds. Unlimited vaccine quantity can be produced from these in limited time; production and management are suitable for developing countries
Safer than conventional vaccines	Lack of contamination with mammalian pathogens
Ideal to face bioweapons	Safety and cost efficiency plant-derived vaccines act as an ideal tool to face bioterrorism
Ideal for veterinary use	Cost affordable and ready for use as food additive

9.5.2 Potato

Transgenic potatoes were created and grown by Charles Arntzen Hugh S. Mason and their colleagues at the Boyce Thompson Institute for Plant Research, an affiliate of Cornell University. Transgenic potatoes containing enterotoxin stimulated strong immune responses in animals. An edible vaccine could stimulate an immune response in humans. Volunteers ate bite-sized pieces of raw potato that had been genetically engineered to produce part of the toxin secreted by the *E. coli* bacterium, which causes diarrhea. Ten of the 11 volunteers (91%) who ingested the transgenic potatoes had four-fold rises in serum antibodies at some point after immunization, and six of the 11 (55%) developed four-fold rises in intestinal antibodies. The potatoes were well tolerated and no one experienced serious adverse side effects (Table 9.2).

9.5.3 Tomato

Tomatoes serve as an ideal candidate for this HIV antigen because unlike other transgenic plants that carry the protein, tomatoes are edible and immune to any thermal process, which helps retain its healing capabilities. Even more importantly, compared to bananas tomatoes were found to grow at a high rate of success in Russia.

TABLE 9.2   Advantages and Disadvantages of Different Plants as Transgenic Bioreactors

Plant/Fruit	Advantage	Disadvantage
Tobacco	• Good model for evaluating recombinant proteins • Low cost preserving system • Easy purification of antibodies stored in the seeds • Large harvests	• Produces toxic compounds* (toxic alkaloids incompatible w/oral delivery) • Potential for outcrossing in field
Potato	• Dominated clinical trials • Easily manipulated/transformed • Easily propagated from its "eyes" • Stored for long periods without refrigeration	• Relatively low tuber protein content • Unpalatable in raw form**; cooking may cause denaturation and poor immunogenicity of vaccine
Banana	• Does not need cooking • Proteins not destroyed even if cooked • Inexpensive • Grown widely in developing countries	• Trees take 2–3 years to mature and transformed trees take about 12 months to bear fruit • Fruits spoil rapidly after ripening and contain very little protein, so unlikely to produce large amounts of recombinant proteins
Tomato	• Grows quickly • Cultivated broadly • High content of vitamin A may boost immune response • Overcomes the spoilage problem by freeze-drying technology • Heat-stable, antigen-containing powders†, made into capsules • Different batches blended to give uniform doses of antigen	• Relatively low fruit protein content • Acidic fruit may be incompatible with some antigens or for delivery to infants • No *in vitro* system to test fruit expression
Rice	• Commonly used in baby food because of low allergenic potential • High expression of proteins/antigens • Easy storage/transportation • Expressed protein is heat stable	• Grows slowly • Requires specialized glasshouse conditions
Lettuce	• Fast growing • Direct consumption	• Spoils readily
Soybean and alfalfa	• Relatively efficient transformation system • High protein content in leaves • Leaves edible uncooked • Ideal system for animal vaccines	• Potential for outcrossing in field • Deep root system problematic for cleaning field
Legumes or cereals	• Production technology widely established • High protein content in seeds • Stable protein in stored seeds • Well suited for animal vaccines • Industrial seed processing well established	• Inefficient transformation systems • Heating or cooking for human use may cause denaturation and poor immunogenicity of vaccine (corn meal is exception) • Potential for outcrossing in field for some species

Currently, therapeutic proteins in tobacco are being produced.
**Some kinds of South American potatoes can be eaten raw. Although some studies show that cooking does not destroy full complement of antigen in potatoes.*
†*Freeze-dried tomato powder containing NV capsid and LT-B was found immunogenic.*

TABLE 9.3   Antigens Produced in Transgenic Plants

Protein	Plant	Carrier
Hepatitis-B surface antigen	Tobacco	–
Rabies virus glycoprotein	Tomato	–
Norwalk virus capside protein	Tobacco	–
E. coli heat labile enterotoxin β-subunit	Potato	–
Cholera toxin β-subunit	Potato, tobacco	–
Mouse glutamate decarboxylase	Potato	–
VPI protein of foot and mouth disease virus	*Arabidopsis*	–
Insulin	Potato	–
Glycoproteins of swine-transmissible gastroenteritis corona virus	*Arabidopsis*	–

9.5.4 Banana

For vaccines or subunit vaccinations, bananas seem to be the desired vector. The advantage of bananas is that they can be eaten raw as compared to potatoes or rice, which need to be cooked, and bananas can also be consumed in a pure form. Research is leaning toward the use of bananas as the vector since most third world countries, which would benefit most from edible vaccines, are in tropical climates that are suitable for growing bananas.

9.5.5 Maize

Egyptian scientists have genetically engineered maize plants to produce a protein used to make the hepatitis-B virus vaccine. A team of researchers led by Hania El-itriby, director of Cairo's Agricultural Genetic Engineering Research Institute, developed genetically modified (GM) maize plants that produce the protein known as HBsAg, which elicits an immune response against the hepatitis-B virus and could be used as a vaccine (Table 9.3).

9.5.6 Rice

When predominant T-cell epitope peptides, which were derived from Japanese cedar pollen allergens, were specifically expressed in rice seed and delivered to the mucosal immune system, the development of an allergic immune response of the allergen-specific Th2 cell was suppressed. Furthermore, not only were specific IgE production and release of histamine from mast cells suppressed, but the inflammatory symptoms of pollinosis, such as sneezing, were also suppressed. These results suggest the feasibility of using an oral immunotherapy agent derived from transgenic plants that accumulate T-cell epitope peptides of allergens for allergy treatment (Table 9.4). When the seed expression system is used as a platform for foreign protein production, substantial amounts of recombinant proteins can be accumulated, because the seed is a natural storage organ for accumulating the starch, protein, and oil required for seedling growth. Also, artificial peptides or proteins accumulate in seed, which is in remarkable contrast with other tissues.

TABLE 9.4   Transient Production of Antigens in Plants After Infection with Plant Virus Expressing Recombinant Gene

Influenza antigen	Tobacco	TMV
Murine zona pellucida antigen	Tobacco	TMV
Rabies antigen	Spinach	AlMV
HIV-1 antigen	Tobacco	AlMV
Mink enteritis virus antigen	Black-eyed bean	CPMV

9.5.7 Safety and Public Acceptance [8–10]

Plant-derived vaccines are free from animal pathogen contaminants. Furthermore, plant DNA is not known to interact with animal DNA and plant viral recombinants does not invade mammalian cells. Further safety of plant-derived vaccines can be achieved by following similar regulations established for traditional vaccines. Nevertheless, the present concern over the use of GM plants is now affecting research in this important field, especially in Europe. One of the fears is that GM pollen may outcross with sexually compatible plants (related crops or weeds) and affect biodiversity. In order to address this alarm, several pollen containment approaches have been developed. These are essentially based on the exploitation of different forms of male sterility (suicide genes, infertility barriers, apomixis). An alternative way of solving the problem is engineering vaccines into the chloroplast DNA (cpDNA), which is not transmitted to the sexual progeny through the pollen grains. An additional safety feature would be the recognition of GM plants that produce vaccines by the addition of genes encoding colored plant pigments. It is important to recognize that plants that produce vaccines are medicinal plants and should be grown, processed, and regulated as pharmaceutical products. In the majority of earlier papers, level of antigen accumulation in the plant organ was in the order of 0.1–0.4% of total soluble protein, while the more recent developments on cpDNA integration promises to increase this value to 30% or more. At the latter value, land requirements for industrial plant-derived vaccine production will be in the order of a few thousand square meters. This will definitely enable vaccine-producing plants to be set apart from field grown crop plants and offer added safety when engineered plant viruses are used for transient antigen expression. A further point of public concern in GM plants is the presence of antibiotic resistance genes (used as selective marker in most transgenic plants). Approaches have now been developed to generate GM plants (with both nuclear or cpDNA integration) that do not carry these genes.

References

[1] Landridge W. Edible vaccines. Scientific Am 2000;283:66–71.
[2] Lal P, Ramachandran VG, Goyal R, Sharma R. Edible vaccines: Current status and future. IJMM 2007;25:93–102.
[3] Giddings G, Allison G, Brooks D, Carter A. Transgenic plants as factories for biopharmaceuticals. Nat Biotechnol 2000;18:1151–5.
[4] Gunn KS, Singh N, Giambrone J, Wu H. Using transgenic plants as bioreactors to produce edible vaccines. J Biotech Research 2012;4:92–9.
[5] Prakash CS. Edible vaccines and antibody producing plants. Biotechnol Develop Monitor 1996;27:10–3.

[6] Daniell H, Streatfield SJ, Wycoff K. Medical molecular farming: production of antibodies, biopharmaceuticals and edible vaccines in plants. Trends Plant Sci 2001;6:219–26.

[7] El Attar AK, Shamloul AM, Shalaby AA, Riad BY, Saad A, Mazyad HM, Keith JM. Expression of chimeric HCV peptide in transgenic tobacco plants infected with recombinant alfalfa mosaic virus for development of a plant-derived vaccine against HCV. African J Biotechnology 2004;3:588–94.

[8] Tacker CO, Mason HS. A review of oral vaccination with transgenic vegetables. Microbes Infect 1999;1:777–83.

[9] Mor TS, Gomez-Lim MA, Palmer KE. Edible vaccines: A concept comes of age. Trends Microbiol 1998;6:449–53.

[10] Korban SS, Krasnyanski SF, Buetow DE. Food as production and delivery vehicles for human vaccine. J Am Coll Nutr 2002;21:212S–7S.

Microenvironmentation in Micropropagation

Saurabh Bhatia, Kiran Sharma

Modern Applications of Plant Biotechnology in Pharmaceutical Sciences. http://dx.doi.org/10.1016/B978-0-12-802221-4.00010-8

10.1 INTRODUCTION

Plant tissue culture is a widely known technique for the production of large numbers of genetically identical plantlets. This technology exhibits several advantages over conventional propagation techniques. Propagules derived from plant tissue culture exhibit several applications in horticulture, crops, and forestry. Genetic expression of such propagules governs their growth and development; however, the environmental conditions have a huge effect on genotype and expression of *in vitro* propagated plant cell/tissue. Utilization of traditional methods to control the physical and chemical environment is time consuming and limited for the large-scale production of propagules. With modernization in technology currently several engineering techniques (robust, automated, and computerized) have been applied to micropropagation with the objective of providing optimum environmental conditions to *in vitro* plant stock at a larger level. Usually *in vitro* propagation is practiced by using three general steps: (i) preparation and sterilization of plant material, (ii) culture medium composition, and (iii) physical environmental conditions in the culture room and culture vessel. Microenvironmentation is essential for the last two steps but especially so for the last step for providing the optimum physical environment to the culture.

Unlike the greenhouse effect where plants have to compromise with environmental conditions, microenvironmentation is investigated in closed plant tissue culture vessels, with their caps or closures, which creates the boundaries between the internal microenvironment and the external environment. This will be helpful in exploring benefits of micropropagation over conventional propagation techniques, such as: rapid clonal propagation, decreasing diseases of plantlets and the period of acclimatization *ex vitro*, cutting down motherstock requirements, improving the survival of micropropagation plantlets after transfer to *ex vitro* conditions, etc., and then reducing the cost of micropropagation plantlets. Physical environmental factors such as temperature, light, air movement, physical boundaries of the culture vessel, and physical characteristics of the culture medium are predetermined and can be maintained constant or varied during the growth cycle. Similarly the chemical environment of the tissue culture is predetermined and variables such as pH and the composition of the medium are maintained in such a way that the optimum conditions are always provided for the nourishment of young propagules. Physical parameters or culture room conditions can be optimized by changing the growth room temperature and humidity, or physically moving the culture to alter growth conditions. High relative humidity, stable temperature, low CO_2 concentration in light and high CO_2 concentration in dark, and high C_2H_4 concentrations are favorable for the proper growth of plant tissue culture [1]. High CO_2 concentrations in the light period inhibit growth of plantlets and induce senescence [2]. High relative humidity reduces the transpiration and induces stomatal malfunction [3].

In addition, the physical properties of the vessels and caps or closures affect the growth microenvironment of plantlets by virtue of the interface between inside and outside environments. The most important specifications for vessels are to provide uniform and adequate light quality, to isolate contamination of microorganisms, and to allow gas exchange. Therefore, growth conditions of plantlets are significantly affected by the inside microenvironment of culture vessels. However, the microenvironment of culture vessels is not easily adjusted. Various essential parameters of microenvironmentation during plant tissue culture are

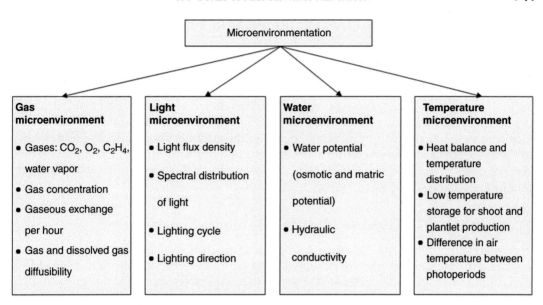

FIGURE 10.1 **Essential parameters of microenvironmentation in plant tissue culture.**

mentioned in Fig. 10.1. In this chapter, environmental factors of microecology *in vitro* and their effects on the growth of plantlets are discussed and developments of environmental control technology and culture facilities are evaluated.

10.2 VARIOUS PROBLEMS FACED DURING MICROENVIRONMENTATION

There are several problems faced during micropropagation such as variation of growth rate at each culture stage, various types of contamination (described in Chapter 13), costings for maintaining physical and chemical parameters either constant or variable and for the significant space acquired by the cultures, screening of live plantlets, disposal of dead tissue, and overproduction or shortage of plantlets.

10.3 GOALS OF MICROENVIRONMENTATION

Development and application of both the automated environmental control system and suitable industrial-scale culture facilities are essential for their commercial application in agriculture. Control of environmental conditions is essential to produce elite propagules. These conditions can be achieved by control of growth and development, control of morphological and physiological characteristics, and reduction of cost, labor, supplies, and consumption in plant tissue culture.

10.4 GAS MICROENVIRONMENT

Concentration and diffusivity are the two main features of the gas microenvironment. Values of these two factors are different between inside the culture vessel and the outside environment. Gas concentration diffusivity differences are attributed to small size of vessel and minimal gas exchange between outside and inside environments. Gas concentration is dependent on the rate of gas exchange and physical properties of the vessel. Diffusion in a culture vessel facilitates gas exchange between the cultures and headspace of the vessel, exchange of solutes between culture and medium, and uniformization of the spatial distributions of gases in the head space and solutes in the medium. Therefore, diffusion is an important process involving mass energy transfer in culture vessels (Fig. 10.1).

10.4.1 Gaseous Transport in Plant Tissue Culture System

Microenvironmental conditions for transplanted explants in small and semiclosed vessels require a microorganism-free environment. Therefore, it is irrational to circulate inside air by ventilation equipment as in greenhouse production. Vessels should be designed in such a way to encourage the exchange of gas between inside and outside environments. For determination of gaseous transfers, the value that gives the number of gases exchanged per minute is a widely used measurement in greenhouse engineering. Volumetric ventilation/air volume of the vessel per hour is defined as the small magnitude of gas exchange of a vessel, the number of exchanges of the vessel per hour [4]. Various factors such as the shape and physical properties of cover and vessel, tightness of the lid, air velocity, and direction outside the vessel, etc. affect these parameters. Further the oxygen transport in plant tissue culture systems can be determined by the presence of oxygen in the gas phase and liquid phase/solid phase. Measurement of oxygen transport at gas/liquid, gas/solid, and solid/liquid interfaces assists in evaluating oxygen mass transfer. Characterization of oxygen mass transfer is essential for the evaluation of optimum value of oxygen required during the whole process.

10.4.2 Effect of Dissolved Oxygen Concentration on Somatic Embryogenesis

To maintain sterility and prevent dehydration of both tissue and medium, a capping system is obligatory in tissue culture. This may restrict the gas exchange between *in vitro* and outer atmosphere; consequently poor plant development occurs with high mortality when relocated to the greenhouse for weaning. Growth and development of plant tissue culture is largely dependent on composition of tissue culture medium and gases present in an *in vitro* environment [5]. There are various designs of capping system and different suitable materials are utilized nowadays. Screw caps, plastic caps, aluminum foil, and transparent films such as propylene films are known examples of capping systems that restrict gaseous exchange and hence affect plant growth [5].

With the development in tissue there has been much interest in the aeration of the culture environment. Such aerated culture vessels have many advantages over conventional air-tight containers, and aeration can be improved by microporous filter membranes, capping with loosely fitted lids, using thin diffusible films, or forced aeration using air pumps [5]. An in-depth understanding of the mechanism of aeration can assist in designing suitable vessels and improving the quality of plantlets. The principle of air mechanisms is mentioned

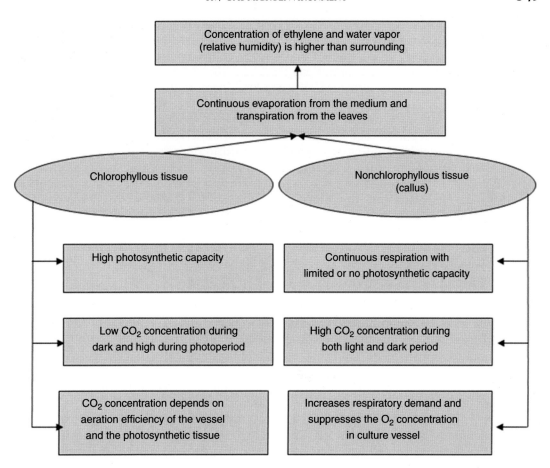

FIGURE 10.2 Differentiation of the microenvironment of chlorophyllous and nonchlorophyllous tissue.

in Fig. 10.2. Aeration in a tissue culture vessel can involve two major processes. The first is bulk flow, humidity-induced and venturi-induced convective flows of air and diffusion of gas molecules. These processes may not be entirely unconnected and commonly can be called natural ventilation. The second is forced ventilation where the outer air is delivered to plant tissues by an external force [5]. The demand for aeration in a tissue culture vessel can be accomplished by providing either or both of the above processes and thus the tissue culture vessel should be designed more efficiently to maximize these processes [5].

10.4.3 Dissolve Oxygen Concentration

Dissolved oxygen concentration is one of the most important environmental factors when growing plants in liquid systems, since oxygen is only slightly soluble in water (8.0 mg/L^{-1} at 25°C, 1 atm, and 21% oxygen at ambient air). The relationship between dissolved oxygen and somatic embryogenesis is not yet clear. Kessel and Carr reported that dissolved oxygen below 16% is essential for somatic embryo production of carrot in a mechanically stirred bioreactor at 90 rpm [6]. Carman reported that low oxygen increases the production of wheat embryo [7]. Stuart et al. reported that higher concentrations of dissolved oxygen increased the regeneration of alfalfa [8]. Jay et al. reported that somatic embryo production can be increased at constant dissolved oxygen concentrations (10% and 100%) [9]. Archambault reported that a constant concentration of dissolved oxygen (20%) increases the somatic embryo production of *Eschscholzia californica* [10]. Okamoto et al. reported that efficiency of regeneration in culture aerated with a mixture of gas (40% of dissolve oxygen) is higher than flask culture [11]. Shigeta et al. reported that 80% concentration of dissolved oxygen is essential for the development of globular and heart stage embryos during the first week of culture. Subsequent development in torpedo stage requires a low level of oxygen. Shimadzu et al. reported that oxygen-enriched aeration provides oxygen to the low oxygen areas in somatic embryos [12]. After the heat-stage embryos, which were grown at the 7% level, were transferred to a flask with ambient, they developed an elongated root part and eventually grew to normal plantlets. Kurta et al. reported that dissolved oxygen is one of the environmental factors that strongly affect the development of somatic embryos in the suspension [12,13].

10.4.4 Humidity Microenvironment

One of the most reliable ways to regulate the internal microclimate of vessels is to adjust the outside environment indirectly. Relative humidity and the air temperature of the culture vessel are important factors that influence plantlet growth. The interactive effect of relative humidity and temperature are optimized and effects are investigated. Owing to the high water content of medium in the culture vessel the relative humidity of the inside air is always higher than that of a greenhouse [14,15]. Several reports available on high relative humidity in culture vessels led to physiological and morphological disorders of plantlets [16,17]. This high relative humidity within the culture vessels results in a poorly developed epicuticular wax layer and malfunctioning stomata of the plantlets. This led to the loss of the normal function (for evaporation) of the stomata. Due to the high relative humidity, plantlets do not have the ability to resist water stress after transplanting from *in vitro* to *ex vitro* conditions. Debergh et al. concluded that high relative humidity was the dominant factor for the hyperhydricity of plantlets [18].

10.4.5 Measurement of Gas Exchange Rates in Plant Tissue Culture Vessels

Aerial microenvironment is dependent on the gas exchange between internal and external environments. This exchange can influence the microenvironment of culture vessels. Therefore, it is necessary to measure the air exchange rate for various vessels. Gaseous influx and efflux has a significant effect on the growth and development of plantlets *in vitro*. There are various inexpensive, rapid, and simple techniques available to determine the air exchange rate of a culture vessel within a short period.

10.5 LIGHT MICROENVIRONMENT

Light-mediated microenvironmental control inside, by regulating light intensity in the culture vessel, affects the growth of regenerated plants. An increase in temperature due to an increase in light intensity suppresses the growth of plant tissue cultures. With respect to the light microenvironment, light flux density, spectral distribution of light, lighting cycle, and lighting direction play an important role in growth and development of cultures (Fig. 10.1).

10.6 WATER MICROENVIRONMENT

Culture media contain large amounts of water. Its abundant availability in media and its free energy status directly promote water transfer, which influences the physiological activities of the cultures. Water potential and hydraulic conductivity are the two main factors affecting water availability in media (Fig. 10.1).

10.7 TEMPERATURE MICROENVIRONMENT

Temperature plays an essential role in the growth and development of *in vitro* plantlets. Heat balance and temperature distribution measurements, difference in air temperature between photoperiod measurements, and evaluation of low temperature storage (for shoot and plantlet production) assist in establishing proper temperature microenvironmental conditions in closed culture vessels (Fig. 10.1).

10.8 PHYSICAL PROPERTIES OF CULTURE VESSELS

Closed vessel transplant production systems with their caps or closures make the boundaries between the internal microenvironment and the external environment of outside air. Physical properties of plant tissue culture vessels influence the growth microenvironment of plantlets by the interface between inside and outside environments. The primary objective of the vessel including caps or closures is to provide uniform and adequate light quality, to avoid microorganisms, and to allow gas exchange. Air exchange rates and transmittance distribution are usually dependent on the physical specification, construction, and shape of the vessel. These vessels are placed on the successive horizontal shelves arranged in the culture room.

Tissue culture plantlets *in vitro* when planted in a culture vessel, internal microclimate conditions such as light quantity and quality, light distribution, and air temperature all decide the growth patterns of plantlets. Robotic adjustment or installing equipment with culture vessels is an impractical approach to adjust the internal microclimate of the culture vessel. One of the promising ways to provide optimum conditions to the internal microclimate of a vessel is to adjust the outside environment of the culture room indirectly. The internal microclimate of culture vessels is usually affected by its material characteristics, which can subsequently affect the spectral irradiance. Several reports based on the relationship between the internal microclimate and other factors have been studied so far [19–22]. Air exchange rate [19–22], transmittance [19,21], and spectral irradiance [23] are the most important physical properties of culture vessels. Regulation of the microenvironment by the optimization of culture room conditions can be attained by altering the interface between inside and outside environments.

Various criteria such as light transmittance, isolation from water loss and contamination, allowance for gas exchange, and provision of adequate growing area are considered during the design and construction of culture vessels [24]. Volumetric ventilation rate per hour divided by the air volume of the vessel gives the actual value of the air exchange rate for the culture vessel [25]. It is impractical to maintain the air exchange rate on the growing conditions of plantlets. Lentini et al. reported that air exchange, humidity build-up, and ethylene were limited by tight closures that adversely affect tissue quality and growth rate [26]. Similarly the contribution of the tight cap to adversely affecting the quality of plantlets was examined by Bottcher et al. [27]. In contrast favorable effects of a sealed Petri dish on bud differentiation in excised cotyledons of *Pinus radiata* in a limited air exchange environment was reported by Kumar et al. [28]. Significant effects of unventilated vessels on the fresh weights and number of shoots of Rhododendron P.J.M were investigated by Walker et al. [29]. Various other reports related to the effect of a closed system on radiations are mentioned in Table 10.1.

TABLE 10.1   Effect of Closed System Design, Construction, and Material on Plantlet Growth

Objectives	Results	References
The effect of force ventilated CO_2 on the growth conditions of *Buddleja alternifolia* was studied	No significant differences between the means of all five CO_2 treatments were found	[30]
Studied cultured leaf of *Dianthus caryophyllus* plantlets in airtight or ventilated vessels	Plantlets grown in ventilated vessels showed better performance of stomatal function than plantlets grown in sealed culture vessels	[31]
Evaluated the effects of ventilation in tissue cultures on ethylene and CO_2 accumulation for *Ficus lyrata* Warb. and *Gerbera jamesonii* Bolus	It was found that poor ventilation assisted in the accumulation of ethylene and CO_2 concentration but then retarded the growth of two kinds of plantlets	[32]
Transmittance of caps and vessel walls affects the irradiance and spectra of light that reach the top of plantlets	Modification in material characteristics improves the light quantity penetrating into vessels	[24]
Investigated the effects of closures and vessels on light transmittance in the culture vessels	Rubber plugs and aluminum foil cap severely reduced the irradiance of the area that was under the closures	[33]
Effects of stainless-steel wire frame stands that were used to support the vessels on irradiance	Reduced the irradiance entering the vessel	[34]
Effect of spectra irradiance on the growth of plantlets has been reviewed	–	[23]
Compared the spectra transmittance of several culture vessels	Glass vessels could transmit the light at wavelengths over 300 nm	[35]
Studied the effect of radiation on medium. Ultraviolet wavelengths and blue wavelengths entered the medium, the formaldehyde production was induced and iron in the medium could be degraded	Caps and walls of vessels exclude the wavelengths between 290 and 450 nm	[36]

10.9 EVALUATION OF PHOTOSYNTHETIC CAPACITY IN MICROPROPAGATED PLANTS BY IMAGE ANALYSIS

Imaging of chlorophyll fluorescence is usually done to evaluate the photosynthetic capacity of plants. This is essential for understanding the light distribution in culture. Light that has been reemitted after being absorbed by chlorophyll molecules of plant leaves can be measured by measuring the intensity and nature of this fluorescence. Flow cytometry can be used to determine the photosynthetic capacity of chlorophyll. In this method, a fluorescence is enhanced in the presence of 3-(3,4-dichlorophenyl)-1,1-dimethylurea, an inhibitor of photosynthetic electron transport. Significant correlations between fluorescence enhancement and photosynthetic capacity can be made by using a mercury–cadmium arc lamp-based flow cytometer. The correlation was dependent on species and growth irradiance. Photosynthetic capacity is a measure of the maximum rate at which leaves are able to fix carbon during photosynthesis. It is typically measured as the amount of CO_2 that is fixed per μmol m^{-2} sec^{-1}. Image analysis-based evaluation can also help in evaluating photosynthetic capacity.

10.10 MONITORING GENE EXPRESSION IN PLANT TISSUE CULTURES

During microenvironmentation there is an automated provision for delivering a gene and examining its expression. Transient and stable transgene expression is the temporary expression of a transformed gene (gene of interest) in the desired target cells over a relatively brief time span. It does not necessarily indicate integration of the gene into the host chromosome and is not passed onto the next generation. Green fluorescent protein (GFP) is usually used to determine the expression of a transformed gene. The green fluorescent protein is a protein that exhibits bright green fluorescence when exposed to light in the blue to ultraviolet range. In cell and molecular biology, the GFP gene is frequently used as a reporter of expression. In modified forms it has been used to make biosensors, and many animals have been created that express GFP as a proof-of-concept that a gene can be expressed throughout a given organism. Image analysis of GFP protein and its quantification *in vivo* assist in determining the localized expression throughout the tissue. Currently development of a robotic GFP image acquisition system is used for the same purpose. For these types of determinations robotic platform, hood modification, microscope and camera, light source and microscope optics, and automated image analysis are required.

10.11 BIOREACTOR DESIGNS

Various types of operating strategies are adopted while using bioreactor. These strategies are dependent on the configuration of bioreactors and impeller designs. Advances in process monitoring by computation or advanced robotics technology are preferred during this process. Based on the nature of cultures, product required, and construction of bioreactors there are many types of bioreactors, e.g., for hairy root, stir tank, airlift, bubble column, liquid dispersed bioreactors, temporary immersion bioreactors, and wave bioreactors. Bioreactor engineering for recombinant protein production using plant cell suspension culture has different considerations from others that are used for secondary metabolite production. Parameters like culture characteristics, cell morphology, degree of aggregation, culture rheology, foaming and wall growth, shear sensitivity, growth rate, oxygen demands and metabolic heat loads, intraphase transport, and ultimately recombinant protein expression can be accessed in the bioreactors that are meant for recombinant protein production.

10.12 INTEGRATING AUTOMATION TECHNOLOGIES WITH COMMERCIAL MICROPROPAGATION

Modern automation technologies with high robotic and computational advancement are required to control the microenvironmental conditions during micropropagation. Large-scale production through such technologies is successful though this would increase the production cost. High cost limits the utilization of such automation technologies, which is ideal for the production of large volumes at economic rates. Automation is always developed after screening of suitable designs and materials used for construction. This practice decreases the cost per plantlet and increases the volumes of plantlets sold. Flexibility in software or hardware modification allows the production of desired volumes of plantlets in micropropagation. Photoautotrophic culture systems generate considerable opportunities in this area. Large-scale biofermenters and other large-scale handling systems are the most reliable technologies for large volume plant producers. Most of the emphasis of micropropagation research has been on multiplication rates and primary cost controlling factors. Once a minimum increase in volume per subculture has been established the final cost per batch can be optimized. Thus, biological, physical, economic, and business parameters that affect automation and mechanization are intensely evaluated for establishing reliability and throughput quality, in order to drive the micropropagation industry to its next level (Fig. 10.3).

10.13 MACHINE VISION AND ROBOTICS FOR THE SEPARATION AND REGENERATION OF PLANT TISSUE CULTURE

During the microenvironmentation plantlets grow either as elongated stems (where identifiable nodes help to determine cutting points) or clumps (e.g., sugarcane, where the separable shoots grow from a single point). These two growth patterns found during microenvironmentation affect the design of the machine vision and robotic mechanisms used to make the transplants. Robotic separation of nodes and clumps is required at this stage. Robotic methods such as arc and the Hugh transform method are good examples for shoot identification. For nodal growth, stems are cut in such a pattern so that each piece bears a leaf node. A prototype robotic unit for cutting and replanting of nodal plants was described by Fujita and Kinase [37].

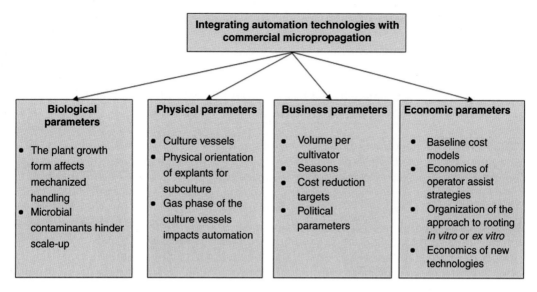

FIGURE 10.3 Illustration of integrated automation technologies accessed to evaluate biological, physical, economic, and business parameters.

10.14 TISSUE CULTURE GEL FIRMNESS: MEASUREMENT AND EFFECTS ON GROWTH

The gel in a solidified tissue culture medium can influence the explant or callus growth and morphology in a concentration-dependent manner. Strength of the gel can be modified by pH, type of carbohydrate, nutrient composition, charcoal concentration, dissolution/autoclaving method, age of the medium, and storage conditions. The most dynamic variable among all of these parameters is the pH of unbuffered gelled media, which is measured prior to the autoclaving. pH values keep on changing during medium preparation (even in the absence of a live culture on the medium). Variation in gel strength causes the most common problem, called syneresis. This process is defined as separation of liquid or "weeping" from the gel [38]. Syneresis occurs due to the contraction or structural changes of the gel matrix. Extended storage and freezing temperature often result in syneresis. Most of the solidifying agents suffer from this problem. Agar is considered to be highly syneretic whereas gellan gum shows slight syneresis. Therefore, selection of solidifying agent and gelling strength plays an important role in deciding the strength of the gel [39]. After solidification the pore size of the matrix decides the extent of diffusion of nutrients from substrate to the explants. Size of the pores is decided by structure and density of the gel matrix. Rigidity and structure-dependent firmness can be assessed by the robotic equipment. Complete characterization of the gel is accomplished by texture profile analysis, using instruments like an Instron tester to measure hardness (rupture strength), firmness (resistance to compression), brittleness (compression distance to the gel's rupture point), and elasticity (height recovery after compression) [40]. Cost of the instrument is expensive; however, provides an accurate and broad description of gel properties for applications like quality control and product development within the food industry. Simpler instruments with more modest and robotic capabilities also are or have been commercially available (e.g., the Marine Colloids Gel Tester).

10.15 COMMERCIALIZED PHOTOAUTOTROPHIC MICROPROPAGATION SYSTEM

A conventional photomixotrophic micropropagation system that utilizes a sugar-containing culture medium is now being replaced by a modern robotic photoautotrophic micropropagation system that uses a sugar-free culture medium (Fig. 10.2). The photoautotrophic micropropagation system has many advantages over the use of large culture vessels with minimum risk of microbial contamination, the enhancement of plantlet growth at a high photosynthetic photon flux (PPF), and a high CO_2 concentration inside the vessel [41–44]. Both natural and forced ventilation methods are used to increase CO_2 concentration in the vessel under pathogen-free conditions. Natural ventilation can be enhanced by placing gas-permeable filter disks over the vessel lid [25]. Forced ventilation can be employed by supplying CO_2-enriched air by air pump, having a gas permeable filter disk to filter the air. An air-flow controller can be used to control the forced ventilation rate while it is difficult to change the natural ventilation rate during the process.

Natural ventilation cannot be maintained in large vessels, thus forced ventilation is more convenient and practical for commercial production especially for large vessels. Several reports promote the utilization of forced ventilation since such utilization considerably enhances the growth of plantlets more than natural ventilation. Application of a photoautotrophic micropropagation system is advantageous to many plants (Table 10.2). In addition, it is advantageous to additional ornamental species such as Calla lily (*Zantedeschia elliottiana*) and China fir (*Cunninghamia lanceolata* (Lamb.) Hook). Nowadays, a photoautotrophic micropropagation system in used in a microenvironmentation, which is a well-equipped, computerized, robotic, and modern system that can be used in cryoengineeering technology (cryopreservation),

TABLE 10.2   Various Applications of Photoautotrophic Growth in Micropropagation

Plant under photoautotrophic growth	Capacity and modification of vessel with forced ventilation	References
Strawberry (*Fragaria* × *ananassa* Duch.)	20-L vessel with forced ventilation	[42]
Potato (*Solanum tuberosum* L.) plantlets	2.6-L vessel with forced ventilation	[45]
Sweet potato (*Ipomoea batatas* (L.) Lam.) plantlets	12.8-L vessel	[46]
Sweet potato plantlets	Vessel of 11 L with air distribution pipes to improve an airflow pattern in the vessel for obtaining uniform growth	[47]
Sweet potato plantlets	Engineered a 3.5-L vessel with units of forced ventilation and sterile nutrient solution supply for uniform and enhanced growth	[48]

controlled rate freezers, cryomicroscopy, and thermal analysis (DSC). In addition, system configuration includes a multishelf unit, culture vessel unit, and provision to control rate or slow cooling.

10.16 CLOSED SYSTEM FOR HIGH QUALITY TRANSPLANTS USING MINIMUM RESOURCES

In microenvironmentation, plants are propagated under aseptic conditions in a closed culture vessel generally under artificial light to produce a number of disease-free transplants. As mentioned above for creating a microenvironment, a photoautotrophic micropropagation method is employed to grow plants photosynthetically under aseptic conditions on the sugar-free culture medium using leafy or chlorophyllous explants in a ventilated culture vessel (Fig. 10.2). Conventional vegetative propagation is conducted mostly under natural light in a greenhouse or a nursery and differs from photoautotrophic micropropagation in size of explants and the degree of asepsis of culture medium and/or plants. Such *in vitro* plants grown on a sugar-containing or sugar-free medium are principally aseptic, but conventionally propagated plants using cuttings are not. The objective of micropropagation or microenvironmentation is not only to produce aseptic plants, but to produce disease-free and physiologically healthy plants, which are tolerant to various kinds of environmental stress. Microorganisms are not the only source of contamination in microenvironmentation, as microorganisms are not necessarily pathogens. Therefore, the closed transplant production system using artificial light is designed in such a way so as to produce disease-free transplants (but not aseptic transplants) at low costs with minimum use of resources. Such a closed system is suitable for microenvironmentation and can be used both for plantlet and seedling production. This closed system comes under the plant propagation and/or transplant production systems in which increased attention is paid to resource saving and environmental conservation than in the photoautotrophic micropropagation system. Such a system is capable of producing high quality transplants at low costs. In addition, it is a resource for saving, environmental conservation, and biomass production.

It has been reported that quality and productivity of transplants are certainly higher and the growth period of transplants can be shortened by more than 30% when produced in the closed system using lamps rather than in the greenhouse using sunlight. In contrast with environmental conditions where lots of water is required for irrigation and energy is required for cooling in summer and for heating in winter, a closed system is energy and material efficient. This ecofriendly system does not release polluted water that contains fertilizers to the outside and seldom requires pesticides and fungicides. Furthermore, its relative low transplant production cost compared to a greenhouse increases its commercialization worldwide. It was first commercialized in Japan in 2002, and in 2004 it was being used at 23 locations in Japan.

The main components that are always considered when designing a closed plant production system are light, gas, air current, temperature, nutrient and irrigation, water and vapor, and medium (substrate). A closed system is characterized on the basis of regulation of these parameters. Such characterization helps in deciding the design and material used in construction. After designing and construction the features of the closed system are compared to a greenhouse. Economic value is again an important parameter evaluated before and after designing of the vessel. To determine the whole cost, some of the factors are initially investigated and compared for large-scale commercial production, such as cost for heating, cooling, electricity, ventilation, CO_2 enrichment, construction material, and disinfectants. Photosynthetically active radiation utilization efficiency of a closed system is again a very important factor evaluated during the process. Safety evaluation should be done after the determination of the aforementioned parameters. Tomato, spinach, sweet potato, and pansy are widely reported and known to be value-added transplants in the closed system.

10.17 OTHER ENVIRONMENT CONTROL SYSTEMS

There are several other examples of environment control systems that acquire the capability to improve plant life by providing a constantly monitored atmosphere, producing a more uniform product. Some of the examples are mentioned below:

- A *greenhouse* is a space of variable size from a small shed to an industrial-sized unit in which plants are grown widely. A greenhouse primarily works by allowing sunlight to warm surfaces inside the structure, but then preventing absorbed heat from leaving the structure through convection.
- *Hydroponics* is a subset of hydroculture and is a method of growing plants using mineral nutrient solutions in water without soil.
- *Aeroponics* is the process of growing plants in an air or mist environment without the use of soil or an aggregate medium (known as geoponics).
- *Aquaponics* is a food production system that combines conventional aquaculture with hydroponics (cultivating plants in water) in a symbiotic environment.

References

[1] Kozai T, Fujiwara K, Kitaya Y. Modeling, measurement and control in plant tissue culture. Acta Hortic 1996;393:63–73.
[2] Buddendorf-Joosten JMC, Woltering EJ. Components of the gaseous environment and their effect on plant growth and development *in vitro*. Plant Growth Reg 1994;15:1–16.
[3] Ghashghaei J, Brenckmann F, Saugier B. Water relations and growth of rose plants cultured *in vitro* under various relative humidities. Plant Cell Tiss Org Cult 1992;30:51–7.
[4] Kozai T, Fujiwara K, Watanabe I. Fundamental studies on environments in plant tissue culture vessels. (2): effects of stoppers and vessels on gas exchange rates between inside and outside of vessels closed with stoppers. J Agric Met 1986;42:119–27. (In Japanese).
[5] Zobayed SMA. Aeration in plant tissue culture. Plan Tiss Cult Eng: Focus on Biotechnol 2006;6:313–27.
[6] Kessell RHJ, Carr AH. The effect of dissolved oxygen concentration on growth and differentiation of carrot (*Daucus carota*) tissue. J Exp Bot 1972;23:996–1007.
[7] Carman JG. Improved somatic embryogenesis in wheat by partial simulation of the *in-ovulo* oxygen, growth-regulator and desiccation environments. Planta 1988;175:417–24.
[8] Stuart DA, Strickland SG, Walker KA. Bioreactor production of alfalfa somatic embryos. Hortscience 1987;22: 800–3.
[9] Jay V, Genestier S, Courduroux JC. Bioreactor studies on the effect of dissolved oxygen concentrations on growth differentiation of carrot (*Daucus carota* L.) cell cultures. Plant Cell Rep 1992;11:605–8.
[10] Archambault J, Williams RD, Lavoie L, Pépin MF, Chavarie C. Production of somatic embryos in a helical ribbon impeller bioreactor. Biotechnol Bioeng 1994;44:930–43.

[11] Shigeta J, Sato K, Mii M. Effects of initial cell density, pH and dissolved oxygen on bioreactor production of carrot somatic embryos. Plant Sci 1996;115:109–14.

[12] Shimazu T, Kurata K. Relationship between production of carrot somatic embryos and dissolved oxygen concentration in liquid culture. Plant Cell Tiss Org Cult 1999;57(1):29–38.

[13] Kurata K, Shimazu T. Effects of dissolved oxygen concentration on somatic embryogenesis. Plan Tiss Cult Eng: Focus on Biotechnol 2006;6:339–53.

[14] Fujiwara K, Kozai T. Physical microenvironment and its effects. In: Aitken-Chistie J, editor. Automation and environmental control in plant tissue culture. Dordrecht, The Netherlands: Kluwer Academic Publishers; 1995. p. 319–69.

[15] Gryze C, De Riek J, Debergh PC. Water relationships in the culture vessel. Acta Horticultura 1995;393:9–44.

[16] Preece JE, Sutter EG. Acclimatization of micropropagated plants to the greenhouse and field. In: Debergh PC, Zimmerman RH, editors. Micropropagation: technology and application. Dordrecht, The Netherlands: Kluwer Academic Publishers; 1990. p. 71–93.

[17] Ziv M. Vitrification: morphological and physiological disorders of in vitro plants. In: Debergh PC, Zimmerman RH, editors. Micropropagation: technology and application. Dordrecht, The Netherlands: Kluwer Academic Publishers; 1990. p. 45–69.

[18] Debergh P, Aitken-Christie J, Cohen D, Grout B, von Arnold S, Zimmerman R, Ziv M. Reconsideration of the term "vitrification" as used in micropropagation. Plant Cell Tiss Org Cult 1992;30:135–40.

[19] Chen C, Chen J. Measurement of gas exchange rates for plant tissue culture vessels. Plant Cell Tiss Org Cult 2002;71(2):103–9.

[20] Chen C. Development of a heat transfer model for plant tissue culture vessels. Biosystems Eng 2003;85(1):67–77.

[21] Chen C. Humidity in plant tissue culture vessels. Biosystems Eng 2004;88(2):231–41.

[22] Chen C. Fluorescent lighting distribution for plant micropropagation. Biosystems Eng 2004;90(3):295–306.

[23] Dooley JH. Influence of lighting spectraon plant tissue culture. ASAE Paper No. 1991:91-7530.

[24] Smith MAL, Spomer L. Vessels, gels, liquid media, and support systems. In: Aitken-Chistie J, editor. Automation and environmental control in plant tissue culture. Dordrecht, The Netherlands: Kluwer Academic Publishers; 1995. p. 371–404.

[25] Kozai T, Kitaya Y, Fujiwara K, Smith MAL, Aitken-Christie J. Environmental measurement and control systems. In: Aitken-Chistie J, editor. Automation and environmental control in plant tissue culture. The Netherlands: Kluwer Academic Publishers; 1995. p. 539–74.

[26] Lentini Z, Mussel H, Mutschler MA, Earle ED. Ethylene generation and reversal of ethylene effects during development in vitro of rapid-cycling Brassica campestris. L Plant Sci 1988;54(1):75–81.

[27] Bottcher I, Zoglauer K, Goring H. Induction and reversion of vitrification of plants cultured in vitro. Physiol Plantarum 1988;72(3):560–4.

[28] Kumar P, Reid D, Thorpe T. The role of ethylene and carbon dioxide in differentiation of shoot buds in excised cotyledons of Pinus radiata in vitro. Physiol Plantarum 1987;69(1):244–51.

[29] Walker P, Heuser C, Heinemann P. Micropropagation: effects of ventilation and carbon dioxide level on Rhododendron "P.J.M". Trans ASAE 1989;32(2):348–52.

[30] Cuello JL, Walker PN, Heuser CW, Heinemann PH. Controlled in vitro environment for stage II micropropagation of Buddleia alternifolia (Butterfly bush). Trans ASAE 1991;34(4):1912–8.

[31] Majada JP, Sierra MI, Sanchez-Tames R. Air exchange rate affects the in vitro developed leaf cuticle of carnation. Sci Hortic-Amsterdam 2001;87(1):121–30.

[32] Jackson MB, Abbott AJ, Belcher AR, Hall KC, Butler R, Cameron J. Ventilation in plant tissue cultures and effects of poor aeration on ethylene and carbon dioxide accumulation, oxygen depletion and explant development. Ann Bot 1991;67(2):229–37.

[33] Fujiwara K, Kozai T, Nakajo Y. Effects of closures and vessels on light intensities in plant tissue culture vessels. J Agr Meteorol 1989;45(3):143–9.

[34] Kozai T, Fujiwara K, Hayashi M, Aitken-Christie J. The in vitro environment and its control in micropropagation. In: Kurata K, Kozai T, editors. Transplant production systems. Dordrecht, The Netherlands: Kluwer Academic Publishers; 1992. p. 247–82.

[35] Stasinopoulos T, Hangarter R. Preventing photochemistry in culture media by long-pass filters alters growth of cultured tissues. Plant Physiol 1990;93(6):1365–9.

[36] Hangarter RP, Stasinopoulos T. Repression of plant tissue culture growth by light is caused by photochemical change in the culture medium. Plant Sci 1991;79(2):253–7.

[37] Fujita N, Kinase A. The use of robotics in automated plant propagation. In: Vasil IK, editor. Scale-up and automation in plant propagation. San Diego: Academic Press, Inc; 1991. p. 231–44.

[38] McNaught AD, Wilkinson A. IUPAC compendium of chemical technology. 2nd ed. Oxford, UK: Blackwell Science; 1997. p. 464. Online at: http://www.nicmila.org/Gold/Output/S06227.xhtml.

[39] Mao R, Tang J, Swanson BG. Water holding capacity and microstructure of gellan gels. Carbohyd Polym 2001;46:365–71.

[40] Whyte JNC, Englar JR, Hosford SPC. Factors affecting texture profile evaluation of agar gels. Bot Mar 1984;27: 63–9.

[41] Kozai T. Photoautotrophic micropropagation. In Vitro Cell Dev Biol-plant 1991;27:47–51.

[42] Fujiwara K, Kozai T, Watanabe I. Development of a photoautotrophic tissue culture system for shoots and/or plantlets at rooting and acclimatization stages. Acta Hort 1988;230:153–8.

[43] Kozai T, Iwanami Y. Effects of CO_2 enrichment and sucrose concentration under high photon fluxes on plantlet growth of Carnation (*Dianthus caryophyllus* L.,) in tissue culture during the preparation stage. J Jpn Soc Hort Sci 1988;57:279–88.

[44] Kubota C. Concepts and background of photoautotrophic micropropagation. In: Morohoshi N, Komamine A, editors. Molecular breeding of woody plants. Amsterdam: Elsevier Science BV; 2001. p. 325–34.

[45] Kubota C, Kozai T. Growth and net photosynthetic rate of *Solanum tuberosum in vitro* under forced ventilation. Hort Sci 1992;27:1312–4.

[46] Heo J, Kozai T. Forced ventilation micropropagation system for enhancing photosynthesis, growth and development of sweet potato plantlets. Environ Contr Biol 1999;37(1):83–92.

[47] Heo J, Wilson SB, Kozai T. A forced ventilation micropropagation system for production of photoautotrophic sweet potato plug plantlets in a scaled-up culture vessel: growth and uniformity. Hort Technol 2000;1:90–4.

[48] Zobayed SMA, Kubota C, Kozai T. Development of a forced ventilation micropropagation system for large-scale photoautotrophic culture and its utilization in sweet potato. In Vitro Cell Dev Biol-plant 1999;34:350–5.

11

Micropropagation

Saurabh Bhatia, Kiran Sharma

11.1 INTRODUCTION

The method for obtaining large numbers of clonal explants in a short duration is called micropropagation. It can also refer to use of a tissue culture technique for clonal propagation of plants. This can be feasible in a short space of time. Micropropagation methods were used in 1960 by George Morel for the production of orchid plants at a commercial level [1]. Generally sexual and asexual methods are used for propagation of plants. Sexual methods of propagation involve pollen grains to fertilize eggs and seeds that are produced at a high degree

Modern Applications of Plant Biotechnology in Pharmaceutical Sciences. http://dx.doi.org/10.1016/B978-0-12-802221-4.00011-X

of heterogeneity. In vegetative propagation or asexual methods mitotic division of plant parts is used for the production of new varieties. In this case, both the new plants and parent plants are genetically identical to each other. Clonal propagation refers to the multiplication of genetically identical copies of plants. A clone is an individual plant obtained by sexual methods. Cutting, budding, and grafting are the usual techniques used in vegetative propagation and together this is known as *in vivo* clonal propagation of plants. *In vivo* clonal propagation is mostly expensive, difficult, and unsuccessful. A better alternative approach for this purpose is tissue culture [2].

The commonly used explants in micropropagation for initiation of the culture are meristem, shoot tip, and axillary buds. The shoot apical portion consists of a group of actively dividing meristematic cells at meristem and shoot tip. Shoot tip and meristem were clearly defined by Cutter in 1965. The terminal portion of the shoot that contains actively dividing meristematic cell mass is the meristem or apical meristem and its length is about 100–250 μm [3].

The terminal meristematic portion with one to three leaf primordia measures about 100–500 μm in length and is referred to as shoot tip and shoot apex. Shoot apex is sufficient explant for *in vitro* clonal propagation, but for the production of disease-free varieties of plants as in meristem cultures, it is important to excise the meristem without any surrounding tissue. The axile portion of the node contains axillary buds, which are made up of meristematic cells and can also be used as explants. Based on the physiological state of the plant they may either be in an active or a dormant state. The axillary bud method was once employed for carnation but is now rarely used. Large-scale micropropagation of gerbera and strawberry is widely done using the axillary method [4]. Several strategies that are currently used in micropropagation and the major steps involved are highlighted in Fig. 11.1.

11.2 TYPES OF EXPLANTS USED IN MICROPROPAGATION

11.2.1 Meristem Culture

Meristem culture is used for shoot apical meristem culture *in vitro*. Meristem culture was developed by Morel and Martin in 1952 for rivers eliminating from *Dahlia* [5]. Orchid *Cymbidium was* micropropagated using meristem culture by Morel in 1965 [6]. An already existing shoot meristem grows in the meristem culture and adventitious roots regenerate from these shoots. In the shoot tip beyond the youngest leaf lies the primordium meristem. It measures up to 250 mm in length and 100 mm in diameter. In addition to the apical meristem one or three leaf primordia would be present in a shoot tip of 100–500 nm. When virus elimination is the objective, to obtain disease-free plants, shoot tips of up to 10 mm are used. For rapid clonal propagation, a shoot-tip culture is followed in which (5–10 mm) explants are used. Hence, the majority of meristem culture are essentially shoot-tip cultures. Various sized nodal explants are also employed for rapid clonal propagation [7].

The size of the shoot tip used for culture is not important when the main objective is micropropagation. But when the objective is to obtain virus-free stock (or stock free from other pathogens) it is necessary for the excision of the apical meristem to be done with a minimum of the surrounding tissue. The shoot tip may be cut into fine pieces in order to obtain more than one plantlet from each shoot tip. Pieces of curd (the inflorescence) are used in some species such as cauliflower. Shoot tips or tissue pieces bearing buds of such stems may be used

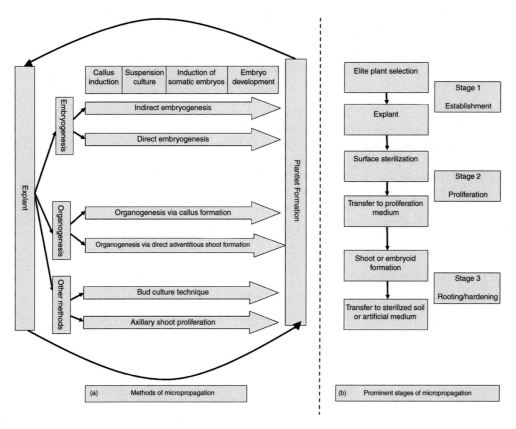

FIGURE 11.1   Illustration of the micropropagation process highlighting methods and major stages.

for those plants having an underground stem. Explants taken from actively growing plants early in the growing season are the most suitable [8].

Explants of meristem are then placed on Murashige and Skoog's (MS) medium, which is considered to be an effective medium for the majority of species. Lower salt concentration is suitable for some species. Fungicides (bavistin) or antibiotics (chloramphenicol/strepto-mycin) can be added to the medium during growth to remove the endophytic contamination. Similarly, meristem culture follows steps similar to micropropagation: (i) initiation of culture, (ii) shoot multiplication, (iii) rooting of the developed shoots, and (iv) transfer of the plantlets to the pots or soil [9].

11.2.2 Shoot-Tip Culture

Explants/shoot tips consist of shoot apical meristem, unexpanded leaves at various development stages, and a number of leaf primordia about 1 cm in length. In shoot-tip culture the explants are inoculated in cytokinin-supplemented media. Suppression of apical dominance is caused by cytokinin and a highly branched shoot system formation is facilitated. Then manipulation of the shootlets is done in the rooting medium to develop plantlets [10].

11.2.3 Seed Culture

The seed culture technique for micropropagation is effective for many dicots and monocots as multiple shoots can be obtained from an embryo instead of single seedlings from a seed [11].

11.2.4 Single-Node Culture

Mature plants or seedlings containing single nodes can be used as explants as nodes contain axillary buds, which when treated with cytokinin in *in vitro* conditions can lead to production of branches. In rooting medium, such axillary shoots produce roots, thus forming a number of plantlets [12].

11.3 METHODS OF PLANTLET PRODUCTION USED IN MICROPROPAGATION

11.3.1 Direct Organogenesis

When axillary or apical meristems are difficult to obtain in culture, the direct organogenesis method may prove to be useful for micropropagation. Any tissue of explants in this method will produce shoots directly, e.g., root, cotyledon, and leaf may be used as the explants and these produce plantlets on inoculation. Explant cells produce plantlets by directly undergoing organogenesis [13].

11.3.2 Indirect Organogenesis

At the cut edges of the explants callus is formed that is known as dedifferentiation callus. Organization of such a callus is done to give a new shoot. Manipulation of phytohormones is required for indirect organogenesis [14].

11.3.3 Axillary Bud Method

In the axillary bud method, isolation of a shoot tip is achieved from which the axils of leaves develop axillary buds under the effect of high concentrations of cytokinin. Apical dominance is suppressed under the effect of high cytokinin concentration and permits the development of axillary buds. If a number of side shoots or axillary shoots have been formed on the shoot tip then their inoculation may be done on the fresh medium containing cytokinin. Often the axillary method is used in combination with the single node method. Certain points must be kept in mind concerning axillary shoot formation [15,16]:

- Often the ratio used in the axillary bud method between cytokinin and auxin is 10:1.
- Concentration of cytokinin is proportional to the developmental stage of the material/culture. Adult material requires more cytokinin than juvenile material.
- Most plants do not react as well to kinetin as they do to 6-benzyladenine. The requirement of cytokinin is therefore variable and must be adjusted according a particular plant species or cultivar.

- Sometimes it is advisable to allow the development of the shoot tip prior to increasing cytokinin concentration in order to induce axillary shoot formation.
- The apical meristem must be removed or killed if development of axillary shoot is unsatisfactory.
- Axillary shoot formation is sometimes promoted by the liquid medium.
- Several substituted pyridylphenylurea compounds and thidiazuron stimulate axillary branching in wide range of species.

11.4 STAGES INVOLVED IN MICROPROPAGATION

The various steps or stages involved in the complex process of *in vitro* clonal propagation or micropropagation are summarized in four stages. The four stages of overall micropropagation were recognized in 1978 by Murashige [17]. Stages I to III were considered under *in vitro* conditions and stage IV under greenhouse conditions. Stage 0 was introduced in the micropropagation system by Debergh and Mane in 1981 [18].

11.4.1 Stage 0: Stock/Elite Plants Selection

The first step in micropropagation is the selection of stock or elite plants having desirable characters for their multiplication on a large scale. After selecting the stock/elite plants they are maintained in controlled environmental conditions of low humidity, irrigation, and without any systemic microbial infection for a period of 3 months for culture initiation.

11.4.2 Stage I: Aseptic Culture Establishment

In this stage, explants selected in Stage 0 are prepared for inoculation after treatment with suitable sterilizing agent and established on a well-defined culture medium. The axillary bud, shoot tip, and meristem are surface sterilized by using various chemicals such as 5% sodium hypochlorite, 0.1% mercuric chloride, or 70% alcohol with various contact times either in combination or alone depending upon the level of surface contamination. After surface sterilization the explants are inoculated onto the MS medium (or any other suitable basal medium) supplemented with various growth regulators, vitamins, and sucrose. For micropropagation, culture medium containing cytokinins (1–3 mg/L 6-benzyl amino purine) with less concentration of auxin (indole-3-acetic acid) was used. The auxin 2,4-dichlorophenoxyacetic acid is good because it suppresses organogenesis and stimulates formation of callus. The cultures are incubated at a 16-h photoperiod at 3000–10,000 flux light intensity.

11.4.3 Stage II: Multiplication of the Explants

Multiplication of explants takes a considerable time through regeneration of shoots from explants. In some cases only single shoots develop from the apical shoots and such shoots are used for excising a number of nodal explants. Further cytokinin-rich media are used to inoculate nodal explants for multiple shoot proliferation. Multiple shoots may also be produced during this process by somatic embryogenesis or organogenesis directly on explants. Each explant produces five to six shoots in a period of 4 to 5 weeks. If all the plants survive, single explants would produce 5^{10}–6^{12} plants in 1 year.

11.4.4 Stage III: Germination of Somatic Embryo or Rooting of Regenerated Shoots

Rooting in fresh medium is induced by multiple shoots produced during stage II. Inoculation of individually separated shoots is done to the rooting medium (with auxins) and in some cases rooting is directly induced in the soil in conditions of high moisture. The rooted plants are highly sensitive and fragile to the moisture. In the case of somatic embryos, germination is allowed to form the plantlets and then they are transferred to the soil. The plantlets, after going through hardening process, are slowly transferred to the soil. The hardening medium should be either pearlite, peat, or vermiculite, holding considerable moisture and maintained at high humidity conditions before it is transferred to the soil.

11.4.5 Stage IV: Hardening

In the hardening stage the plantlets of stage III are prepared for external soil conditions from their *in vitro* conditions. This involves the plants becoming resistant to stress, moisture, and disease resulting in the autotrophic nature of plants from the heterotrophic nature in *in vitro* culture conditions. Protection must be given to plantlets from direct sunlight and a decrease in relative humidity should be done over a period of time. Well-developed roots are formed by the plantlets during this acclimatization period and cuticular wax is also formed in the aerial tissues. After this the plantlets become suitable for transfer to the open fields [19].

In some cases vitrification is observed under *in vitro* conditions where some species or shoots appear brittle, glossy, and water soaked. Vitrification is due to abnormal functioning of stomata, poorly developed vascular bundles, and abnormal wax quality resulting in loss of plantlets. This condition can be overcome by use of growth retardants, bottom cooling of culture tubes, addition of high concentration of agar (1%), and addition of hydrolysate compounds [20].

11.5 ECONOMIC SIGNIFICANCE

Throughout the world interest in natural drugs is increasing. The market for flavors, pharmaceuticals, fragrances, and colors derived from natural plants is worth several billion dollars per year. Vincristine, vinblastine, colchicine, taxol, forskolin, artemisinin, saponins, etc. are phytochemicals of interest in medicine and biology and it has been possible to produce these phytochemical compounds using plant tissue culture techniques such as micropropagation in short periods. Hence, the advanced plant tissue culture techniques serve to satisfy the ever-growing needs of the commercial market for herbal drugs [21].

11.6 APPLICATIONS AND MERITS OF MICROPROPAGATION OVER CONVENTIONAL PLANT BREEDING [22–24]

The various applications of micropropagation are:

- Plant tissue in small amounts is sufficient for the production of millions of clones in a year using micropropagation. It would take a great deal of time to produce an equal number of plants using conventional methods.
- The technique of micropropagation provides a good alternative for those plant species that show resistance to practices of conventional bulk propagation.
- An alternative method of vegetative propagation for mass propagation is offered through micropropagation. Plants in large numbers can be produced in a short period. Any particular variety may be produced in large quantities and the time to develop new varieties is reduced by 50%.
- Large amounts of plants can be maintained in small spaces. This helps to save endangered species and the storage of germplasm.
- The micropropagation method produces plants free of diseases. Hence, disease-free varieties are obtained through this technique by using meristem tip culture.
- Proliferation of *in vitro* stocks can be done at any time of the year. Also, a nursery can produce fruit, ornamental, and tree species throughout the year.
- Increased yield of plants and increased vigor in floriculture species are achieved.
- Fast international exchange of plant material without the risk of disease introduction is provided. The time required for quarantine is lessened by this method.
- The micropropagation technique is also useful for seed production in certain crops as the requirement of genetic conservation to a high degree is important for seed production.
- Through somatic embryogenesis production of synthetic artificial seeds is becoming popular nowadays.

With micropropagation having various advantages over conventional methods of propagation, this method holds better scope and future for production of important plant-based phytopharmaceuticals. Independent of availability of plants, micropropagation offers a lucrative alternative approach to conventional methods in producing controlled amounts of biochemicals. Therefore, intense and continuous efforts in this field will direct controlled and successful production of valuable, specific, and yet undiscovered plant chemicals.

References

[1] Morel G. Producing virus free cymbidiums. Am Orchid Soc 1960;25:495–7.
[2] Saxena S, Bopana N. *In vitro* clonal propagation of *Asparagus racemosus*, a high value medicinal plant. Methods Mol Biol 2009;547:179–89.
[3] June IM. Vegetative apical meristems. Plant Cell 1992;4:1029–39.
[4] Sateesh MK. Biotechnology – 5: Animal cells. Immunol Plant Biotechnol 2003;155–60.
[5] Morel GM, Martin C. Guerison de dahlias atteints d'une maladie A virus. Comptes rendus hebdomaire des séances de l'Academie des Sciences, Paris 1952;235:1324–5.
[6] Morel G. Clonal propagation of orchids by meristem culture. Cymbidium Soc News 1965;20:3–11.
[7] Banerjee N, Langhe E. A tissue culture technique for rapid clonal propagation and storage under minimal growth conditions of Musa (Banana and Plantain). Plant Cell Rep 1985;4:351–4.

 [8] Cimen A, Ozgee C. Micropropagation of *Anthurium andraeanum* from leaf explants. Pak J Bot 2009;41(3):1155–61.

 [9] Gray DJ, Benton CM. *In vitro* micropropagation and plant establishment of muscadine grape cultivars (*Vitis rotundifolia*). Plant Cell Tiss Org Cult 1991;27:7–14.

[10] Saeed NA, Zafar Y, Malik KA. A simple procedure of *Gossypium* meristem shoots tip culture. Plant Cell Tiss Org Cult 1997;51(3):201–7.

[11] Amrane A. Seed culture and its effect on the growth and lactic acid production of Lactobacillus helveticus. J Gen Appl Microbiol 2003;49(1):21–7.

[12] Barna KS, Wakhlu AK. Modified single node culture method – a new micropropagation method for chickpea. *In Vitro* Cell Dev Biol Plant 1995;31(3):150–2.

[13] Kumari KG, Ganesan M, Jayabalan N. Somatic embryogenesis and plant regeneration in *Ricinus communis*. Biol Plantarum 2008;52(1):17–25.

[14] Kumar SR, Krishna V, Pradeepa K, Kumar KG, Gnanesh AU. Direct and indirect method regeneration from root explants Caesalpinia bonduc (L.) Roxb. – a threatened medicinal plant of Western Ghats. Ind J Exp Biol 2012;50:910–7.

[15] Abhyankar G, Reddy VD. Rapid micropropagation via axillary bud proliferation of *Adhatoda vasica* Nees from nodal segments. Ind J Exp Biol 2007;45:268–71.

[16] Annarita L. Morphological evaluation of olive plants *in vitro* culture through axillary buds and somatic embryogenesis methods. Afr J Plant Sci 2009;3(3):037–43.

[17] Murashige T. Impact of plant tissue culture on agriculture. In: Thorpe, TA, editor. Frontiers of plant tissue culture; 1978. p. 15-26 and 518-524. The International Association for Plant Tissue Culture. Calgary. p. 556.

[18] Debergh PC, Mane LJ. A scheme of commercial propagation of ornamental plants by tissue culture. Sci Hortic 1981;14:335–45.

[19] Gaspar T. Vitrification in micropropagation. Biotechnol Agr Forest 1991;17:116–26.

[20] Ziv M. Quality of micropropagated plants – vitrification. *In Vitro* Cell Dev Biol 1991;27(2):64–9.

[21] Ozdemir FA, Yildirim MU, Kahriz MP. Efficient micropropagation of highly economic, medicinal and ornamental plant Lallemantia iberica (Bieb.) Fisch. and C.A. Mey. Biomed Res Int 2014; http//:dx.doi.org/10.1155/2014/476346.

[22] Thorpe TA, Harry IS, Kumar PP. Application of micropropagation to forestry. Micropropagation. Netherlands: Springer; 1991. p. 311-336.

[23] Torress KC. Application of tissue culture techniques to horticultural crops. USA: Springer; 1989. p. 66-69.

[24] Debnath M, Malik CP, Bisen PS. Micropropagation: a tool for the production of high quality plant-based medicines. Curr Pharm Biotechnol 2006;7:33–49.

CHAPTER

12

Laws in Plant Biotechnology

Saurabh Bhatia, Randhir Dahiya

OUTLINE

Modern Applications of Plant Biotechnology in Pharmaceutical Sciences. http://dx.doi.org/10.1016/B978-0-12-802221-4.00012-1

12.1 INTRODUCTION

Development in biotechnology brings attention to issues such as the legal characterization of new inventions. Therefore, currently the major concern of the biotechnology industry is toward legal characterization of innovation and technologies through patenting or intellectual property rights (IPR). Generally intellectual property (IP) is defined as a product of the mind. It is intangible in contrast to real property or physical property, which one can see, feel, and use. With any type of property there are property rights. When IPR are expressed in a tangible form, they can also be protected.

12.2 INTELLECTUAL PROPERTY RIGHT PROTECTION

IP has been created to protect the right of individuals to have the benefit of their creations and discoveries. IPR is a broad term that covers several forms of protection. These several forms of protection are governed by a number of organizations. Forms of protection like patent and copyright are known to be the most prominent laws that are frequently utilized in IPR. Copyright is a right to protect the form of expression; however, subject matter in this right is not protected. On the contrary, a patent permits the protection of those subject matters that are legally permissible under this law. Another form of protection called trademark is a symbolic representation of the product to distinguish the proprietary product from others, which clearly describes the source of the product. Trademark itself is a protection, though it does not provide security to the product that represents the trademark. There are various others forms of protection such as geographical indications (GIs), data protection, trade secrets, and layout of integrated circuits, which generally provide protection in a different manner. All these forms of protection are governed by the World Trade Organization (WTO), the Agreement on Trade-Related Aspects of Intellectual Property (TRIPS), the World Intellectual Property Organization (WIPO), and the International Convention for the Protection of New Varieties of Plants (UPOV). The General Agreement on Tariffs and Trade (GATT) was signed in 1947 and lasted until 1994, when it was replaced by the WTO in 1995. GATT held a total of nine rounds. There are a total of 157 member countries in the WTO, with Russia and Vanuatu being new members as of 2012.

12.2.1 Forms of Protection (Fig. 12.1)

12.2.1.1 Copyright, Trademark, and Patent

Copyrights, trademarks, and patents are all forms of legal protection provided by a government entity to inventors, musicians, businesses, and many others. Each offers a unique set of rights and protections but differs in what they cover, as well as how long these protections last. In general, a copyright protects written or artistic works, like books, plays, musical compositions, and paintings; trademarks protect brand names and symbols, like logos; and patents protect inventions, including processes, devices, designs, and even plants. Copyright protects the form of expression rather than the subject matter. A patent is an exclusive right given to an inventor to exclude all others from making, using, selling, or offering to sell the

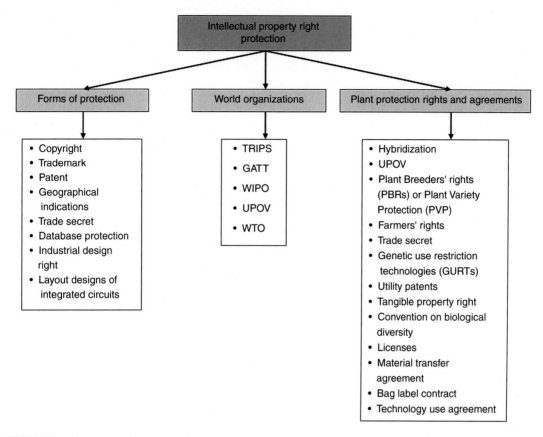

FIGURE 12.1 Forms of protection that come under intellectual property rights (IPR).

invention in the country that granted the patent right, and importing it into that country. A patent temporarily protects the subject matter with a condition that the subject comes under patent-eligible subject matter. Patentable, statutory, or patent-eligible subject matter is subject matter that is susceptible to patent protection. In agricultural biotechnology, patents may cover, for example, plant transformation methods, vectors, genes, etc., and in countries that allow patenting of higher life forms, transgenic plants or animals are also covered under them. Patents are the most critical form of protection for agricultural biotechnology and are considered to be the most powerful in the IP system. Patents are temporary, generally for about 20 years, and are country specific. The granting of a patent is subject to the fulfillment of three conditions:

- Usefulness or industrial application
- Newness or novelty, in the sense that the invention was not previously known to the public
- Nonobviousness, or inventive step, so that the invention constitutes an acknowledged extension of prior knowledge

Trademark is a word, name, or symbol used in the trade to indicate the source of the goods and to distinguish them from others. The words trademark or trademark law are frequently used generically to encompass similar identifiers of origin such as service marks, collective marks, certification marks, trade dress, and trade names. The primary purpose of the trademark laws is to prevent unfair competition by applying a test of consumer confusion and providing rights and remedies to the owner of the trademark. In contrast, copyrights do not generally protect individual words or slogans but will protect creative designs. Therefore, a logo design could be protected by both copyright law and trademark law.

12.2.1.2 Trade Secrets

These consist of commercially valuable information about production methods, business plans, clientele, etc. They are protected as long as they remain secret by laws that prevent acquisition by commercially unfair means and unauthorized disclosure.

12.2.1.3 Database Protection

The European Union (EU) has adopted legislation to provide *sui generis* protection in respect of databases, preventing unauthorized use of data compilations even if nonoriginal. Exclusive rights to extract or utilize all or a substantial part of the contents of the protected database are granted.

Over the last two decades there has been an unprecedented increase in the level, scope, territorial extent, and role of IP protection in crop biosafety and biosecurity, which includes the following trends:

- The patenting of living things and materials found in nature, as opposed to man-made products and processes more readily recognizable to the layman as inventions;
- The modification of protection regimes to accommodate new technologies (particularly biotechnology and information technology);
- A new emphasis on the protection of new knowledge and technologies used in the public sector;
- The focus on the relationship between IP protection and traditional knowledge (TK), folklore, and genetic resources;
- The geographical extension of minimum standards for IP protection through the TRIPS agreement and of higher standards through bilateral and regional trade and investment agreements; and
- The widening of exclusive rights, extension of the duration of protection, and strengthening of enforcement mechanisms.

12.2.1.4 Geographical Indications (GIs)

GIs identify the specific geographical origin of a product, and the associated qualities, reputation, or other characteristics and usually consist of the name of the place of origin. For example, food products sometimes have qualities that derive from their place of production and local environmental factors. The GI prevents unauthorized parties from using a protected GI for products not from that region or from misleading the public as to the true origin of the product.

12.2.1.5 *Industrial Design Right*

Industrial design right is a form of IPR. These rights protect the visual design of objects. An industrial design consists of the creation of a shape, configuration, or composition of pattern or color, containing esthetic value. Industrial designs help make any product or item more beautiful and appealing. When a new and original design is created, applied to a product, and commercialized, if it obtains a certain level of commercial success, it is very important to protect the design legally. This is because if a third party (normally a competitor) manufactures, uses, or sells products with the same design or a very similar one that can be confused with the original, it will be highly detrimental for the creator of the design.

12.3 ORGANIZATION IN INTELLECTUAL PROPERTY RIGHT PROTECTION

Plant variety protection in the form of plant breeders' rights (PBRs) has been in existence in industrialized countries for a long time. From the 1920s a number of European countries have recognized various kinds of PBRs. From the 1930s, plant varieties were admitted to patent protection in the United States and Germany and subsequently many developed countries. At the international level, UPOV was first adopted in 1961 and subsequently revised in 1972, 1978, and 1991 to recognize the need to protect varieties of plants for the interest of breeders [1,2]. The introduction of IPR, as one of the new issues in the Uruguay Round GATT negotiations, was approved at the ministerial meeting held in Punta del Este in 1986. The WTO TRIPS Agreement, one of the results of the Uruguay Round, states that:

> WTO members shall provide for the protection of plant varieties either by patents or by effective *sui generis* system or by any combination thereof.

The obligation to introduce plant variety protection in developing countries is a novelty for all but a few. It will bring fundamental changes to their legal system and constitute significant departure from previous practices, which generally empathized the free sharing of knowledge at all levels. Moreover, it affects access to propagating material (seeds) by local or rural communities where most of the population meets their basic needs largely from traditional farming. Farming communities have a well-established practice of saving, exchanging, and replanting seeds, which may be restricted under PBRs. Accordingly, the recognition and the grant of an IPR to the breeder of a new plant variety is not welcomed in a large number of developing countries [3].

The TRIPs agreement leaves to each country's discretion whether to protect new plant varieties by means of patent, by an effective *sui generis* system, or by any combination thereof. TRIPS contain no further standard as to what constitutes an effective *sui generis* system, nor does it mention UPOV. Thus, developing countries are not obliged to provide for the protection of plant varieties under patents or to comply with UPOV provisions; instead, they may prefer to develop their own *sui generis* system of protection. However, major developed countries, especially the United States, are applying unilateral pressure to force developing countries to go beyond the TRIPS standards in order to safeguard the interest of their multinational corporations.

On the other hand, developing countries are rich in biodiversity; much of the germplasm of the world comes from such countries. Farmers in developing countries usually possess

TK and use traditional techniques to manage and develop new crop types and biodiversity conservation. They play a major role in the conservation of plant genetic resources (PGR) and transmission of these resources to seed companies, plant breeders, and research institutions. At one time, it was acceptable to collect germplasm freely in any nation, including developing nations, and use it in breeding. However, when developed nations moved quite strongly toward adopting plant variety protection, there arose concerns, based on the perception that it was unfair for the source material contributed by developing countries to be transferred freely while breeding activities contributed by developed nations were being rewarded with IPR. Traditional farmers and indigenous people around the world have seen their PGRs and TK monopolized by private enterprises under patents and PBRs and have not been receiving their equitable share of benefits for their contribution [4].

These concerns led to the adoption of two United Nations binding international treaties, the Convention on Biological Diversity (CBD), the first global agreement on the conservation and sustainable use of biological diversity, signed at the 1992 Earth Summit in Rio de Janeiro, and the International Treaty on Plant Genetic Resources for Food and Agriculture, adopted on November 3, 2001 under the auspices of the Food and Agricultural Organization, which recognizes the enormous contribution that farmers and their communities have made and continue to make to the conservation and development of genetic resources.

The TRIPS Agreement established minimum standards for protection and enforcement of IPR. As laid out in Article 7, which indicates the TRIPS Agreement objectives:

> The protection and enforcement of intellectual property rights should contribute to the promotion of technological innovation and to the transfer and dissemination of technology, to the mutual advantage of producers and users of technological knowledge and in a manner conducive to social and economic welfare, and to a balance of rights and obligations.

Article 27(3)(b) of the TRIPS Agreement allows WTO members to exclude from patentability:

> ... (b) plants and animals other than micro-organisms, and essentially biological processes for the production of plants or animals other than non-biological and microbiological processes. However, this provision makes it mandatory for WTO members to provide for the protection of plant varieties either by patents or by an effective *sui generis* system or by any combination thereof.

The wording of this obligation, which leaves the choice of the protection system entirely to the members, reflects the differences between the existing legal systems, ranging from the highest level of protection in the United States, where plant varieties may be protected by patents or by specific plant variety protection rights or even by special plant patents, to EU countries, where plant variety protection is confined to specific variety protection systems only [5].

If a state chooses to implement its obligation under Article 27.3(b) by means of a *sui generis* system that system would have to be effective. It should be noted that while the TRIPS agreement contains a minimum standard of protection for patents, it contains no further standard as to what constitutes an effective *sui generis* system, nor does it mention UPOV. Therefore, WTO members that have not acceded UPOV are not obliged to comply with UPOV provisions, and may prefer to develop their own *sui generis* system of protection.

In developing countries, the issue has been how to balance the interest of "breeders" and "farmers" while providing protection to new varieties of plants. The protection of plant varieties under patent would be the worst solution for developing countries, as patent is the most powerful mean of protection.

In most patent laws, in effect, there is no exception similar to the "breeders exemption" under plant breeder rights regimes. Hence, the patentee may, in principle, prevent a third party from using the patented variety for further research and breeding. For instance, multiplication of the variety, even for experimental purposes, can also be prevented. The claims in a variety patent may cover inbred lines or hybrids, seeds or plants, and attempt to extend to progeny. Since a plant variety "is characterized by essentially all of its genes" the patenting of plant varieties may restrict the access to and use of the whole combination of genes that constitutes a variety, and prevent the development of new combinations of such genes.

The possibility of excluding plant varieties from patent protection as permitted under the TRIPS agreement and the previous resistance of many developing countries to provide any protection at all in this field will most likely result in either the adherence of those countries to the UPOV Convention or the creation of *sui generis* protection according to their own concepts.

The experience of a few developing countries that have become party to the UPOV is limited since they have joined the UPOV relatively recently. However, Cullet has reported that

> Limited lessons can be learnt from the experience of Kenya and Zimbabwe, which already have plant variety protection regimes in place. In both cases, the introduction of plant variety protection has not substantially fostered the development of new food crops. On the contrary, in Kenya, out of 136 applications filed and tested since 1997, only one was a food crop while most concerned cash crops such as ornamentals or sugarcane and more than half concerned rose varieties [6]

There is a requirement for plant protection under TRIPS and members of the WTO are bound by their membership to adhere to the TRIPS. The agreement sets out the minimum standards of IP protection the member countries are required to provide.

One of the most controversial provisions of the agreement surrounds protection of plant varieties. Article 27(3)(b) of the agreement allows countries to exclude plants and essentially biological processes for their production from their patent system of protection. The same Article, however, states that countries must

> ... provide for the protection of plant varieties either by patents or by an effective *sui generis* system or by any combination thereof.

Under the agreement, a country can implement more than one form of plant protection.

The meaning of *"sui generis"* is one of the contentious issues surrounding the agreement. It is generally believed that the term enables member countries to design their own system of protection for plant varieties if they have selected not to use their patent system for plant protection.

12.3.1 International Union for the Protection of New Varieties of Plants

UPOV is the only international treaty focusing on plant variety protection. The Convention was first adopted in Paris in 1961 and entered into force in 1968. It has been revised three times in 1972, 1978, and 1991. It established the International Union for the Protection of New Varieties of Plants, which has the mandate to enforce the Convention. Its main goal is to encourage the development of new varieties of plants, for the benefit of society through the grant of protection, which serves as an incentive to those who engage in commercial plant breeding.

On April 24, 1999, the 1991 Act entered into force in accordance with Article 37(1), which states that

> This Convention shall enter into force one month after five States have deposited their instruments of ratification.

The provision of Article 37(3) ensured that the 1978 Act of the Convention is closed to further accession. By virtue of the TRIPS Agreement, member states of the WTO are obliged to provide for the protection of plant varieties. To bring the TRIPS patent provisions into line with the UPOV Convention on the protection of plant varieties, Article 27.3(b) permits members to provide for the protection of plant varieties. As most developing countries are yet to adopt some form of plant variety protection, the need to adopt a system that would comply with their international obligations and also adapt to their national circumstances in recent times has come to the fore and triggered discussions focusing on the salient features of the UPOV Convention. This is due to the fact that UPOV is an intergovernmental organization and not a "treaty" as such.

Countries are not obliged to join UPOV as a result of their affiliation with any other organization or the ratification of any specific treaty. Membership is purely voluntary. Each member of the organization becomes bound to the UPOV Convention. The Convention requires member countries to provide an IPR specifically for plant varieties. This form of IP protection is often referred to as plant breeders' rights (PBRs). As a result of PBRs, plant breeders are granted a legal monopoly over the commercialization of their plant varieties. Protection allows breeders to try to recover the costs associated with the development of the variety. By conferring protection on plant varieties, UPOV also aims to provide an incentive to individuals or companies to invest in plant breeding, thereby providing a positive stimulus in the plant breeding industry. The rights granted are for a specific time only (depending on the plant variety), and upon expiration of the time period, the protected variety passes into the public domain.

The UPOV Convention has been revised three times; however, not all member countries are bound by the latest Convention (1991). Approximately 26 countries remain bound by the 1978 Convention, while Spain and Belgium are bound by the original Convention (1961). The main differences in the two latest agreements can be seen in Table 12.1.

The requirements for protection under UPOV require clarity. The variety must be distinguishable from any other variety that is publicly known at the time of filing the application. The variety must have predictable characteristics and be able to be reliably reproduced.

TABLE 12.1 The Main Differences in the Two Latest Agreements

UPOV convention	1978	1991
Requirements	Distinct, uniform, and stable	Distinct, uniform, stable, new
Protects	Commercial use of reproductive material of the variety	All plant varieties and products including plants that are derived
Duration of protection	15 years from application date for most species. 18 years for trees and vines	20 years from application date for most species. 25 years for trees and vines
Breeder's exemption	Yes. Acts for breeding and development of other varieties are not prohibited	Optional. The decision to include an exemption is dependent on each member's national legislation

The additional requirement under the 1991 Convention states that the variety must be "new." The word "new" is held to mean that the variety has not been sold or otherwise disposed of by the breeder for commercial purposes prior to filing for protection. However, similarly to a utility patent, natural source material is not protectable. The UPOV Convention does allow a 12-month "grace period" for sales of the new variety before protection is no longer available (Article 6(1b)).

The latest convention protects all plant varieties including those that are "essentially derived," i.e., plants that require the protected variety for their production. The protection offered to the plant variety is an exclusionary right [7].

Protection confers the right to exclude others from:

- Producing or reproducing
- Propagating
- Offering for sale
- Selling or other marketing
- Exporting
- Importing
- Stocking the protected variety for any of the mentioned purposes

However, the protected plant can be used for noncommercial acts (provided they are done privately) and for experimental purposes without infringement.

Considering that many UPOV members are also bound to the TRIPS Agreement (due to their WTO membership), UPOV provides a framework by which countries can implement a protection system that generally fulfills the TRIPS requirement of providing "an effective *sui generis* system."

12.3.2 WTO Agreement on Trade-Related Aspects of Intellectual Property Rights

The TRIPS Agreement, adopted in 1994, requires that

> ... patents shall be available for any inventions, whether products or processes, in all fields of technology.

However, it allows countries to exclude from protection "plants and animals other than micro-organisms." It does require that countries provide for the protection of plant varieties either by patents or by an effective *sui generis* system (i.e., plant variety protection (PVP)) or both. The TRIPS agreement permits countries some flexibility in the precise form and extent of protection and promotes the fundamental idea of extending IPRs to agricultural genetic resources. The general objectives of the TRIPS Agreement are the protection and enforcement of IPRs, the promotion of technological innovation, and the transfer and dissemination of technology. A WTO member country must be nondiscriminatory and extend the same treatment to all other members that it affords one member. Most developing countries are opposed to the use of patent systems in agriculture.

There are several objectives of the TRIPS Convention: the conservation of biodiversity, the sustainable use of the components of genetic resources like crops, forest plants, and animals, and the fair and equitable sharing of the benefits arising out of the utilization of generic resources.

All the commitments such as general measures for conservation and sustainable use, *in situ* and *ex situ* conservation and sustainable use of the components of biological diversity, access to genetic resources, access to and transfer of technology, handling of biotechnology and distribution of benefits, and financial mechanisms are governed by objectives that are interrelated to each other [8].

Article (6) obligates contracting parties to develop and adopt a national strategy for the conservation and distribution of benefits, sustainable use of biological diversity, and also to integrate the conservation and sustainable use of biological diversity into relevant sectoral or cross-sectoral plans, programs, and policies. This should be done in accordance with each party's particular conditions and capabilities.

Article (6) provides the basis for Article (10), which contains more concrete provisions related to national strategy and commitments to avoid or minimize the adverse impact on biological diversity, and to protect and encourage customary and traditional culture.

Regarding crop biosecurity, the TRIPS Agreement under the Article 27.3(b) imposes on all member states the introduction of plant variety protection either through patents or an alternative *sui generis* system [9,10].

12.3.3 Plant Protection Rights and Agreements

12.3.3.1 *Hybridization*

Prior to the 1980s, even if legal protection had been given to seed producers against unauthorized use of new varieties, enforcement would have been hampered by the difficulty of identifying proprietary germplasm as the parent of a new commercial variety. Until the advent of biotechnology, only hybrid seeds, which do not breed true upon replanting, were protected against this type of misappropriation. With the case of corn in the United States as the most prominent example, protection via hybridization was strong enough to foster the growth of a profitable private agricultural seed breeding industry in 1930s, well before the effective strengthening of legal IP protection for these types of plants. In developing countries, such as India, hybridization offers less protection because parent lines cannot be effectively protected from misappropriation for more than a few years. In the twentieth century, a major innovation in IPR for germplasm was the US Plant Patent Act of 1930, which gave protection from unauthorized use of many kinds of clonally propagated plants for the life of the patent. This form of protection was useful principally in horticulture, and has been important, for example, for strawberry breeding at the University of California. In many other countries, protection of clones has since become available via PBRs, which, like plant patents (but unlike utility patents), do not protect against use of the protected material for sexual reproduction or use of germplasm to breed new cultivars, if that is possible.

In some cases, specialized plant breeding can present an alternative to IP protection. Breeders often select individual plants that display beneficial or attractive traits such as a fast growth rate in comparison to other plants or an increase in either herbicide or disease resistance, etc. The breeder then crosses these plants with individual plants of different varieties that also demonstrate attractive traits. The resulting progeny are called hybrids. Seeds resulting from hybrids show an extremely poor ability to reliably reproduce the trait of interest in their progeny or next generation. It therefore becomes necessary for the farmer to purchase new seed for subsequent plantings. Hybrid selection therefore becomes a way for plant breeders to protect their varieties from exploitation, as they are safe in the knowledge that the farmer or purchaser can only access the trait reliably for one generation. Farmers and others must obtain more seed from the breeder if they wish to continue to use the same hybrid plants. Hybridization therefore serves as a way of not only creating new plant varieties with attractive traits but ensuring some sort of protection for new commercial plant varieties. Although this method of protection is inexpensive and is not subject to legal requirements or restrictions, breeders have no enforceable remedy available to them, except under trade secret law or by contractual agreement [11].

12.3.3.2 *Plant Breeders' Rights or Plant Variety Protection*

While in the United States plant varieties can be protected under the patent system, in the majority of jurisdictions including Australia, the protection of plant varieties under patent legislation is not permitted. Having a form of protection in place that is available to new plant varieties is thought to be important in order to encourage and promote plant breeding, import of foreign varieties, promote the exportation of plant varieties, and benefit the market. The term plant breeders' rights is synonymous with plant variety protection. Plant breeders' rights include protection provided to plant breeders by nations, almost all of whom are members of UPOV, founded in 1961. PBRs protect varieties that are deemed new, uniform, stable, and distinct against unauthorized sale for replanting. In one notorious US case, a soybean cultivar was approved as distinct based only on its blue flower color, a trait not generally considered meaningful in commercial soybeans. Use of germplasm as breeding stock for producing new varieties is not prohibited. An exception introduced in the 1991 version of UPOV is the breeding of a variety "essentially derived" from a protected parent. This exception might cover a similar cultivar derived from a simple back-cross, differing by a small amount of transgenic DNA, but its scope is yet to be legally established. It is not well recognized that the requirements for evaluation in each country, and the need for local legal representation, can render broad international application for PBRs comparable in cost to patents, and it is time consuming.

In the United States, restrictions are placed on the use of sexually propagated seed germplasm for reproduction by way of Plant Variety Protection Certificates (PVPCs). PVPCs are administered by the US Department of Agriculture under the legal authority of the Plant Variety Protection Act of 1970, which had liberal provisions for saving and replanting of seed by farmers. Restrictions on replanting saved seed by producers have been strengthened over time in the United States, but are still difficult to enforce. Other countries have enacted much more liberal versions of PBRs. In India and Thailand, indigenous varieties are covered, and contain clauses for "benefit sharing" with local communities when land races are used in commercial breeding. Indian PBRs appear to allow farmers to sell unlimited quantities of what in the United States are called "brown bag" seeds, unidentified by variety or registration.

The PBRs allow for the protection of new plant varieties for a term of 20 years (25 for tree crops). A country can develop its own system of protection, referred to as a *sui generis* system, i.e., a system of rights designed to fit a particular context and need that is a unique alternative to standard patent protection. Patent law was originally considered unsuitable for protecting new plant varieties developed by traditional breeding methods. Some countries therefore introduced special national laws for PVR in the 1960s, as did UPOV. These rights are granted by the state to plant breeders to exclude others from producing or commercializing material of a specific plant variety for a minimum of 15 to 20 years. To be eligible for PVR, the variety must be novel, distinct from existing varieties, and uniform and stable in its essential characteristics. At first, this form of legal protection was limited to commercializing reproductive or vegetatively propagated material taken from a new variety. It was implied or specified that certain exemptions were allowed to farmers and researchers (breeders). Such exemptions under PVR systems are termed farmers' privilege and breeders' privilege (or research exemption) [12,13].

12.3.4 Farmers' Rights

The Plant Variety Protection Act recognizes the farmer not just as a cultivator but also as a conserver of the agricultural gene pool and a breeder who has bred several successful varieties. The Act makes provisions for such farmers' varieties to be registered with the help of nongovernmental organizations (NGOs) so that they are protected against being scavenged by formal sector breeders. The rights of rural communities are acknowledged as well. Farmers' rights are defined in the following way: The farmer shall be deemed to be entitled to save, use, sow, resow, exchange, share, or sell his farm produce including seed of a variety protected under this Act in the same manner as he was entitled before the coming into force of this Act, provided that the farmer shall not be entitled to sell branded seed of a variety protected under this Act.

This formulation allows the farmer to sell seed in the way he has always done, with the restriction that this seed cannot be branded with the breeder's registered name. In this way, both farmers' and breeders' rights are protected. The breeder is rewarded for his innovation by having control of the commercial marketplace but without being able to threaten the farmers' ability to independently engage in his livelihood, and supporting the livelihood of other farmers. The pivotal importance of the farmer having the right to sell (not save or exchange, but sell) seed has to be seen in the context of seed production in India. In India, the farming community is the largest seed producer, providing about 87% of the country's annual requirement of over 60 lakh tons. If the farmer were to be denied the right to sell, it would not only result in a substantial loss of income for him but far more importantly, such a step would displace the farming community as the country's major seed provider. Weak farmers' rights, including denial of right to sell seed, will allow seed corporations to dominate the seed market since farmers will be denied the right to function as seed producers. The space vacated by them will be taken by the seed industries since public sector institutions have been so weakened by budget cuts that they could not compete. The seed industry would then become the dominant source of seed. Strong farmers' rights, allowing the farmer to continue to be a significant supplier of seed, make the farming community a viable competitor and an effective deterrent to the takeover of the seed market by the corporate sector. Control over seed production is central to food security, which is in the forefront of national security [14].

12.3.5 Contributions of International Agreements on Crop Biosecurity

The CBD was adopted at the Rio de Janeiro Earth Summit, in June 1992. Over 150 governments signed the documents at the Rio conference, and since then more than 175 countries have ratified the Convention. The main objectives of the Convention as indicated in Article 1 are: (i) the conservation of biological diversity; (ii) sustainable use of its components; and (iii) sharing the benefits arising from the utilization of generic resources in a fair and equitable way. Under Article 2 of the Convention "biological diversity" means the variability among living organisms from all sources including, *inter alia*, terrestrial, marine, and other aquatic ecosystems and the ecological complexes of which they are part; this includes diversity within species, between species, and of ecosystems.

During the last three decades, there have been numerous meetings and consultations at the international level for streamlining the availability and utilization of existing biological resources in an equitable manner. This has been necessitated by revolutionary developments in the life sciences and possibilities of generating immense economic benefits. This situation is in contrast to the era of the Green Revolution when all the germplasm developed was easily available throughout the world and many developing countries greatly benefited from it. At that time no issues regarding IPRs were raised. However, now that the world situation has changed with the "free market economy" as the dominant force, agriculture is viewed as an industry or business subject to all the regulatory measures. It is in this context that agriculture figures prominently in all the deliberations of the WTO wherein various aspects have been strongly contested between countries of different blocks with different interests [15].

The main international agreements that impact on IP for crop biosecurity are as follows.

12.3.6 Trade Secrets

A trade secret is confidential information. A trade secret is commonly regarded as any formula, pattern, device, or compilation of information that is used in a business and gives that business an opportunity to obtain advantages over competitors. The information is kept from the public and from competitors, usually by the use of confidentiality agreements with employees. These agreements confer an obligation on the employees to keep the information secret. These agreements can be enforced by the court. Generally, for a trade secret to exist there must have been:

Secrecy: In the form of a confidentiality agreement or covenant. External forms of protection such as security systems, etc., also impart the necessary requirement of secrecy.

Novelty: The subject of the secrecy must have been novel.

Value: The subject of the trade secret must be of some value or give some advantage over competitors.

For a breach of a trade secret to occur, there must have been an improper taking. That is there must have been a breach of the secrecy whether by theft or the breaking of a confidentiality agreement. One advantage of using trade secret law to protect an invention is the unlimited time for protection. Some disadvantages, however, are that trade secret protection does not prevent competitors from legally reverse engineering a product to determine the secret or from independently duplicating the information. Inventions involving the use of DNA are now unlikely to be protected by trade secrets due to the ability to reverse engineer. Trade secret laws can be used to protect plants. Plants can be protected provided that reasonable efforts have been made to keep the plant variety confidential, secret, and out of the public domain. In the United States, trade secrets have been used for decades to protect parental lines of hybrid corn. Recently a US court recognized that "genetic messages" of inbred plant varietal lines may be protected by trade secret law subject to the provision that reasonable effort has been taken to preserve the secrecy of the gene sequence (the Pioneer Hi-Bred case). In the Pioneer Hi-Bred case, it was held that the accidental inclusion of inbred seed in bags of commercially available first generation seed by Pioneer Hi-Bred was not enough to destroy the secrecy surrounding its "genetic message." Reasonable precaution had been taken to keep the "genetic message" contained in the inbred seed out of the public domain. Under Australian law, it is theoretically possible that specific varieties of plants may be afforded protection under the doctrine of confidential information or trade secrets; however, to date, no cases involving the doctrine and plant varieties have been brought before the courts. As a result it is currently unclear as to the extent of protection available under the doctrine of trade secrets.

12.3.7 Genetic Use Restriction Technologies

Genetic use restriction technologies (GURTs) is a group of tools that allows the control of gene expression of an organism, further allowing constraints or restrictions on the use of the organism or trait. The term GURT was developed by the lead author (Cambia's CEO) of the first study commissioned by the United Nations Convention on Biological Diversity.

There are two main types of GURT: variety-level GURT (v-GURT) and trait-level GURT (t-GURT). v-GURT causes the seeds of the affected plant variety to be sterile in contrast to t-GURT, which results in the expression of a selected trait. t-GURT introduces a mechanism for trait expression into the variety, which can only be turned on, or off, by treatment with specific chemical inducers. The gene of interest can thus be expressed at particular stages or generations of the crop.

In addition to IPR, plant breeders in principle are able to use GURTs to strengthen the protection of newly developed plant varieties. The use of v-GURTs requires farmers to buy seeds from the breeder each season and therefore could be used as a way of avoiding the farmers' privilege exception to patentability that exists in Europe. However, in some situations v-GURTs are advantageous to farmers as they reduce the need for tillage and do not sprout inappropriately. t-GURTs require the farmer to purchase chemical inducers from the breeder in order for the farmer to be able to make use of the specific traits of the variety, i.e., herbicide resistance [16–18].

12.3.8 A *Sui Generis* System (India)

Many developing countries have an agricultural economy that is geared toward the domestic as opposed to the export market. Such an economy is dependent upon farmer-produced seed of varieties that are both maintained and further adapted to their local growing conditions by small-scale farmers. Developing countries with such an economy want to acknowledge the rights of farmers arising from their contribution to crop conservation and development and the sharing of their knowledge on adaptive traits. They also want to encourage farmer-to-farmer exchange of new crop/plant varieties that are adapted to the local growing conditions. As a result, some developing countries have chosen a *sui generis* system of plant protection that is not compliant with UPOV in that it allows farmers to improve and adapt the seed in order to make it more successful in the local conditions.

Under the Indian Protection of Plant Varieties and Farmers' Rights Act 2001, plants are divided into four main classes: new varieties, extant varieties, essentially derived varieties, and farmer's varieties. The regime for plant protection is similar to that set out by UPOV and the requirements for protection are novelty, distinctness, uniformity, and stability. Under Article 39(iv) the farmer is entitled to save, use, sow, resow, exchange, share, or sell his farm product including seed of a protected variety. However, he is unable to sell seed that is branded with the breeder's name. In this way the breeder has control of the commercial marketplace without threatening the farmer's ability to practice his livelihood.

The Indian Act also contains provisions for "benefit sharing" whereby the local communities are acknowledged as contributors of land races and farmer varieties in the breeding of "new" plant varieties. It is these extra provisions granting rights to both breeders and farmers that make the Indian system a *sui generis* method of protection. China and Thailand are other examples of countries that do not implement UPOV-style protection system [19].

12.3.9 Community Plant Variety Rights (EU)

Plant variety protection in the EU is a result of the European Convention (Regulation 2100/94/EC), which is based on the 1991 UPOV Convention. It was introduced in order to harmonize and streamline the method of plant variety protection available throughout Europe. The Community protection of plant varieties (CPVR – Community Plant Variety Right) enables applicants, on the basis of one application, to be granted a single IPR that is operative throughout all countries who are members of the EU. A CPVR can only be transferred or ceased within the EU Community on a uniform basis. That is, a CPVR is valid (or cancelled) across all EU countries only, not individual countries.

The CPVR exists alongside individual European countries' national plant protection legislation as an alternative form of protection. As a result, it is not possible to hold protection for the same plant variety under both the Community and a national system at the same time. Where a CPVR is granted in relation to a variety for which a national right has already been granted, the national right is suspended for the duration of the CPVR.

The CPVR confers protection to all "new" botanical genera and species, including their hybrids, provided that the varieties meet exactly the same requirements as outlined under the UPOV Convention. A CPVR is issued by the Community Plant Variety Office in Angers, France [20].

12.3.10 Plant Breeders' Rights (Australia)

Similarly to the United States, Australia is both a WTO and UPOV member and has implemented the UPOV protection system as a mechanism for complying with TRIPS. Australia is signed to the 1991 Convention. As a result, plant varieties are protected in Australia by a PBR under the Plant Breeder's Rights Act (1994). The requirements, terms, and rights conferred by the UPOV Convention are implemented under the Plant Breeder's Rights Act.

In Australia, a PBR is obtained from and administered by the Plant Breeder's Rights Office, in contrast to patents that are granted by IP Australia. Recently the Plant Breeder's Rights Office was brought within IP Australia.

A choice is usually made between the two protection systems depending on the level of protection sought and the ability to satisfy the necessary requirements. PBRs are generally obtained much faster than a patent due to the lack of examination and are also much cheaper. They are therefore desirable when protection is required for a short period of time and there is no need to acquire rights over the use of the variety for noncommercial purposes. Where comprehensive exclusive rights are desired, protection under the patent system would be more suitable.

12.3.11 Plant Variety Protection Certificates (United States)

The United States is bound by the TRIPS Agreement and is also a UPOV member. Because the United States offers patents for plant varieties, technically it does not need to also provide a *sui generis* system. In the United States, the UPOV Convention is implemented by the Plant Variety Protection Act (1970). Changes to the Act made by Amendments in 1994 extended statutory protection to F1 hybrids and tuber propagated plants and generally brought the United States into compliance with the 1991 UPOV Convention. The Plant Variety Protection Act is administered by the US Department of Agriculture, which issues PVPCs for qualifying plant varieties.

The Plant Variety Protection Act protects sexually reproduced plants, including first generation (F1) hybrids and tuber propagated plants (e.g., potato varieties). The requirements and terms of this protection offered are exactly the same as those outlined in the UPOV Convention.

The Plant Variety Protection Act requires that a deposit of seeds of the new variety be made at an authorized depository, and in the case of F1 hybrids, seeds of the parents must also be deposited.

The United States has in its national legislation only a limited farmers' exemption. In the case of farmers, protected seed may be "saved" for replanting on their own individual holdings provided that it is not sold to any third parties who use it for reproductive purposes.

Simultaneous protection by both a utility patent and a PVPC is allowed. Any variety that was protected prior to the 1994 amendments is subject to the original Plant Variety Protection Act (1970), which only provides 18 years of protection for nonwoody plants. However, applications submitted prior to April 4, 1995 (effective amendment date) might be resubmitted in order to secure the extended term of protection provided by the amendments.

12.3.11.1 *Utility Patents*

Patents protect inventions of both processes and products (composition of matter) that must be embodied in tangible things. They confer a legally enforceable right allowing the owner of a patent to exclude others from practicing the invention as described and claimed in the patent document. However, these property rights apply only for a limited period of time, generally 20 years from the date of filing, and only in a specific jurisdiction. The scope of the property rights is circumscribed by the claims made in the patent, which, in the event of litigation, may be subject to interpretation by the court of law. In agricultural biotechnology, utility patents now cover many kinds of different innovations including research tools, transformation processes, vectors, components of vectors such as markers, promoters, and genes of interest, as well as organisms and their parts.

Although international treaties and conventions govern international aspects of patenting, patents are awarded by national governments, and the protection conferred by a patent extends only to the national jurisdiction in which the patent is awarded. To protect an innovation in more than one country, a patent must be obtained in each. Applications in more than one country are facilitated by the Patent Cooperation Treaty, administered by WIPO. Applications in multiple European countries can be lodged in each country or be sent for examination by the European Patent Office (EPO) with subsequent registration on a country-by-country basis. English-speaking African nations that are members of the African Regional Industrial Property Office (ARIPO) headquartered in Harare can file patents through that office subject to confirmation. Similarly, Francophone African members of the Yaoundé, Cameroon-based organization Africaine de la Propriété Intellectualle (OAPI), can file a single application with designations to member states. The cost of obtaining a patent varies from country to country; the cost of obtaining protection in all important markets can be very substantial, reaching hundreds of thousands of US dollars. Beyond the actual filing fees for each country, translation and local legal fees are important components of this cost. The EPO, ARIPO, and OAPI are means of reducing the transaction costs associated with patenting in multiple international jurisdictions. In jurisdictions covered by TRIPS, inventions, not discoveries, are patentable. Inventions have the legal requirements of utility (i.e., have an industrial application), novelty, and nonobviousness and must be adequately described and disclosed to enable the making and using of the invention by a person ordinarily skilled in the relevant arts. These criteria and their implementation vary among countries.

In 1980, the US Supreme Court ruled that utility patents could apply to life forms. Then in 1985, the US Patent Office Board of Appeals ruled that this utility patent protection could be applied to sexually propagated seeds, plants, and cultured tissue. Now, in the United States, DNA sequences and transgenic animals are also patentable. In Europe, the EPO has ruled that plant varieties are not patentable, although it has also held that transgenic methods and plants are not *per se* unpatentable [21]. DNA sequences and amino acid sequences corresponding to the peptides or proteins produced by a naturally occurring organism are unpatentable in a number of countries including Brazil, Cameroon, Colombia, Cuba, Guatemala, and Uzbekistan (Thambisetty, 2002). The distribution of patents by value is highly skewed. While, for example, the widely-licensed Cohen-Boyer patent earned more than $200 million in royalties, most patents generate values ranging from zero to just tens of thousands of dollars. It is not surprising then, that most inventions are patented in just one or a few developed countries with large markets.

The chance that relevant biotech patents have been protected in developing countries is currently quite small, even where patenting of the relevant type of technology is available. For example, *Agrobacterium* technology is patented or pending in more than four jurisdictions outside Europe, while the very popular CaMV 35S promoter is patented only in European countries and the United States (Pardey et al., 2003). Utility patent grants in the United States show strong growth trends in all four technology categories examined, including plant cell and tissue culture technologies, enabling plant biotechnologies, genetic traits, and germplasm.

By contrast, Europe and Japan show significantly less utility patenting of enabling biotechnologies and genetic traits and none whatsoever of plant germplasm. The WIPO (WO) applications are utility patent applications filed in more than one country through the application process of the Patent Cooperation Treaty. The numbers of these WIPO applications tend to follow US patent granting trends, with the notable exception of germplasm where multiple country filings are limited. These PCT filings reflect the activity of US firms filing at home and abroad as well as European and Japanese firms filing at their home offices and in the United States. Interestingly, plant cell culture technologies are more intensively patented in Japan than anywhere else in the world, while in the other three plant technology categories the Japanese patent office shows very little or no activity.

12.3.12 Utility Patents and Plant Patent

The term "utility patent" is used to distinguish between patents and other specific forms of IP claims that exist in some jurisdictions, i.e., "plant/petty/innovation patents." Utility patents in the United States are comparable to the standard patents that are awarded both in Australia (under the Patents Act (1990)) and in Europe. In the United States, any living organism that is the product of human intervention (such as by some breeding process or laboratory-based alteration) qualifies as a composition of matter, which is patentable. As a result, plants are patentable subject matter. Furthermore, the United States has extended patent protection to plants produced by either sexual or asexual reproduction and to plant parts including seeds and tissue cultures. In Australia, the Patent Act (1990) allows all technologies to be patented (except "human beings and the biological processes for their production") provided that there is an "invention," defined as "an innovative idea which provides a practical solution to a technological problem." Utility and standard patents may be used to claim exclusionary rights in:

- New varieties of plants (United States only);
- Transgenic plants, plant groups;
- Individual plants and their descendants, particular plant traits;
- Plant parts, plant components (e.g., specific genes or chromosomes), plant products (e.g., fruit, oils, pharmaceuticals);
- Plant material used in industrial processes (e.g., cell lines used in cultivation methods);
- Reproductive material (e.g., seeds or cuttings), plant culture cells, plant breeding methodologies, and vectors and processes involved in the production of transgenic plants.

Natural source material should *not* be coverable by patents as exclusionary rights in any country in the world, because natural source material is not novel. In the United States and Australia individual plant varieties are patentable. In Europe, individual plant varieties *per se* are *not* patentable; however, a plant that is characterized by a particular gene (as opposed to its whole genome) is not included in the definition of a plant variety and *is* therefore patentable. In Europe, transgenic plants are patentable if they are not restricted to a specific plant variety, but represent a broader plant grouping. The EU Directive considers plant cells to be "microbiological products" and as a result are patentable. The EU Directive 98/44/EC provides a "farmer's privilege." Under the Directive, farmers are allowed to use patent protected seeds freely for their own use and the resulting plant material is free from protection. Farmers are not permitted, however, to resell the patented seed.

The Plant Patent Act was enacted by US Congress in 1930. It was introduced primarily to benefit the horticulture industry by encouraging plant breeding and increasing plant genetic diversity. Limited types of plants are eligible for protection. The Plant Patent Act 1930 provides for patent protection of all asexually reproduced plants *except* tuber propagated plants and plants found in an uncultivated state.

Plant patents encompass newly found plant varieties as well as cultivated spores, mutants, hybrids, and newly found seedlings on the provison that they reproduce asexually. Asexual reproduction is defined as any reproductive process that does not involve the union of individuals or germ cells. It is the propagation of a plant to multiply the plant without the use of genetic seeds. Modes of asexual reproduction in plants include grafting, bulbs, apomictic seeds, rhizomes, and tissue culture. Specifically excluded from protection under the Plant Patent Act are tuber propagated plants and plants found in an uncultivated state. The requirements that must be fulfilled in order to obtain a plant patent are the same as those for utility patents. However, the implementation of these requirements is less stringent. A plant patent gives the patent holder the right to: *exclude* others from asexually reproducing, using, selling, offering for sale, or importing into the United States the reproduced plant (or any of its parts) for a period of 20 years. In contrast to utility patents, plant patents only protect a single plant or genome and the protection conferred is quite limited. It does not protect the plant characteristics, mutants of the patented plant, nor technologies associated with its cultivation. Because plant patents are granted on the entire plant, it follows that only one claim per plant patent is permitted.

The Plant Patent Act was amended on October 27, 1998 to extend the exclusive right to plant parts obtained from protected varieties but it is not applied retroactively. A utility patent and a plant patent can both be obtained to protect the same plant. It is possible to obtain protection for the same plant under both a utility patent and a plant patent in the United States at the same time, provided that the requirements for patentability for both types of patents are fulfilled.

It should be emphasized that at the time of editing (2007) there are no commercial examples of GURTs known anywhere in the world, apart from one civil society organization who has applied patent application that had not reduced the technology to commercial practice.

12.3.13 Contracts

The following types of agreements are all governed by contract law as opposed to IP law. There are no international agreements that regulate the law of contracts.

12.3.14 Material Transfer Agreements

Material transfer agreements (MTAs) are legal agreements made between a provider and a recipient party when research material is being transferred between institutions.

Material most often transferred includes plant varieties, transgenic plants, cell lines, germplasm, vectors, chemicals, equipment, or software.

The MTA itself contains a written description of the material to be transferred and any limits on the material that the provider wishes. For example, some providers may limit the use of the transferred material to noncommercial situations or to a specific field of research. In some cases, where publication of results occurs, which involves the material, it may be necessary to acknowledge the source of the material. The terms and conditions of the MTA also usually outline the ownership rights, confidentiality provisions, and any third party transfer restrictions that the provider of the material wishes to impose. The agreement acts as a contractual agreement that is often used to protect the rights of ownership of the provider and also to protect the material from unauthorized use.

12.3.15 Bag Label Contract

Bag label contracts are another form of legal protection that can be applied to plants, especially seeds. An explicit contract is described on a bag label, which is normally sewn into the seal of a bag. By opening the bag and breaking the seal, the purchaser agrees to comply with the contract.

12.3.16 Technology Use Agreements

A technology use agreement is an agreement most commonly used between technology suppliers and farmers, which usually control the right to plant a given seed on a specific area of land often for a certain period of time. The agreement provisions can also include restrictions on the use of proprietary traits in the creation of new varieties and also gives permission for the technology supplier to access the farmer's property to check for violations. This form of property right enforcement has been implemented by producers of agronomic traits in the United States and other countries. In some cases, the producers reserve the right to inspect the field of the contracting farmer and to take samples to ensure the compliance of the farmer with the technology use agreement.

A breach of a technology use agreement gives rise to a claim for damages if a breach of contract occurs.

12.4 CONTROVERSIAL PATENT CASES INVOLVING TRADITIONAL KNOWLEDGE AND GENETIC RESOURCES

Some cases of biopiracy relating to patents of agricultural crops are listed to illustrate the issues faced by current IPR regulations.

12.4.1 Rice

The "Battle for Basmati," an aromatic variety of rice, started in 1997 when US rice breeding firm RiceTec Inc. was awarded a patent (US5663484) relating to plants and seeds, seeking a monopoly over various rice lines including some having characteristics similar to basmati lines. Concerned about the potential effect on exports, India requested a reexamination of this patent in 2000. The patentee in response to this request withdrew a number of claims including those covering basmati-type lines. Further claims were also withdrawn following concerns raised by the US Patent and Trademark Office (USPTO). The dispute has, however, moved on from the patent to the misuse of the name "basmati" [20,21].

12.4.2 Turmeric

Turmeric (*Curcuma longa*), a plant of the ginger family yielding saffron colored rhizomes used as a spice in cooking, has properties that make it an effective ingredient in medicines, cosmetics, and as a color dye. As a traditional medicine, it is used to heal wounds and rashes. In 1995, two Indian nationals at the University of Mississippi Medical Center were granted US patent no. 5,401,504 on "use of turmeric in wound healing." The Indian Council of Scientific and Industrial Research (CSIR) requested the USPTO to reexamine the patent. CSIR argued that turmeric has been used for thousands of years for healing wounds and rashes and its medicinal use was not novel as per documentary evidence of TK, including an ancient Sanskrit text and a paper published in 1953 in the *Journal of the Indian Medical Association*. Despite arguments by the patentees, the USPTO upheld the CSIR objections and revoked the patent. The turmeric case was a landmark case as it was the first time that a patent based on the TK of a developing country had been successfully challenged [22].

12.4.3 Neem

Neem (*Azadirachta indica*) is a tree from South and Southeast Asia now planted across the tropics because of its properties as a natural medicine, pesticide, and fertilizer. Neem extracts can be used against hundreds of pests and fungal diseases that attack food crops. Oil extract from its seeds is used to treat colds and influenza; and when used in soap, seemingly, offers low-cost relief from malaria, skin diseases, and even meningitis. In 1994, the EPO granted European Patent No. 0436257 to the US corporation W.R. Grace and USDA for a "method for controlling fungi on plants by the aid of hydrophobic extracted neem oil." In 1995, a group of international NGOs and representatives of Indian farmers filed a legal opposition against the patent with evidence that the fungicidal effect of extracts of neem seeds had been known and used for centuries in South Asian agriculture to protect crops, thus indicating the invention claimed in EP257 was not novel [23]. In 1999, the EPO determined that according to the evidence "all features of the present claim have been disclosed to the public prior to the patent application ... and [the patent] was considered not to involve an inventive step." The patent was revoked by the EPO in 2000.

12.4.4 Ayahuasca

For generations, shamans of indigenous tribes throughout the Amazon Basin have processed the bark of *Banisteriopsis caapi* to produce a ceremonial drink called "ayahuasca." The shamans use ayahuasca or "vine of the soul" in religious and healing ceremonies to diagnose and treat illnesses, meet with spirits, and divine the future. A US national, Loren Miller, obtained US Plant Patent 5,751 in June 1986, granting him rights over an alleged variety of *B. caapi* he had called "Da Vine." The patent description stated that the "plant was discovered growing in a domestic garden in the Amazon rain-forest of South America." The patentee claimed that Da Vine represented a new and distinct variety of *B. caapi*, primarily because of the flower color. The Coordinating Body of Indigenous Organizations of the Amazon Basin (COICA) – an umbrella organization representing over 400 indigenous groups – learned of the patent in 1994. On their behalf the Center for International Environmental Law (CIEL) filed a reexamination request on the patent. CIEL protested that a review of the prior art revealed that Da Vine was neither new nor distinct and argued that the granting of the patent would be contrary to the public and morality aspects of the Patent Act because of the sacred nature of *B. caapi* throughout the Amazon region. Extensive, new prior art was presented by CIEL, and in November 1999, the USPTO rejected the patent claim agreeing that Da Vine was not distinguishable from the prior art presented by CIEL and therefore the patent should never have been issued. However, further arguments by the patentee persuaded the USPTO to reverse its decision and announce in early 2001 that the patent should stand.

12.4.5 *Hoodia* Cactus

The San, who live around the Kalahari Desert in southern Africa, have traditionally eaten the *Hoodia* cactus to stave off hunger and thirst on long hunting trips. In 1937, a Dutch anthropologist studying the San noted this use of *Hoodia*. Scientists at the South African CSIR only recently found his report and began studying the plant. In 1995, CSIR patented *Hoodia*'s appetite-suppressing element (P57) and in 1997 licensed P57 to the UK biotech company Phytopharm. In 1998, the Intellectual Property Rights and Crop Biosecurity 30 Asian Biotechnology and Development Review pharmaceutical company Pfizer acquired the rights to develop and market P57 as a potential slimming drug and cure for obesity (with a market worth more than £6 billion) from Phytopharm for up to $32 million in royalty and milestone payments. On hearing of possible exploitation of their TK, the San people threatened legal action against the CSIR on grounds of "biopiracy" and claimed that their TK had been stolen, and that the CSIR had failed to comply with the rules of the CBD, which requires the prior informed consent of all stakeholders, including the original discoverers and users. Phytopharm had conducted extensive enquiries but were unable to find any of the "knowledge holders." The remaining San were apparently at the time living in a tented camp 1500 miles from their tribal lands. The CSIR claimed they had planned to inform the San of the research and share the benefits, but first wanted to make sure the drug proved successful. In March 2002, an understanding was reached between the CSIR and the San whereby the San, recognized as the custodians of TK associated with the *Hoodia* plant, will receive a share of any future royalties [24].

References

[1] Price SC. Public and private plant breeding. Nat Biotechnol 1999;17:938–9.
[2] Article 15 Exceptions to the breeder's right. In Union International pour la Protection des Obtentions Végétales (UPOV) International Convention for the Protection of New Varieties of Plants of December 2, 1961, as revised in Geneva on November 10, 1972, on October 23, 1978, and on March 19, 1991. UPOV Publication No. 221(E), ISBN 92-805-0332-4.
[3] Blakeney M. Protection of plant varieties and farmers' rights. European Intellect Prop Rev 2002;24:9–19.
[4] Crucible Group. People, Plants and Patents: The Impact of Intellectual Property on Trade, Plant Biodiversity, and Rural Society. International Development Research Centre, Ottawa, Canada; 1994.
[5] Article 27(3)(b). In Agreement on Trade Related Aspects of Intellectual Property Rights (TRIPS), World Intellectual Property Office (WIPO) Publication No. 223(E) (1996). ISBN 92-805-0640-4.
[6] Cullet P. Revision of the TRIPS agreement concerning the protection of plant varieties – lessons from India concerning the development of a *sui generis* system. J. World Intellectual Property 1999;2:617–56.
[7] Lettington RJL. The international undertaking on plant genetic resources in the context of TRIPS and the CBD. Bridges: Between Trade and Sustainable Development, International Center for Trade and Sustainable Development 2001;5(6):11–3.

[8] Agreement on Trade Related Aspects of Intellectual Property Rights (TRIPS) World Intellectual Property Office (WIPO) Publication No. 223(E) (1996). ISBN 92-805-0640-4.

[9] Article 27(1). In Agreement on Trade Related Aspects of Intellectual Property Rights (TRIPS), World Intellectual Property Office (WIPO) Publication No. 223(E) (1996). ISBN 92-805-0640-4.

[10] Article 27(2) and (3). In Agreement on Trade Related Aspects of Intellectual Property Rights (TRIPS), World Intellectual Property Office (WIPO) Publication No. 223(E) (1996). ISBN 92-805-0640-4.

[11] UPOV. States parties to the International Convention for the Protection of New Varieties of Plants, Status on 6 August 2001.

[12] Barry Greengrass. UPOV and the protection of plant breeders – past development, future perspectives. IIC, 1989; 20(5):622–36.

[13] Barry Greengrass. The 1991 Act of the UPOV Convention, Seminar on the Nature and Rationale of Plant Varieties under the UPOV Convention, UPOV, Geneva; 1993.

[14] Wright BD, Pardey PG, Nottenburg C, Koo B. Agricultural innovation: economic incentives and institutions. In: Evenson RE, Pingali P, Schultz TP, editors. Handbook of agricultural economics, 3. Amsterdam: Elsevier; 2005.

[15] African Model Legislation for the Protection of the Rights of Local Communities, Farmers and Breeders, and for the Regulation of Access to Biological Resources; 1998.

[16] Goeschl T, Swanson T. The development impact of genetic use restriction technologies: a forecast based on the hybrid crop experience. Environ Devel Econ 2003;8:149–65.

[17] Mascia PN, Flavell RB. Safe and acceptable strategies for producing foreign molecules in plants. Curr Opin Plant Biol 2004;7:189–95.

[18] Daniell H. Molecular strategies for gene containment in transgenic crops. Nat Biotechnol 2002;20:581–7.

[19] Esquinas Alcazar J. The realization of farmer's right. In: Swaminathan MS, editor. Agro-biodiversity and farmer's rights, vol 2; 1996.

[20] European Commission Directorate-General for Trade. Communication by the European Communities and their Member States to the TRIPs Council on the Review of Article 27.3(b) of the TRIPs Agreement, and the Relationship Between the TRIPs Agreement and the Convention on Biological Diversity (CBD) and the Protection of Traditional Knowledge and Folklore: "A Concept Paper," 12 September 2002.

[21] Sumathi S. Reaping what they sow: the basmati rice controversy and strategies for protecting traditional knowledge, Boston College International and Company Law Reviews 2004;27:529.

[22] Shiva V. The turmeric patent is just the first step in stopping biopiracy. Third World Network 1997;86.

[23] Shiva V. Piracy by patent: the case of the neem tree. In: Mander J, Goldsmith E, editors. The case against the global economy and for a turn towards the local, San Franciso: Sierra Club Books; 1996. p. 154.

[24] Arunachalam V. The science behind tradition. Curr Sci 2000;80:1272–5.

Technical Glitches in Micropropagation

Saurabh Bhatia, Kiran Sharma

13.1 INTRODUCTION

Contamination is defined as the accidental introduction of undesirable bacterial, fungal, and algal microorganisms and vectors or sources of pathogens into a culture medium. There are various sources of contaminants. Various sterilization procedures and aseptic techniques used for eliminating the contamination problems are highlighted in Fig. 13.1 and Table 13.1. A high concentration of sugar in plant tissue culture media supports the growth of microorganisms

Modern Applications of Plant Biotechnology in Pharmaceutical Sciences. http://dx.doi.org/10.1016/B978-0-12-802221-4.00013-3

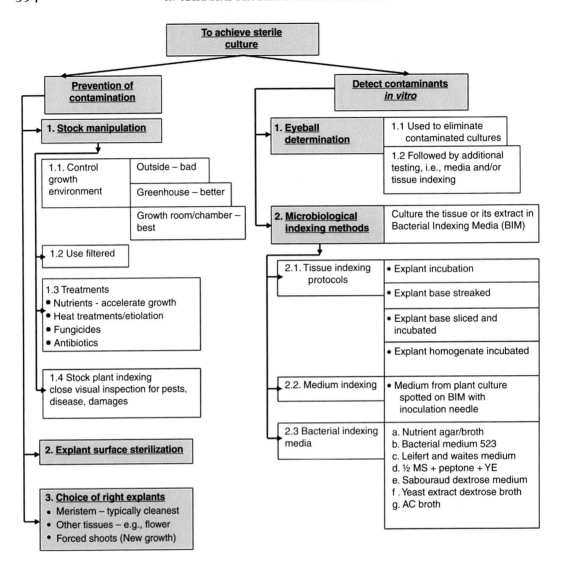

FIGURE 13.1   Protocols to achieve sterile culture.

like bacteria and fungi. Explant is known to be the major source of contamination. Contaminants that are associated with explant are often more epiphytic than endophytic [1]. Various sterilization protocols are utilized to remove several types of contaminants (Fig. 13.2). When plant is in its native state, the growth of microorganisms is suppressed by the defense mechanism and dry environment. But when plant is brought into *in vitro* conditions its molecular pathways, which are essential for the production of optimum amounts of secondary metabolites, are disturbed. In addition, plant cell/tissue/organ is exposed to high levels of moist conditions that may favor the growth of microorganisms in the culture medium. These

TABLE 13.1 Different Types of Sterilization Strategies Used in Plant Tissue Culture

Type of sterilization	Features		Specifications
Sterilization by heat	Heat is the most widely used lethal agent for sterilization.	Dry heat (oven)	170°C for 120 minutes.
		Moist heat (autoclave)	121°C at 15 lb for 15–20 min.
Sterilization by filtration	A liquid medium or solution that contains microorganisms can be sterilized by passing through a filter.	Filters may have different sizes and pores.	0.2 μm (pore size)
Tyndallization	Fractionated discontinuous method of sterilization.	Media is heated in water bath for 1 h for 3 consecutive days and kept at normal room temperature for two successive instances of boiling.	At 100°C for 15 min/day up to 3 consecutive days.
Air sterilization	Laminar air flow cabinet equipped with high efficiency particulate air filters (HEPA), blower is used to blow the air through the HEPA filters	A manometer is fitted with the instrument to check the air pressure. Pressure more than 13 bars can choke the filter UV light provides additional sterilization.	HEPA prevents all sorts of microorganisms larger than 0.3 μm with 99% efficiency.
Surface sterilization of the explants	Mercuric chloride Bromine water Sodium hypochlorite Calcium hypochlorite Silver nitrate Hydrogen peroxide Bromine water Antibiotics: tetracycline, ciprofloxacin Ethanol	Sodium hypochlorite can be used for any material. Mercuric chloride is most toxic material. Combinations of antibiotics are beneficial.	Time of treatment (5–50 min).

microorganisms when inside the medium grow faster than plant cells and multiply up to several fold by depleting carbohydrate sources and producing phytotoxic fermentation products such as ethanol and acetic acid. Plant cells in this starvation state become stressed and produce high levels of secondary metabolites, which are toxic for plant tissue. In addition to microbial contamination there are various other contaminations caused during micropropagation, e.g., chemical, radiation, and gas contamination. However, the frequency of these contaminations is considerably lower than microbial contamination. Browning of the medium or phenolic exudation in response to biotic and abiotic stresses is again a major constraint as this may lead to oxidation of leached phenolic contents causing darkening or browning of the media, which may further block the uptake of nutrients, ultimately leading to death of the explants. Similarly

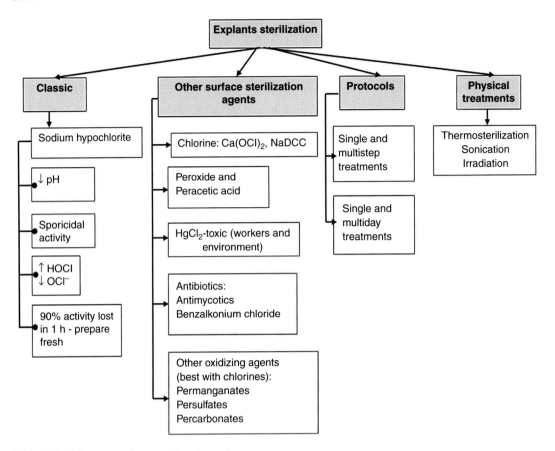

FIGURE 13.2   **Protocols to sterilize the explants.**

absence of rooting and acclimatization, hyperhydricity, shoot-tip necrosis, habituation, and tissue proliferation also suppress the growth of the tissue under *in vitro* conditions. This chapter describes various types of contamination sources and the alternative strategies to produce a contamination-free environment.

13.2 MICROBIAL CONTAMINATION

Microbial contamination is a big problem in plant tissue culture practices. Bacteria, fungi, molds, and yeast are common contaminating microorganisms found in plant tissue culture practices. Microorganisms and their reproductive structures are ubiquitous although their relative abundance may vary considerably with environment and season. Microorganisms are found inside and on the surface of the plants. Microbial contamination of plant tissue culture is due to the high nutrient availability in the almost universally used culture medium. In recent years, it has been shown that many plants, especially perennials, are at least locally endophytically colonized intercellularly by bacteria [2]. The intracellular pathogenic bacteria and viruses/viroids may pass latently into culture and be spread horizontally and vertically in cultures. Growth of some potentially cultivable endophytes may be suppressed by the high salt and sugar content of the Murashige and Skoog basal medium and suboptimal temperatures for their growth in plant tissue growth rooms. The management of contamination in tissue culture involves three stages: disease screening of the stock plants with disease and endophyte elimination; pathogen and contaminant screening of established initial cultures; and observation, random sampling, and culture screening for microorganisms in multiplication and stored cultures. The increasing accessibility of both broad-spectrum and specific molecular diagnostics has resulted in advances in multiple pathogen and latent contaminant detection. The hazard analysis critical control point management strategy for tissue culture laboratories is underpinned by staff training in aseptic techniques and good laboratory practices. The ideal procedure for preventing bacterial growth includes the following steps:

- Indexing explants and cultures for contaminants
- Identifying the source of those contaminants
- Identifying or characterizing the contaminants
- Eliminating the contaminating organism with improved cultural practices such as antibiotics (aminoglycosides, quinolones, β-lactams, glycopeptides, polymyxins, macrolides, and lincosamides) [3] or other chemical agent treatment

Bacterial contaminants may affect *in vitro* plant growth negatively, positively, or not at all. Bacterial growth may be suppressed in plant media by high salts, high sucrose, pH, temperature, tannins in explant sap, and appropriate nutrients not present in tissue culture media, e.g., pseudomonads, xanthomonads, and corynebacteria. In plants, bacteria may be endophytes, which can become pathogenic *in vitro* (*in vitro* pathogens = "vitropaths"), and *in vivo* pathogens, which can become saprophytes *in vitro*.

Bacteria are the most frequent contaminants. They are usually introduced with the explants and may survive even after surface sterilization of the explants because they are in the interior tissues. Bacteria can be recognized by a characteristic ooze. This ooze can be of many colors including white, pink, creamish, and yellow. Fungi may enter cultures on explants or the spore may be airborne. Fungi may be recognized by their fuzzy appearance and they occur in a multitude of colors. Yeast is a common contaminant of plant cultures. Yeast lives on the external surfaces of the plants as well as in the air. Viruses, mycoplasma-like organisms, spiroplasms, and rickettsias are not easily detected but they do form a source of serious contamination in cultures. Several insects are particularly troublesome in plant cultures including ants, thripes, and mites.

13.3 GASEOUS CONTAMINATION

Apart from the various contaminations caused by microorganisms, gaseous contamination also influences the growth of the culture. Culture ventilation is necessary to facilitate the gaseous exchange with the atmosphere and to allow ethylene to escape from the vessels. This problem can be overcome by using gas permeable filters as lid seals or by replacing the lid or wrapping the open-lidded vessel in gas permeable plastic film [4,5]. There is a wide range of transparent plastic wrapping materials that can be used instead of a conventional lid or the film can be wrapped around an open lidded vessel with the provision that the film be adequately permeable to oxygen, carbon dioxide, and ethylene to allow equilibration with the ambient atmosphere. If replacing the lid with a plastic film, the permeability of the film to water vapor should be chosen such that the cultures do not dry out [4,5].

13.4 CROSS-CULTURE CONTAMINATION

This generally occurs when a different cell type is inadvertently introduced into the cells that are being cultured. This is a significant problem because the new type of cell could have different morphology and function and react differently to any experimental conditions that are applied. Cross-contamination voids the experiment because results cannot be valid or credible, as the effect of the contaminating cells is unknown.

13.5 BROWNING OF THE MEDIUM OR PHENOLIC EXUDATION

Secondary metabolites like phenolic compounds in the plants are produced in response to biotic and abiotic stresses. These are basically involved in the defense mechanism of plants. However, leaching of phenolics contents from the explants of most woody and some herbaceous plants often produce lethal effects for the growing cells or tissues. This problem appears in tissue culture when explants are excised during the preparation of the cultures, which leads to stimulation of phenolic exudation. Oxidation of these exuded phenolic contents causes darkening or browning of the media, which blocks the uptake of nutrients and ultimately leads to death of the explants. Browning did not affect the growth of roots and shoots when explants were cultured in a large volume of medium, but in a small volume it was lethal. Various absorbents and antioxidants can be used to minimize this exudation problem. Alternatives used to minimize this type of problem are:

- Frequent subculturing of explants.
- Use of antioxidant compounds like ascorbic acid, butylated hydroxyl anisole, or butylated hydroxyl toluene; citric acid may prevent the oxidation of phenolic compounds.
- Use of adsorbents (like activated charcoal or PVP) to adsorb polyphenols secreted in the medium.
- Culturing in the dark to prevent polyphenolic oxidation as light enhances it.
- Soaking in water after excision to reduce the browning effect.
- After excision, when the explants are being transferred to nutrient media, the positioning of explants on medium have a considerable effect, e.g., some woody herbaceous plants produce more shoots when placed horizontally instead of vertically on the nutrient medium.
- A brief period of culture in liquid medium (3–7 days) to remove phenolics and other substances.
- Control of phenolic oxidation by the supplementation of certain compounds to the medium, e.g., adenine sulfate and $300 \, mg \, L^{-1}$ polyvinylpyrrolidone (PVP).
- Sealing the cut ends with paraffin wax to control browning by preventing exudation [6].

13.6 ABSENCE OF ROOTING AND ACCLIMATIZATION

Rooting is a critical phase since it depends on the genotype and physiological condition at the time of root induction [7]. This stage is followed by a process called acclimatization and is essential because the *in vitro* plants are cultivated under heterotrophic conditions [8]. Morphological anomalies, such as nonfunctional stomata, and physiological anomalies, such as a decrease in photosynthesis, might occur during this process [9]. These anomalies interfere with plant survival in the greenhouse or field. Therefore, acclimatization is critical for the transition of micropropagated plants from *in vitro* cultivation to *ex vitro* cultivation. The explants can naturally form roots during propagation without the additional rooting stage as with the potato but some species may show root production deficiency. Rooting may be induced by incorporating auxins and carbon in the culture medium. Extent of proper rooting varies species to species. To overcome this, the following critical growth regulators are added: 1-naphthalene acetic acid, indole-3-butyric acid, picloram, 2,4-dichlorophenoxyacetic acid (2,4-D), etc. These *in vitro* plants are sensitive to the external environment, so maintenance of relatively high humidity is required. Due to the high sensitivity of *in vitro* plants they should never be transplanted directly to open fields. Acclimatization is a key step to successful production. Tissue cultured plants may develop water stress upon transfer out of the test tube. Plants that do not acclimatize to the greenhouse die quickly. Leaves wilt, shrivel, and fall off. Root tips may turn brown and shrivel. The complete plant may turn brown after several days. Water stress is caused by many anatomical and physiological reasons. The main reason for short-term water loss is the lack of stomatal closure in unacclimatized tissue cultured plants. No worry methods, mist bench/polytent method, humidification chamber method, are the best solution for acclimatization.

13.7 HYPERHYDRICITY

In general terms, swelling/thickening of the tissue, just like callus, is called vitrification or hyperhydricity. In many species, vitrification may be represented by symptoms not visible to the naked eye. It is a physiological malformation that results in excessive hydration, low lignification, poorly developed vascular bundles, impaired stomatal function, and reduced mechanical strength of tissue culture-generated plants [10]. In vitrification, tissue becomes water soaked and translucent, which is mainly caused by excessive water uptake. It is usually controlled by changing agar concentration or source. The consequence is poor regeneration of such plants without intensive greenhouse acclimation for outdoor growth. Additionally, it may also lead to leaf-tip and bud necrosis in some cases, which often leads to loss of apical dominance in the shoots. In general, the main symptoms of hyperhydricity are translucent characteristics signified by a shortage of chlorophyll and high water content [10]. Specifically, the presence of a thin or lack of a cuticular layer, reduced number of palisade cells, irregular stomata, less developed cell wall, and large intracellular spaces in the mesophyll cell layer have been described as some of the anatomic changes associated with hyperhydricity.

13.7.1 The Main Causes of Hyperhydricity in Plant Tissue Culture

- Oxidative stresses as a result of high salt concentration
- The type of explants utilized

- The concentrations of microelement and hormonal imbalances
- Low light intensity
- High relative humidity
- Gas accumulation in the atmosphere of the jar
- Length of time intervals between subcultures
- Number of subcultures
- Concentration and type of gelling agent
- High ammonium concentration
- Evident in liquid culture-grown plants or when there is a low concentration of gelling agent

13.7.2 Control of Hyperhydricity

- Monitoring the modified atmosphere of the culture vessels.
- Adjusting the relative humidity in the vessel.
- Use of gas-permeable membranes to increase exchange of water vapor and other gases such as ethylene with the surrounding environment.
- Use of higher concentration of a gelling agent to reduce the risk of hyperhydricity.
- Addition of agar hydrolysate.
- Use of growth retardants and osmotic agents.
- Use of bottom cooling, which allows water to condense on the medium.
- Use of cytokinin-meta-topolin (6-(3-hydroxybenzylamino)purine).
- Combination of lower cytokinin content and ammonium nitrate in the media.
- Use of nitrate or glutamine as the sole nitrogen source.
- Decreasing the ratio of ammonium: nitrate in the medium.

13.8 SHOOT-TIP NECROSIS

Shoot-tip necrosis can be a major obstruction in the successful propagation of certain species by tissue culture. The symptoms of shoot-tip necrosis are browning and die-back of buds and the youngest leaves [11]. Shoot-tip necrosis occurs in some woody perennial tissue cultures when actively growing shoot tips develop tip die-back. This condition is usually caused by a calcium deficiency in the medium. The first assumption in seeing shoot-tip necrosis is that it is caused by nutrient deficiency [11]. The symptoms of nutrient deficiency of less mobile elements such as calcium (Ca) and boron (B) first appear in the meristematic regions and young leaves whereas symptoms of excessive amounts of these minerals are first observed on the older leaves. However, in *in vitro* systems, shoot-tip necrosis is caused by a complex set of factors rather than just nutrient deficiency [11].

13.9 HABITUATION

Plant tissue culture usually requires sources of the growth hormones auxin and cytokinin for continuous proliferation in culture. In 1942, Gautheret reported that carrot tissue can gradually lose its requirement for exogenous auxin. He called this phenomenon auxin habituation.

It was soon recognized that similar variation can occur for cytokinins and more rarely for some other hormones. Thus, habituation is when a culture continues to develop in the absence of auxin or cytokinin. For example, shoot cultures habituated for cytokinin would continue to produce new shoots on a cytokinin-free medium. Hormone habituation is a phenomenon by which plant cells and tissues lose the requirement of exogenous hormones to sustain cell division and development upon continuous culture [12].

13.10 TISSUE PROLIFERATION

Tissue proliferation may be the expression of naturally occurring growths in plants like Rhododendron induced by the tissue culture environment. Variation in micropropagated plants is one of the greatest problems faced by tissue culture during micropropagation. There are many types of variation that cause several problems during tissue proliferation, which can further create a great problem in defining the genotype of new variants [13].

13.10.1 Genetic or Chimeral Variation or Somaclonal Variation

Somaclonal variation is the variation seen in plants that have been produced by plant tissue culture. Chromosomal rearrangements are an important source of this variation. Somaclonal variation is not restricted to, but is particularly common in, plants regenerated from callus. The variations can be genotypic or phenotypic, which in the latter case can be either genetic or epigenetic in origin. Typical genetic alterations are: changes in chromosome numbers (polyploidy and aneuploidy), chromosome structure (translocations, deletions, insertions, and duplications), and DNA sequence (base mutations) [13]. Typical epigenetic-related events are gene amplification and gene methylation. If no visual, morphogenic changes are apparent, other plant screening procedures must be applied. There are both benefits and disadvantages to somaclonal variation. The phenomenon of high variability in individuals from plant cell cultures or adventitious shoots is called somaclonal variation [13]. Therefore, it can be defined as the variation that occurs because of genetic mutation caused by *in vitro* conditions or by chimeral separation. Somaclonal variation is usually undesirable. In some cases, somaclonal variation can lead to new cultivars (e.g., disease resistance, new leave pattern) that may have desirable ornamental characteristics or increased pest resistance.

The occurrence of somaclonal variation can be reduced by:

- Avoiding long-term cultures.
- Using axillary shoot induction systems where possible.
- Propagating chimeras by other clonal systems.
- It is well known that increasing numbers of subcultures increase the likelihood of somaclonal variation, so the number of subcultures in micropropagation protocols should be kept to a minimum.
- Regularly reinitiating clones from new explants, which might reduce variability over time.
- Avoiding 2,4-D in the culture medium, as this hormone is known to introduce variation.

13.10.2 Transient Phenotypic Variation

Plant populations show phenotypic diversity, which may be caused by genetic and epigenetic variation. It has recently been shown that new epigenetic variants are generated at a higher rate than genetic variants and several studies have shown that epigenetic variation can be influenced by the environment. Although the heritability of environmentally induced epigenetic traits has gained increasing interest in past years, it is still not clear whether and to what extent induced epigenetic changes have a role in ecology and evolution. Some reports on model and nonmodel species support the possibility of adaptive epigenetic alleles, indicating that epigenetic variants are subject to natural selection. However, most of these studies rely solely on phenotypic data and no information is available about the underlying mechanisms. Thus, the role of inherited epigenetic variation for plant adaptation is unclear and further investigations are required to gain insights into the significance of epigenetic variation for ecological and evolutionary processes.

13.10.3 Epigenetic Variation

In general terms, epigenetics can be defined as the study of changes in gene expression or cellular phenotype, caused by mechanisms other than changes in the underlying DNA sequence, hence the name *epi-* (Greek: επί-, over, above, outer) *genetics*. Some of these changes have been shown to be heritable. It refers to functionally relevant modifications to the genome that do not involve a change in the nucleotide sequence [13]. Examples of such modifications are DNA methylation and histone modification, both of which serve to regulate gene expression without altering the underlying DNA sequence. In tissue culture, new plants may be generated by outgrowth of axillary buds or by adventitious regeneration. Researchers expected initially that these clonally propagated plants would be exact copies of the parent plant, but frequently aberrant plants were observed. Various causes have been established:

- Genetic changes (also referred to as somaclonal variation): changes in the DNA sequence.
- Epigenetic variation: long-lasting changes in the expression of the information in the genome.
- Chimeral segregation and loss of pathogens in particular viruses.

Epigenetic changes are caused by changes in the expression of the information in the DNA brought about by alterations in DNA methylation, in histones, or in both [13]. These modifications may influence gene transcription. Epigenetic changes are often temporary and plants may revert to the normal phenotype relatively easily, but some can be long lasting and may even be transferred during sexual propagation.

13.11 DETECTION OF THE CONTAMINANTS

Contaminants may be introduced with the explants or during manipulation in the laboratory. They may express themselves immediately or remain latent for long periods of time. Eyeball determination method (visual determination method), stock plant indexing (taking part of the plant and transferring to media that are specific for bacteria and fungi, e.g., potato

TABLE 13.2 Identification and Characterization of Bacterial Contaminants

Test	Procedure	Reference
TRADITIONAL TESTS		
Biochemical tests	Gram stain, motility, gelatinase, oxidase, and oxidation/ fermentation	[20]
Bergey's Manual of Systematic Bacteriology	Descriptions of genera and species, which are helpful for identifying bacteria	[21]
CONTEMPORARY TESTS		
Tetrazolium dye test	Reduction of tetrazolium dye in response to cellular respiration and results are compared with standard database	[22]
The API identification system	Carbon source utilization test: relies on visual detection of the test bacterium	[23]
Fatty acid analysis profiles test	Fatty acid methyl esters with those of known organisms	[24]
Probe test	DNA probes and 16S rRNA use PCR amplification and probes for known sequences	[25]

dextrose agar and NB broth), semiselective media, and polymerase chain reaction (PCR)-based molecular techniques are usually used for the detection of the contaminants. Hazard analysis critical control point systems are used in commercial plant tissue culture laboratories. Several detection strategies are highlighted in Fig. 13.1.

Visual inspection of the medium may provide evidence of some contaminants but it is not adequate for slow growing bacteria, e.g., endophytes, or those bacteria that do not grow on plant tissue culture media [14]. There are various screening methods reported for the identification of many contaminants [14–17]. Some bacteria require specialized media and some contaminants can be easily detected by screening on two or three commercially available bacteriological media [18,19]. For indexing microbes, plant tissue can be inoculated into liquid and agar solidified yeast extract glucose, Sabouraud glucose, and AC media and incubated for 3 weeks at 30°C. This procedure is reported for indexing microbes in woody plant species. This can be further utilized by growing explants in a liquid culture system at pH 6.9. There might be chances of increase in expression of pathogens under greenhouse conditions. Therefore, such cultured batches should be separately placed to avoid multiplication of contaminants among healthy propagates. Various strategies for identification and characterization of bacterial contaminants are highlighted in Table 13.2.

References

[1] Fogh Jørgen, Holmgren NB, Ludovici PP. A review of cell culture contaminants. In Vitro 1971;7(1):26–41.
[2] Cassells AC. Problems in tissue culture: culture contamination. In: Debergh PC, Zimmerman RH, editors. Micropropagation technology and application. Dordrecht, Netherlands: Kluwer Academic Publishers; 1991. p. 31–44.
[3] Falkiner FR. The criteria for choosing an antibiotic for control of bacteria in plant tissue culture. Newsletter International Association for Plant Tissue Culture 1990;60:13–23.
[4] Marino G, Altan AD, Biavati B. The effect of bacterial contamination on the growth and gas evolution of *in vitro* cultured apricot shoots. In Vitro Plant 1996;32(1):51–6.

[5] Odutayo OI, Amusa NA, Okutade OO, Ogunsanwo YR. Sources of microbial contamination in tissue culture laboratories in southwestern Nigeria. Afr J Agr Res 2007;2(3):067–72.

[6] Bhat SR, Chandel KP. A novel technique to overcome browning in tissue culture. Plant Cell Rep 1991;10(6-7):358–61.

[7] Martins L, Pedrotti EL. Enraizamento *in vitro* e *ex vitro* dos porta-enxertos de macieira M7, M9 e Marubakaido. Rev Bras Frutic 2001;23(1):11–6.

[8] Hazarika BN. Acclimatization of tissue-cultured plants. Curr Sci 2003;85(12):1704–12.

[9] Rogalski M, Moraes LKA, Felisbino C, Crestani L, Guerra MP, Silva AL. Aclimatização de porta-enxertos de Prunus sp. micropropagados. Rev Bras Frutic 2003;25(2):279–81.

[10] Kevers C, Franck T, Strasser RJ, Dommes J, Gaspar T. Hyperhydricity of micropropagated shoots: a typically stress-induced change of physiological state. Plant Cell Tiss Org Cult 2004;77(2):181–91.

[11] Bairu MW, Stirk WA, Staden JV. Factors contributing to *in vitro* shoot-tip necrosis and their physiological interactions. Plant Cell Tiss Org Cult 2009;98(3):239–48.

[12] Meins F. Habituation: heritable variation in the requirement of cultured plant cells for hormones. Annu Rev Genet 1989;23:395–408.

[13] Neelakandan AK, Wang K. Recent progress in the understanding of tissue culture-induced genome level changes in plants and potential applications. Plant Cell Rep 2012;31:597–620.

[14] Kane ME. Indexing explants and cultures to maintain clean stock. In Vitro 1995;31:25A.

[15] Reed BM, Buckley PM, DeWilde TN. Detection and eradication of endophytic bacteria from micropropagated mint plants. In Vitro Cell Dev Biol 1995;31:53–7.

[16] Leifen C, Camotla H, Wailes WM. Effect of combinations of antibiotics on micro-propagated Clematis, Delphinium, Hosta, Iris, and Photinia. Plant Cell Tiss Org Cult 1992;29:153–60.

[17] Holland MA, Polacco JC. PPFMs and or her covert contaminants: is there more to plant physiology than just plant? Annu Rev Plant Physiol Mol Biol 1994;45:197–209.

[18] George KL, Falkinham JO. Selective medium for the isolation and enumeration of *Mycobacterium avium-intracellulare* and *M. scrofulaceum*. Can J Microbiol 1986;32:10–4.

[19] Gunson HE, Spencer-Phillips PTN. Latent bacterial infections: epiphytes and endophytes as contaminants of micropropagated plants. In: Nicholas JR, editor. Physiology, growth and development of plants in culture. Dordrecht, Netherlands: Kluwer Academic Publishers; 1994. p. 379–96.

[20] Klement Z, Rudolph K, Sands DC, editors. Methods in phytobacteriology. Budapest: Akademiai Kiado; 1990.

[21] Krieg NR, Holt JG, editors. Bergey's manual of systematic bacteriology, Vol. I. Baltimore: Williams and Wilkens; 1984.

[22] Jones JB, Chase AR, Harris GK. Evaluation of the Biolog GN MicroPlate system for identification of some plant-pathogenic bacteria. Plant Dis 1993;77:553–8.

[23] Leifert C, Waites WM, Nicholas JR. Bacterial contamination of micropropagated plant tissue cultures. J Appl Bact 1989;67:353–61.

[24] Chase AR, Stall RE, Hodge NC, Jones JB. Characterization of *Xanthomonas campestris* strains from aroids using physiological, pathological, and fatty acid analysis. Phytopathology 1992;82:754–9.

[25] KJijn N, Weerkamp AH, deVos WM. Identification of mesophilic lactic acid bacteria by using polymerase chain reaction-amplified variable regions of 16s rRNA and specific DNA probes. Appl Environ Microbiol 1991;57:3390–3.

Plant Tissue Culture-Based Industries

Saurabh Bhatia, Kiran Sharma

14.1 INTRODUCTION

Plant biotechnology is a powerful tool for the development of new plant traits and varieties. Such new varieties must be produced on a large scale to achieve commercial success and to satisfy the demand from growers. Traditionally, new varieties were achieved by the seed propagation method. Currently, micropropagation-produced plantlets offer a practical alternative for many plant species. Micropropagation is labor intensive although the time needed to commercialize new varieties and permit the production of disease-free plants is reduced. Recent developments in genetic engineering and molecular biology techniques allowed the production of improved and new agricultural products in several countries worldwide. This is only possible with the evolution of tissue culture techniques, which provide the platform for the introduction of genetic information into plant cells.

Current plant biotechnology has developed as a new age of science and technology where production of secondary metabolites, valuable plant genetics improvements, germplasm conservation, and production of large numbers of disease-free and new varieties are preferred. Production of artificial seeds, biopharmaceuticals, plant-made pharmaceuticals, recombinant or other therapeutic proteins, transgenic plants, and plant-made vaccines or antibodies

Modern Applications of Plant Biotechnology in Pharmaceutical Sciences. http://dx.doi.org/10.1016/B978-0-12-802221-4.00014-5

(plantibodies) is part of the current research work in plant tissue culture science. Most of the plant tissue culture industries are exploiting the fundamental property of regeneration of plant cells for rapid production of elite varieties with superior genotypes on a large scale in a comparatively short time.

The current plant tissue culture industry is estimated to be worth around US$150 billion (50–60% of the agriculture industry). Annual demand of tissue culture-raised products is about 10% of the total estimated value (US$15 billion with growth rate of 15%) [1]. Most of the plant tissue culture-based industries are limiting the time-consuming labor or manual processes fully by transforming into more automated and robust technologies. The introduction of such robust and automated technologies has led to rapid multiplication of plantlets at a larger level. In this chapter, we discuss national and international scenarios of various plant tissue culture-based industries equipped with recent technologies used nowadays to make the process more suitable for large-scale production.

14.2 INTERNATIONAL SCENARIO

Based on plant tissue culture science, large-scale production of plant material was initially revolutionized in the United States with micropropagation of orchids in the 1970s. Most of the initial research was focused on crop improvement. International Agricultural Research Centers (IARCs) were established in different parts of the world to collaborate plant research and to explore the mutual benefits to the participants and the positive effect of research in developing countries (Table 14.1). Currently, these centers are emphasizing various plant tissue culture-based researches such as anther culture, somaclonal variation, meristem culture, rapid clonal propagation, *in vitro* germplasm conservation, pathogen-free plant production,

TABLE 14.1 International Location of the CGIAR-Supported Centers [2]

Centers		Location
WARDA	West African Rice Development Association	Liberia
ISNAR	International Service for National Agricultural Research	Netherlands
IRRI	International Rice Research Institute	Philippines
ILRAD	International Laboratory for Research on Animal Diseases	Kenya
ILCA	International Livestock Center for Africa	Ethiopia
IITA	International Institute of Tropical Agriculture	Nigeria
IFPRI	International Food Policy Research Institute	USA
ICRISAT	International Crops Research Institute for the Semi-Arid Tropics	India
ICARDA	International Center for Agricultural Research in the Dry Areas	Syria
IBPGR	International Board for Plant Genetic Resources	Italy
CIP	International Potato Center	Peru
CIMMYT	International Maize and Wheat Improvement Center	Mexico
CIAT	Centro Internacional de Agricultura Tropical	Colombia

molecular diagnostics (nucleic acid probes, monoclonal antibodies, ELISA), embryo rescue, and genetic engineering [3]. Plant tissue culture-based research at the Consultative Group for International Agricultural Research (CGIAR) centers is frequently executed in conjunction with traditional crop improvement programs such as germplasm-related activities (conservation, evaluation, prebreeding), breeding, testing, and distribution of plant and seed material [4]. IARCs also promote more competent means of assessment, conservation, and distribution of germplasm. Technology acquisition and integration and access to such technologies to developing countries require the procurement of various national programs (IARCs and indigenous private sector). Identification of donor agency support and collaborative partners promotes the mutual biotechnological research more smoothly.

During 1986–1993, the international production of cultured plants was increased by 50% (Table 14.2). In 1990, it was estimated that production of only ornamental plants reached 130 million units per annum. The whole production was later estimated at 663 million plants in 1993 and 800 million plants in 1997. Afterwards, demand for genetically engineered plants has considerably increased. *In vitro* culture techniques required for the production of such genetically modified (GM) plants established a platform for the production of biopharmaceuticals and transgenic plants. Presently, plant tissue culture-based industries represent a billion

TABLE 14.2 Growth of Plant Tissue Culture-Based Industries at Global and National Levels [5]

Year	Global status		India status	
	No. of plants produced	No. of plants produced	Number of commercial (tissue culture units)	Installed capacity (million plants/year)
1986	130.00	0.5	1.00	1.00
1987	180.00	2.5	1.00	4.00
1988	240.00	–	–	
1989	300.00	5.00	3.00	10.00
1990	390.00	–	–	
1991	513.00	10.00	17.00	
1992	562.00	–	–	
1993	663.00	–	–	
1994	680.00	15.00	21.00	80.00
1995	722.00	–	–	
1996	783.00	22.00	51.00	210.00
1997	800.00	–	–	
1998	822.00	15.00	51.00	210.00
1999	865.00	20.00	57.00	225.00
2000	900.00	25.00	61.00	255.00
2001	815.00	22.00	69.00	280.00
2002	865.00	30.00	76.00	300.00
2003	922.00	50.00	76.00	300.00

dollar industry where 500 million to 1.0 billion plantlets are produced annually [6]. In 2007, it was reported that 23 countries were involved in the planting of biotech crops. Based on international standards, some of companies have been approved by the Department of Agriculture (Australia) to export high health tissue cultures free of media to Australia (Table 14.3). India, the largest cotton growing country in the world, showed the highest proportional increase of any biotech crop country in the world with an extraordinary gain of 63% in 2007 [8]. The cause of this impressive growth in Bt cotton was that it had constantly distributed exceptional benefits to farmers and to the nation. In 2006, the income from Bt cotton was estimated at US$840 million and has since been raised to US$1.7 billion [8]. Production was almost doubled, and India is now an exporter rather than an importer of cotton.

TABLE 14.3 List of the Companies that are Approved by the Department of Agriculture (Australia) to Export High Health Tissue Cultures Free of Media to Australia [7]

Source	Address	Country
Ankur Biotech	B60b, KSSIDC Industrial Area, Industrial Estate Bommasandra, Anekal Taluk, Bangalore 560 099	India
Anthura BV	Anthuriumweg 7-9, 2665 KV Bleiswijk	The Netherlands
Bangalore Horti Tech	1. No. 39, 8th Cross, Shanthi Layout, Ramamurthy Nagar, Bangalore 560016 2. No. 57, 8th Cross, Shanthi Layout, Ramamurthy Nagar, Bangalore 560016 3. Kuyampu Nagara, Doddakkallasandra, Kanakapura Road, Bangalore 560062 4. Narayanan Agar 2nd block, Tippasandra Village, Kanakapura Road, Bangalore 560062 5. Bolare Village, Kanakapura Main Road, Bangalore 560084	India
Bock Bio Science GmbH	Butemdieker, Landstrasse 49A, D-2800 Bremen 33	Germany
Eastern Green Fields Co., Ltd	27/7 Moo 2, LiabKhlong Sam, Khlong Sam, Khlong Luang, PathumTha Ni 12120	Thailand
Florist Holland BV	Dwarsweg 15, 1424 PL De Kwakel	The Netherlands
Foshan Sanshui Youngplants Co., Ltd	Bagang Village, Lubao Town, Sanshui District, Foshan City, Guangdong Province 528139	China
Gadera Ltd	Unit 1, IDA Industrial Estate, Dublin Road, Enniscorthy, Co. Wexford	Ireland
Grand Biotechnology	No. 2 Industry E Road Science Based Industrial Park, Hsinchu	Taiwan
Hayleys Agro Biotech (Pvt) Ltd	400 Dean Road, Colombo-10	Sri Lanka
K.F. Bioplants Pvt Ltd	1. Survey no. 129/1 to 3 C Manjri Budruk, Taluka Haveli, Pune, 411307, Maharashtra, India 2. Survey no. 178m Kirtane Baug, Mundwa Road, Magarpatta, Hadpasar, Pune, 411036, India	India
Konst Alstroemeria BV	Nieuwveens Jaagpad 93, 2441 GA, Nieuwveen	The Netherlands

TABLE 14.3 List of the Companies that are Approved by the Department of Agriculture (Australia) to Export High Health Tissue Cultures Free of Media to Australia [7] *(cont.)*

Source	Address	Country
Kunming Taikoo Young Plants Ltd	Ha Hou Village, Xiao Jie Town, Song Ming County, Kun Min City	China
L.J. International Ltd	Plot No. 10 & 11, C.S. E Z, Kakkanad, Cochin-30	India
Lifetech Laboratories Ltd	224 Albany Highway, Albany, Auckland 0632	New Zealand
Lowes TCI Tissue Culture (India) Private Limited	12/44, Rajiv Gandhi Nagar Bommanahalli, Bangalore, 560068	India
Malesiana Tropicals	Lot 8, Jalan Jugan-Buso, Buso 94000, Kuching Sarawak	Malaysia
Mike Biotech Asia (Pvt)	No. 65/13, Orchid Place, Off Swarnadisi Place, Koswatta, Nawala, Rajagiriya	Sri Lanka
North American Plants, LLC	3367 St. Joseph Road, McMinnville, Oregon 97128	USA
Oglesby Plants International Inc.	26664 SR 71N, Altha, Florida 32421	USA
Plantek International	23 Pattanagere, Next to Global Village, Rajarajeswary Nagar, Bangalore 560 098	India
PT Monfori Nusantara	Jl. Raya Jampang Karihkil Km. 4, Desa Tegal Kemang, Parung-Bogor 16310	Indonesia
PT. Bambu Nusa Verde	Jl. Mangunan, Tebonan, Harjobinangun, Pakem, Sleman, Yogyakarta 55585	Indonesia
Ramya Horticulture Pvt Ltd	459/1, Kandy Road, Rammuthugala, Kadawata, Sri Lanka	Sri Lanka
Rise n' Shine Biotech Pvt Ltd	301/2, Metro House, Mangaldas Road, Pune	India
Royal Van Zanten	Portion 375 Farm, Zoutpansdrift (along R511), Thabazunbi Road, Brits 0250	South Africa
SBW International BV	Sotaweg 29, 2371 GA Roelofarendsveen	The Netherlands
Sunshine Horticulture Co., Ltd	North Sunshine Road, Shuangyang Town, Luojiang, Quanzhou, Fujian	China
Thai Orchids Lab Co., Ltd	10/14–16 Moo 5, Thakham, Sampran, Nakorn Pathom 73110	Thailand
Twyford International Inc.	100 mts Oeste del Super La Canastita, La Guacima de Alajuela, Apartado 429-4005, San Antonio de Belen, Heredia	Costa Rica
Vitro Ferns BV	Kalslagerweg 20, 1424 PM De Kwakel	The Netherlands
Vitrocom Holland BV	Broekpolderlaan 40, 2675 LJ Honselersdijk	The Netherlands
Vitroflora	Laboratorium Kultur Tkankowych Agnieszka-Pawlak Anhalt, Ul. Bukowa 3-86-065 Lochowo	Poland
Wolfgang Bock	Butemdieker, Landstrasse 49A, D-28357 Bremen	Germany

The biggest producer of cotton in the world is China, which introduced Bt cotton in 1996/1997, 6 years ahead of India. In total, of the 5.5 million hectares of all cotton planted in China, 3.8 million hectares gave resource to poor farmers [8]. In China, numerous large-scale local companies are involved in plant seedling biotechnology and their major products (Table 14.4). Argentina, which commercialized RR® soybean in 1996, has now become the second largest grower of biotech crops in the world, growing 19.1 million hectares in 2007 [8]. In 2007, Brazil maintained its position as the third largest adopter of biotech crops globally, projected at 15.0 million hectares (14.5 million hectares for RR soybean and 500,000 hectares planted for gene Bt cotton) [8]. South Africa is positioned at number eight internationally with a total biotech crop of 1.8 million hectares in 2007 [8]. The international market in biotech crops in 2007 was US$6.9 billion, representing 16% of the US$42.2 billion global crop production market. Out of the US$6.9 billion biotech crop market, US$3.2 billion is for biotech maize, US$2.6 billion for biotech soybean, US$0.9 billion for biotech cotton (13%), and US$0.2 billion for biotech canola (3%) [8]. In addition, of the US$6.9 billion biotech crop market, US$5.2 billion (76%) was in industrialized countries and US$1.6 billion (24%) was in

TABLE 14.4 Large-Scale Local Taiwan Companies Involved in Plant Seedling Biotechnology and Their Major Products [9]

Company name	No. of operational units	Major species produced
I-Hsin Biotech Corporation	120	*Phalaenopsis cadmium, Oncidium, Cymbidium*
Perfect Butterfly Orchid Service Center	65	*P. cadmium*
Yu Pin Biotech Corporation	55	*P. cadmium*
Sogo Team Co., Ltd	43	*P. cadmium*
Grand Biotech, Inc.	40	*P. cadmium*, cut flowers, ornamental plants, garden bulbs
King Car Biotech Corporation	32	*P. cadmium*
Chung Hun Biotech Corporation	31	*P. cadmium, Oncidium, Cymbidium*, Chinese orchids
Pao Lung Biotech Corporation	25	*P. cadmium, Oncidium*, Chinese orchids, *Cypripedioideae*, cut flowers, ornamental plants, garden bulbs, wasabi, etc.
San Ho National Arts Workshop	24	*P. cadmium, Cattleya* orchids, *Dendrobium, Oncidium, Cymbidium*, Chinese orchids
Taida Horticultural Co., Ltd	23	*P. cadmium, Oncidium, Cattleya* orchids, Chinese orchids
Feng Yuan Orchidarium	20	*Oncidium, P. cadmium, Cymbidium*
Luxe Enterprises Ltd	17	*P. cadmium*
S & B Biological Technologies	15	*Oncidium, P. cadmium*, banana seedlings
Gin-Sheng Orchidarium	15	*P. cadmium*
Chia-Chang Orchidarium	15	*P. cadmium, Cattleya* orchids, *Dendrobium*

developing countries. The international value of the biotech crop market was about US$7.5 billion in 2008.

Recently, commercialization of GM crops, including the four main crops of soybeans, corn, cotton, and canola, was studied. An annual report has showed significant net economic benefits at the farm level amounting to $18.8 billion in 2012 and $116.6 billion for the 17-year period 1996–2012 (in nominal terms) [10]. It was also reported that GM technology has also made important contributions to increasing global production levels of the four main crops, having added 122 million tonnes and 230 million tonnes, respectively, since the introduction of the technology in the mid-1990s [10].

Various micropropagation techniques available worldwide are being practiced at the industrial level for the production of commercial crops, medicinal plants, ornamental crops (rosa, dahalia, freesia, hyacinth, iris, begonia), and horticultural or agricultural crops (alfalfa, asparagus, banana, citrus, grapevine, cucumber, groundnut, maize, strawberry, sugarcane, tobacco, and tomato).

14.3 PLANT TISSUE CULTURE-BASED INDUSTRIES IN INDIA

Currently, India maintains a unique position globally for establishing micropropagation industries throughout the nation. Economic growth of the Indian market based on plant tissue culture has risen dramatically in last few years. This might be due to the availability of skilled labor at much cheaper rates. During 1987–1993, micropropagation-based industries expanded in India exponentially. A.V. Thomas and Co. (Cochin) was the first Indian commercial plant unit to be set up in 1987–1988 [11]. The company has an export processing zone with a 5 million capacity. Later, several venture capitalists and industrialists were attracted to this growing business and started expanding the commercialization of micropropagation throughout the nation. During this period, several units have been established with production capacities reaching 200 million plants per annum [11]. Twenty-one commercial plant propagation units were set up in 1994, with an objective of producing 80 million plants annually. However, as these units did not achieve this target, in 1996 30 more units were set up with a target of producing 210 million plants annually. During the period of 1986–1989 the targets achieved were 50% of the installed capacity. In 1996, owing to the drastic reduction in the number of units, the whole production was reduced to a mere 7% of the targeted volume. From 1991 to 1994 and in 1998 there was a gradual decrease in the production rate, but this rate was increased again from 1999 to 2001 [11]. From this period, the number of units increased and there was a noticeable 35% of increase in tissue culture production. In 2002, new facilities were installed with the advantage of computer automation with better robotics technologies to achieve a target production rate of 300 million plants per annum.

There are a number of priority crops being targeted by the majority of these plant tissue culture-based industries. Most industries have as their primary concern agricultural crops such as wheat, maize, soybean, cotton, etc., whereas others have concentrated on the floriculture sector including several ornamental plants, and some are covering food and vegetables. These industries mainly are located in Maharashtra, Andhra Pradesh, Karnataka, and Kerala. It has been proven that currently most of the Indian plant tissue culture-based industries are involved in micropropagation of ornamental plants making a profit of 6–7 million, followed by the trees (1.0–2.0 million), fruit species (0.5–1.0 million), and other plants (less than 0.5 million) [11].

14.3.1 Organizations that are Engaged in Commercial Micropropagation

ICAR institutes and organizations have given a platform to the micropropagation of several crops such as potato, sweet potato, garlic, lemon, banana, mango, and various citrus varieties. Several other disease crops such as coffee, tea, and pepper are also produced. The revolution of commercialization of plant tissue culture at a national level was first brought about by A.V. Thomas and Co. Ltd in Cochin, India, with a 5 million capacity annually. Later on, various industries followed suit (Table 14.5). Research and development related with biotechnology is governed and funded by the Department of Biotechnology, under the Ministry of Science and Technology, India (established since 1986). Tissue culture pilot plants (the

TABLE 14.5   List of India-Based Plant Tissue Culture Industries and Their Products [11]

Company name	Location	Products
A.V. Thomas & Co. Ltd	Cochin, Kerela	Banana, pineapple, cardamom, ginger, turmeric, vanilla, black pepper, tea, rose, *Gerbera*, lily
Beena Nursery Ltd	Trivandrum	Orchids
Cadila Pharmaceutical Ltd	Ahmedabad, Gujarat	*Calathea*, banana, sugarcane, etc.
Dhampur Sugar Mills and EID Parry	Dhampur and Chennai	Sugarcane
Godrej Plant Biotech Ltd	Medak, Andhra Pradesh	Banana, pineapple, strawberry, lily, ornamental bamboo
Gujarat State Fertilizers and Chemicals Ltd	Vadodara, Gujarat	Roses, *Alocasia*, banana, ginger, turmeric stevia, *Withania*, aloe, *Brahmi*, etc.
Harrisons Malyalam Ltd	Bangalore	Mango, cashew, teak, rosewood
Hindustan Lever Ltd	Mumbai, Maharashtra	Coffee, tea, eucalyptus, etc.
In Vitro International Pvt Ltd	Bangalore, Karnataka	*Anthurium*, yucca, cordyline, *Alocasia*, *Lilium*, etc.
Indo American Hybrid Seeds	Bangalore, Karnataka	*Alpinia*, *Calathea*, Calla lily, chrysanthemum, iris, rose, strawberry, cardamom, teak, peach, ginger, etc.
Nath Biotechnologies	Aurangabad, Maharashtra	Banana, pineapple, ficus, etc.
National Agricultural and Scientific Foundation	Kolkata, West Bengal	Tea, jaboba, *Ficus*, orchids, etc.
Reliance Life Sciences	Navi Mumbai, Maharashtra	Banana, pomegranate, potato, aloe, *Stevia*, *Alpenia ficus*, etc.
Southern Petrochemicals Industries Corporation Ltd	Chennai, Tamil Nadu	Cardamom, vanilla, banana, mango, female papaya, etc.
Sun Agrigenetics	Vadodara, Gujarat	Sugarcane, banana, etc.
Vasantdada Sugar Institute	Pune, Maharashtra	Sugarcane

National Chemical Laboratory, Pune, and the Energy Research Institute, New Delhi) were also set up for large-scale multiplication of plantlets. Biotech Consortium India Ltd, promoted by the Department of Biotechnology, Government of India, was introduced in 1990 with the objective of providing necessary linkages among different stakeholders to facilitate accelerated commercialization of biotechnology.

14.4 RECENT TECHNOLOGIES

Current plant tissue culture-based industries use several technologies for the regulation of developmental cell fate *in vitro*. Such strategies include QTL analysis, biochemical studies, global expression profiling [12], and candidate gene analysis. These techniques are used to study molecular mechanisms during callus initiation, embryogenesis, and organogenesis in different species. To analyze relative protein expression levels, quantitative proteomics techniques such as stable isotope labeling by amino acids in cell culture have been recently utilized in *Arabidopsis* suspension cell culture systems [13]. To simultaneously identify and monitor a large number of RNAs/proteins and their expression changes *in vitro*, techniques like high-throughput transcriptomics [14], proteomic techniques [15], state-of-the-art protein analysis techniques such as liquid chromatography, mass spectrometry, and multidimensional protein identification technology are exploited. Various techniques used for analyzing the genetic variations under *in vitro* culture conditions are mentioned in Table 14.6. Other modern technologies that are used for plant tissue cultures are discussed in Chapter 4.

TABLE 14.6 Types of Cell Culture-Induced Genetic Variation and Their Respective Detection Techniques

Type of variation	Technique	Example reference
DNA sequence-specific changes	Inter retrotransposon amplified polymorphism	[16]
	Sequence-specific amplification polymorphism	[17]
	Transposon display	[18]
Chromatin modification	Chromatin Immunoprecipitation analysis	[19]
Chromosome level changes	Flow cytometry	[15]
Isozyme pattern changes	Starch gel electrophoresis and staining	[20]
Metabolite changes	Nuclear magnetic resonance spectroscopy	[21]
Small RNA expression changes	MicroRNA array hybridization	[22]
	Cloning and quantitative reverse transcription polymerase chain reaction (qRT-PCR)	[23]
	Cloning and northern analysis	[24]
	Cloning and deep sequencing of small RNA libraries	[25]
Chromatin condensation	Fluorescent *in situ* hybridization	[26]

(Continued)

TABLE 14.6 Types of Cell Culture-Induced Genetic Variation and Their Respective Detection Techniques *(cont.)*

Type of variation	Technique	Example reference
DNA methylation changes	Based on bisulfite treatment, which changes un-methylated cytosines into uracil, and sequencing	[18]
	Based on treatment with the restriction enzyme McrBC, which only cleaves DNA at 5-methylcy-tosine	[25]
	DNA degradation followed by high performance capillary electrophoresis	[27]
	DNA degradation followed by reversed-phase high-performance liquid chromatography (RP-HPLC)	[28]
	Methylation-sensitive amplification polymorphism	[17]
	Methylation-sensitive restriction fragment length polymorphism	[29]
	Methylation-sensitive restriction fragment length polymorphism	[30]
	Transposon methylation display	[31]
RNA expression changes	cDNA macroarray hybridization	[32]
	Differential display	[33]
	EST array or Genechip hybridization	[12]
	Genome-scale microarray hybridization	[14]
	Suppression subtractive hybridization	[34]
DNA sequence changes	Fluorescent *in situ* hybridization	[35]
	Amplified fragment length polymorphism	[36]
	Inter-simple sequence repeats markers	[37]
	Microsatellites or simple sequence repeat	[38]
	Next generation sequencing of genomic DNA libraries	[39]
	Polymerase chain reaction–restriction fragment length polymorphism	[17]
	Random amplified polymorphic DNA	[38]
	Restriction fragment length polymorphism	[40]
Protein expression changes	Two-dimensional gel electrophoresis	[15]
	Stable isotope labeling of amino acids in cell culture	[13]
	Sodium dodecyl sulfate-polyacrylamide gel electrophoresis	[41]

14.5 VARIOUS PROBLEMS FACED DURING MICROPROPAGATION

Some protocols that are utilized in plant tissue sometimes fail to generate technology suitable for large-scale propagation.

- Cost consideration: For achieving large-scale propagation in plant tissue culture science, currently most of the industries are emphasizing the introduction of various automated and robotics processes that can be monitored by high-quality computer software. The scale-up technique (bioreactors) and microenvironmentation require more automation than others. But these sophisticated technologies have a high cost consideration. In addition, most of the costs associated with micropropagation are also related to manual labor.
- Protocol efficiency: Protocols that have less than threefold efficiency in multiplication of plantlets are unacceptable. Thus, a high multiplication rate is required for governing large-scale propagation. Protocol efficiency is essential for reducing the number of subculturing processes and hence cuts the cost of labor.
- Contamination: Various types of contamination with their suitable sterilization procedures are discussed in Chapter 13.
- Variability in cultures: Somaclonal variation caused during *in vitro* practice on plant cells leads to generic variation. Thus, the primary objective of micropropagation studies is to maintain the genetic fidelity of plantlets. Therefore, only those techniques that are able to maintain the genetic fidelity of plantlets are preferred.
- Microbial infection: This subject is discussed in Chapter 13.

References

[1] Govil S, Gupta SC. Commercialization of plant tissue culture in India. Plant Cell Tiss Org Cult 1997;51(1):65–73.
[2] Cohen IJ. Biotechnology research for the developing world. Tibtech 1989;(7):296–303.
[3] Smuckler RH, Berg RJ, Gordon DF. New challenges, new opportunities: US cooperation for international growth and development in the 1990s. East Lansing, Michigan: Michigan State University Press; 1988.
[4] Cohen JI Strengthening collaboration in biotechnology: international agricultural research and the private sector. In: Cohen JI, editor. AID, 1989, Washington, DC.
[5] Singh G, Shetty S. Impact of tissue culture on agriculture in India. Biotechnol Bioinf Bioeng 2011;1(2):147–58.
[6] Brookes G, Barfoot P. GM crops: global socio-economic and environmental impacts. UK: PG Economics Ltd; 1996-2010.
[7] http://www.agriculture.gov.au/biosecurity/import/plants-grains-hort/daff-approved-sources-of-tissue-cultures-free-of-media
[8] ISAAA Brief 37-2007: Executive Summary, Global Status of Commercialized Biotech/GM Crops: 2007, http://www.isaaa.org/resources/publications/briefs/37/executivesummary.
[9] http://eng.coa.gov.tw/content_view.php?catid=9142&hot_new=8856
[10] Brookes G, Barfoot P. Economic impact of GM crops: the global income and production effects 1996-2012. GM Crops Food 2014;5(1):65–75.
[11] Purohit SD. Introduction to plant cell, tissue and organ culture. Delhi: PHI Learning Private Ltd; 2013. 253-271.
[12] Che P, Love TM, Frame BR, Wang K, Carriquiry AL, Howell SH. Gene expression patterns during somatic embryo development and germination in maize Hi II callus culture. Plant Mol Biol 2006;62:1–14.
[13] Schütz W, Hausmann N, Krug K, Hampp R, Macek B. Extending SILAC to proteomics of plant cell lines. Plant Cell 2011;23:1701–5.
[14] Bao Y, Dharmawardhana P, Mockler TC, Strauss SH. Genome scale transcriptome analysis of shoot organogenesis in Populus. BMC Plant Biol 2009;9:132–46.
[15] Yin L, Tao Y, Zhao K, Shao J, Li X, Liu G, et al. Proteomic and transcriptomic analysis of rice mature seed derived callus differentiation. Proteomics 2007;7:755–68.

[16] Smákal P, Valledor L, Rodráguez R, Griga M. Assessment of genetic and epigenetic stability in long-term in vitro shoot culture of pea (*Pisum sativum* L.). Plant Cell Rep 2007;26:1985–98.

[17] Kour GL, Kour B, Kaul S, Dhar MK. Genetic and epigenetic instability of amplification-prone sequences of a novel B chromosome induced by tissue culture in *Plantago lagopus*. Plant Cell Rep 2009;28:1857–67.

[18] Ngezahayo F, Xu C, Wang H, Jiang L, Pang J, Liu B. Tissue culture-induced transpositional activity of mPing is correlated with cytosine methylation in rice. BMC Plant Biol 2009;9:91–105.

[19] Grafi G, Ben-Meir H, Avivi Y, Moshe M, Dahan Y, Zemach A. Histone methylation controls telomerase-independent telomere lengthening in cells undergoing dedifferentiation. Dev Biol 2007;306:838–46.

[20] Mangolin CA, Prioli AJ, Machado MF. Isozyme patterns in callus cultures and in plants regenerated from calli of *Cereus peruvianus* (Cactaceae). Biochem Genet 1994;32:237–47.

[21] Palama TL, Menard P, Fock I, Choi YH, Bourdon E, Govinden- Soulange J, et al. Shoot differentiation from protocorm callus cultures of *Vanilla planifolia* (Orchidaceae): proteomic and metabolic responses at early stage. BMC Plant Biol 2010;10:82.

[22] Zhang S, Zhou J, Han S, Yang W, Li W, Wei H, et al. Four abiotic stress-induced miRNA families differentially regulated in the embryogenic and non-embryogenic callus tissues of *Larix leptolepis*. Biochem Biophys Res Commun 2010;398:355–60.

[23] Wu XM, Liu MY, Ge XX, Xu Q, Guo WW. Stage and tissue-specific modulation of ten conserved miRNAs and their targets during somatic embryogenesis of Valencia sweet orange. Planta 2011;233:495–505.

[24] Luo YC, Zhou H, Li Y, Chen JY, Yang JH, Chen YQ, et al. Rice embryogenic calli express a unique set of microRNAs, suggesting regulatory roles of microRNAs in plant postembryogenic development. FEBS Lett 2006;580:5111–6.

[25] Tanurdzic M, Vaughn MW, Jiang H, Lee TJ, Slotkin RK, Sosinski B, et al. Epigenomic consequences of immortalized plant cell suspension culture. PLoS Biol 2008;6:2880–95.

[26] Koukalova B, Fojtova M, Lim KY, Fulnecek J, Leitch AR, Kovarik A. Dedifferentiation of tobacco cells is associated with ribosomal RNA gene hypomethylation, increased transcription, and chromatin alterations. Plant Physiol 2005;139:275–86.

[27] Berdasco M, Alcázar R, Garcáa-Ortiz MV, Ballestar E, Fernández AF, Roldán-Arjona T, Tiburcio AF, et al. Promoter DNA hypermethylation and gene repression in undifferentiated Arabidopsis cells. PLoS One 2008;3:e3306.

[28] Kubis SE, Castilho AM, Vershinin AV, Heslop-Harrison JS. Retroelements, transposons and methylation status in the genome of oil palm (*Elaeis guineensis*) and the relationship to somaclonal variation. Plant Mol Biol 2003;52:69–79.

[29] Bednarek PT, Orłowska R, Koebner RMD, Zimny J. Quantification of the tissue-culture induced variation in barley (*Hordeum vulgare* L.). BMC Plant Biol 2007;7:10–8.

[30] Kaeppler SM, Phillips RL. DNA methylation and tissue culture-induced variation in plants. In Vitro Cell Dev Biol 1993;29P:125–30.

[31] Ngezahayo F, Xu C, Wang H, Jiang L, Pang J, Liu B. Tissue culture-induced transpositional activity of mPing is correlated with cytosine methylation in rice. BMC Plant Biol 2009;9:91–105.

[32] Singla B, Tyagi AK, Khurana JP, Khurana P. Analysis of expression profile of selected genes expressed during auxin-induced somatic embryogenesis in leaf base system of wheat (*Triticum aestivum*) and their possible interactions. Plant Mol Biol 2007;65:677–92.

[33] Linkiewicz A, Filipeck M, Tomczak A, Grabowska A, Malepszy S. The cloning of sequences differentially transcribed during the induction of somatic embryogenesis in cucumber (*Cucumis sativus* L.). Cell Mol Biol Lett 2004;9:795–804.

[34] Zeng F, Zhang X, Zhu L, Tu L, Guo X, Nie Y. Isolation and characterization of genes associated to cotton somatic embryogenesis by suppression subtractive hybridization and macroarray. Plant Mol Biol 2006;60:167–83.

[35] Gernand D, Golczyk H, Rutten T, Ilnicki T, Houben A, Joachimiak AJ. Tissue culture triggers chromosome alterations, amplification, and transposition of repeat sequences in *Allium fistulosum*. Genome 2007;50:435–42.

[36] Li X, Yu X, Wang N, Feng Q, Dong Z, Liu L, et al. Genetic and epigenetic instabilities induced by tissue culture in wild barley (*Hordeum brevisubulatum* (Trin.) Link). Plant Cell Tiss Org Cult 2007;90:153–68.

[37] Sreedhar RV, Venkatachalam L, Bhagyalakshmi N. Genetic fidelity of long-term micropropagated shoot cultures of vanilla (Vanilla planifolia Andrews) as assessed by molecular markers. Biotechnol J 2007;2:1007–13.

[38] Jin S, Mushke R, Zhu H, Tu L, Lin Z, Zhang Y, et al. Detection of somaclonal variation of cotton (*Gossypium hirsutum*) using cytogenetics, flow cytometry and molecular markers. Plant Cell Rep 2008;27:1303–16.

[39] Jiang C, Mithani A, Gan X, Belfield EJ, Klingler JP, Zhu JK, et al. Regenerant Arabidopsis lineages display a distinct genome-wide spectrum of mutations conferring variant phenotypes. Curr Biol 2011;21:1385–90.

[40] Andreev O, Spiridonova KV, Solovyan VT, Kunakh VA. Variability of ribosomal RNA genes in Rauwolfia species: parallelism between tissue culture-induced rearrangements and interspecies polymorphism. Cell Biol Int 2005;29:21–7.

[41] Krsnik-Rasol M. Peroxidase as a developmental marker in plant tissue culture. Int J Dev Biol 1991;35:259–63.

Subject Index